T0227185

# Non-Spine Ablation Procedures

*Editor*

## SANTOS F. MARTINEZ

# PHYSICAL MEDICINE AND REHABILITATION CLINICS OF NORTH AMERICA

www.pmr.theclinics.com

*Consulting Editor*
## SANTOS F. MARTINEZ

November 2021 • Volume 32 • Number 4

**ELSEVIER**

1600 John F. Kennedy Boulevard • Suite 1800 • Philadelphia, Pennsylvania, 19103-2899

http://www.theclinics.com

**PHYSICAL MEDICINE AND REHABILITATION CLINICS OF NORTH AMERICA Volume 32, Number 4**
**November 2021 ISSN 1047-9651, 978-0-323-79228-8**

Editor: Lauren Boyle
Developmental Editor: Diana Grace Ang

*Reprints.* For copies of 100 or more of articles in this publication, please contact the Commercial Reprints Department, Elsevier Inc., 360 Park Avenue South, New York, NY 10010-1710. Tel.: 212-633-3874; Fax: 212-633-3820; E-mail: reprints@elsevier.com.

*Physical Medicine and Rehabilitation Clinics of North America* (ISSN 1047-9651) is published quarterly by Elsevier Inc., 360 Park Avenue South, New York, NY 10010-1710. Months of issue are February, May, August, and November. Business and Editorial Offices: 1600 John F. Kennedy Blvd., Suite 1800, Philadelphia, PA 19103-2899. Customer Service Office: 3251 Riverport Lane, Maryland Heights, MO 63043. Periodicals postage paid at New York, NY and additional mailing offices. Subscription price per year is $322.00 (US individuals), $879.00 (US institutions), $100.00 (US students), $366.00 (Canadian individuals), $923.00 (Canadian institutions), $100.00 (Canadian students), $463.00 (foreign individuals), $923.00 (foreign institutions), and $210.00 (foreign students). Foreign air speed delivery is included in all *Clinics* subscription prices. All prices are subject to change without notice. **POSTMASTER:** Send address changes to *Physical Medicine and Rehabilitation Clinics of North America*, Customer Service Office: Elsevier Health Sciences Division, Subscription Customer Service, 3251 Riverport Lane, Maryland Heights, MO 63043. **Customer Service: 1-800-654-2452 (US). From outside of the United States, call 314-447-8871. Fax: 314-447-8029. E-mail: JournalsCustomer Service-usa@elsevier.com (for print support); JournalsOnlineSupport-usa@elsevier.com (for online support).**

*Physical Medicine and Rehabilitation Clinics of North America* is indexed in *Excerpta Medica, MEDLINE/ PubMed (Index Medicus), Cinahl,* and *Cumulative Index to Nursing and Allied Health Literature.*

# Contributors

## CONSULTING EDITOR

**SANTOS F. MARTINEZ, MD, MS**
Diplomate, American Academy of Physical Medicine and Rehabilitation; Certificate of
Added Qualification Sports Medicine, Assistant Professor, Department of
Orthopaedics,Campbell Clinic Orthopaedics, University of Tennessee, Memphis,
Tennessee, USA

## EDITOR

**SANTOS F. MARTINEZ, MD, MS**
Diplomate, American Academy of Physical Medicine and Rehabilitation; Certificate of
Added Qualification Sports Medicine, Assistant Professor, Department of
Orthopaedics,Campbell Clinic Orthopaedics, University of Tennessee, Memphis,
Tennessee, USA

## AUTHORS

**ALAA ABD-ELSAYED, MD, MPH**
Medical Director, UW Health Pain Services, Associate Professor, Department of
Anesthesiology, Division of Pain Medicine, University of Wisconsin-Madison School of
Medicine and Public Health, Madison, Wisconsin, USA

**ANNE M.R. AGUR, BSc(OT), MSc, PhD**
Professor, Division of Anatomy, Department of Surgery, Temerty Faculty of Medicine,
University of Toronto, Toronto, Ontario, Canada

**JESSI JO G. BARNETT, BSc (Hon)**
School of Medicine, St. George's University, Grenada, West Indies; Division of Anatomy,
Department of Surgery, Temerty Faculty of Medicine, University of Toronto, Toronto,
Ontario, Canada

**NAHUM M. BEARD, MD, CAQSM**
Faculty, Campbell Clinic Sports Medicine Fellowship, Department of Orthopaedic Surgery
and Rehabilitation, Department of Family Medicine, University of Tennessee Health
Science Center, Germantown, Tennessee, USA

**ROBERT S. BURNHAM, MSc, MD, FRCPC**
Associate Clinical Professor, Division of Physical Medicine and Rehabilitation, Faculty of
Medicine and Dentistry, University of Alberta, Edmonton, Alberta, Canada; Central Alberta
Pain and Rehabilitation Institute, Lacombe, Alberta, Canada; Vivo Cura Health, Calgary,
Alberta, Canada

**TAYLOR R. BURNHAM, MD, MSCI**
Assistant Professor, Division of Physical Medicine and Rehabilitation, University of Utah,
Salt Lake City, Utah, USA

**MICHAEL CATAPANO, BHSc, MD, FRCPC**
Division of Physical Medicine and Rehabilitation, Department of Medicine, University of Toronto, Toronto Rehabilitation Institute, Toronto, Ontario, Canada

**VINCENT W.S. CHAN, MD, FRCPC**
Professor, Department of Anesthesia and Pain Management, Toronto Western Hospital, University of Toronto, Toronto, Ontario, Canada

**B. RYDER CONNOLLY, MD**
Department of Rehabilitation Medicine, The University of Texas Health Science Center at San Antonio, San Antonio, Texas, USA

**GUY FEIGIN, MD**
Clinical Fellow, Attending Anesthesiologist, Department of Anesthesia and Pain Management, University of Toronto, Toronto Western Hospital, Women's College Hospital, Wasser Pain Management Clinic, Mount Sinai Hospital, Toronto, Ontario, Canada; Department of Anesthesiology, Critical Care and Pain Management, Meir Medical Center, Kfar Saba, Israel

**JONATHAN M. HAGEDORN, MD**
Department of Anesthesiology and Perioperative Medicine, Division of Pain Medicine, Mayo Clinic, Rochester, Minnesota, USA

**JOHN R. HAN, BPHE, BA(Hons)**
Division of Anatomy, Department of Surgery, Temerty Faculty of Medicine, University of Toronto, Toronto, Ontario, Canada

**KENDALL HULK, DO**
Department of Rehabilitation Medicine, The University of Texas Health Science Center at San Antonio, San Antonio, Texas, USA

**JAY KARRI, MD, MPH**
Department of Physical Medicine and Rehabilitation, Baylor College of Medicine, Houston, Texas, USA

**LAURA LACHMAN, MD**
Department of Physical Medicine and Rehabilitation, Baylor College of Medicine, Houston, Texas, USA

**ELDON LOH, MD, FRCPC**
Associate Professor, Department of Physical Medicine and Rehabilitation, Schulich School of Medicine and Dentistry, Western University, Parkwood Institute Research, Lawson Health Research Institute, London, Ontario, Canada

**NIMISH MITTAL, MBBS, MD, MSc**
Assistant Professor, Division of Physical Medicine and Rehabilitation, Department of Medicine, University of Toronto, Toronto Rehabilitation Institute, Toronto, Ontario, Canada

**AMEET S. NAGPAL, MD, MS, MEd**
Department of Anesthesiology, The University of Texas Health Science Center at San Antonio, San Antonio, Texas, USA

**CHARLES A. ODONKOR, MD, MA**
Department of Orthoapaedic Surgery, Division of Physical Medicine and Rehabilitation, Yale School of Medicine, Yale New Haven Hospital, New Haven, Connecticut, USA; Yale School of Medicine, Old Saybrook, Connecticut, USA

**VWAIRE ORHURHU, MD, MPH**
Department of Anesthesia, Critical Care and Pain Medicine, Division of Pain, Massachusetts General Hospital, Harvard Medical School, Boston, Massachusetts, USA; University of Pittsburgh Medical Center, Williamsport, Pennsylvania, USA

**PHILIP W.H. PENG, MBBS, FRCPC, Founder (Pain Medicine)**
Professor, Department of Anesthesia and Pain Management, University of Toronto, University Health Network, Toronto Western Hospital, Women's College Hospital, Wasser Pain Management Clinic, Mount Sinai Hospital, Toronto, Ontario, Canada

**JACOB ROBERTS, MD**
Johns Hopkins School of Medicine, Baltimore, Maryland, USA

**SHANNON L. ROBERTS, PhD**
Toronto, Ontario, Canada

**ANGELA SAMAAN, DO**
Department of Rehabilitation and Human Performance, Icahn School of Medicine at Mount Sinai, New York, New York, USA

**CALEB SEALE, MD**
Department of Rehabilitation Medicine, The University of Texas Health Science Center at San Antonio, San Antonio, Texas, USA

**SHAYAN SHAKERI, BSc (Hon)**
School of Medicine, St. George's University, Grenada, West Indies; Division of Anatomy, Department of Surgery, Temerty Faculty of Medicine, University of Toronto, Toronto, Ontario, Canada

**SHAWN SIDHARTHAN, MD**
Department of Neurology, Northwell Health–Northshore-LIJ, Manhasset, New York, USA

**MANI SINGH, MD**
Department of Rehabilitation Medicine, Weill Cornell Medical Center, New York, New York, USA

**DAVID SPINNER, DO, RMSK, CIPS, FAAPMR**
Department of Rehabilitation and Human Performance, Icahn School of Medicine at Mount Sinai, New York, New York, USA

**SHARON SWITZER-MCINTYRE, BPE, BScPT, MEd, PhD**
Associate Professor, Department of Physical Therapy, Temerty Faculty of Medicine, University of Toronto, Toronto, Ontario, Canada

**JOHN TRAN, HBSc, PhD**
Postdoctoral Fellow, Division of Anatomy, Department of Surgery, Temerty Faculty of Medicine, University of Toronto, Toronto, Ontario, Canada.

**NELLY UMUKORO, MD**
Department of Anesthesia, Riley Hospital for Children, Indiana University Health, Indianapolis, Indiana, USA

**GREGORY G. YU, MD, PharmD, MBA, MPH**
Department of Anesthesiology, The University of Texas Health Science Center at San Antonio, San Antonio, Texas, USA

# Contents

> Headache disorders and trigeminal neuralgia are common conditions rep-
> resenting the types of craniofacial pain syndrome that can significantly
> impact quality of life. Many cases are refractory to traditional pharmaco-
> logic treatments, whether oral or intravenous. Radiofrequency ablation
> has been increasingly used as a tool to treat resistant, chronic pain of
> both of these disorders. Multiple studies have been reported that illustrate
> the efficacy of radiofrequency ablation in the treatment of the numerous
> headache subtypes and trigeminal neuralgia.

> Chronic thoracic pain and chronic abdominal pain are common conditions
> that can significantly affect quality of life. Pain syndromes encompassing a
> variety of causes, including cancer pain, neuritis, and postsurgical pain,
> are traditionally managed by the use of pharmacologic therapy; however,
> many cases are refractory to these conservative methods. Radiofrequency
> ablation (RFA) has been increasingly used as a tool to treat resistant,
> chronic pain of both thoracic and abdominal origin. Multiple cases and tri-
> als have been reported that show the efficacy of RFA in the treatment of
> these chronic pain conditions.

> Detailed understanding of the course and location of articular nerves sup-
> plying the shoulder joint is paramount to the successful utilization of
> image-guided radiofrequency ablation to manage chronic shoulder pain.
> In this article, the origin, course, and relationship to anatomic landmarks
> of articular nerves supplying the shoulder and acromioclavicular joints
> are discussed. The shoulder joint capsule was consistently reported to
> receive innervation from multiple sources including the suprascapular,
> axillary, subscapular, and lateral pectoral nerves. The acromioclavicular
> joint received innervation from suprascapular and lateral pectoral nerves.
> The consistent relationship of articular branches to anatomic landmarks
> provides the basis for specific image-guided targeting.

The shoulder is structurally and functionally complex. Shoulder pain may be refractory to conventional treatments, such as physical therapy, pharmacotherapy, and corticosteroid injections. In such cases, radiofrequency ablation may serve as an alternative treatment plan. Current literature has demonstrated 4 target nerves for ablative therapy: the suprascapular nerve, axillary nerve, lateral pectoral nerve, and subscapular nerve. Special caution is needed when targeting these nerves in order to avoid motor denervation. This article summarizes the current evidence for radiofrequency ablation as a useful treatment option for chronic shoulder pain as well as the described techniques for performing this promising procedure.

Radiofrequency ablation (RFA) is a procedure in which radio waves are used to destroy abnormal or dysfunctional tissue. It has been an increasingly utilized treatment option for a variety of medical conditions, such as chronic pain, wherein sensory nerves are targeted and ablated, eliminating their ability to transmit pain signals to the brain. There is a lack of clarity regarding the indications, technique, and efficacy of RFA for chronic pelvic pain. This article reviews recent literature and discusses these topics, including adverse events for different pelvic ablation and pulsed radiofrequency treatment of chronic pelvic pain.

 Video content accompanies this article at http://www.pmr.theclinics. com.

The sacroiliac joint can be a source of low back pain. This review article summarizes current anatomic evidence of the innervation of the intraarticular and extraarticular parts of the sacroiliac joint relative to bony landmarks identifiable with fluoroscopy and ultrasound. This article aims to provide clinicians with an anatomic basis for clinical application to diagnostic blocks and radiofrequency ablation for sacroiliac pain to optimize clinical outcomes.

Radiofrequency ablation (RFA) is a potential treatment for those with sacroiliac joint (SIJ) pain. There is no consensus on the optimal procedural techniques for SIJ diagnostic blocks, or RFA. This article describes different techniques for SIJ diagnostic blocks and RFA, including the relevant innervation that underlies these techniques. SIJ RFA techniques differ in important ways, including lesioning techniques, needle placements, and type of RFA cannula used. Clinicians utilize a variety of image guidance modalities for SIJ RFA; fluoroscopic guidance is standard, although endoscopic and ultrasound-guided techniques are described. Additional studies are necessary to delineate potential differences between SIJ RFA techniques.

The innervation of the hip joint has been investigated for over 200 years by anatomists and clinicians. Knowledge of the distribution and location of these nerves relative to anatomic landmarks visible with image guidance is important for optimizing nerve blocks and radiofrequency ablation procedures. In this article, the innervation of the anterior and posterior hip joint is reviewed, focusing on the source of articular branches, their course, termination, and relationship to anatomic landmarks. The innervation of the hip joint is multifaceted, with articular nerves originating from many sources in close proximity to and distant from the hip joint.

Radiofrequency ablation (RFA) is still an emergent technique for the management of chronic hip pain. Although the ablation technique for facet articular branches of lumbar and cervical spine was already established, the literature on the targets and technique of needle placement for hip denervation are evolving. This article summarizes the current understanding of the anatomy of the articular branches, sonoanatomy, and the suggested techniques for the RFA of the hip. It also reviews the literature on the clinical studies.

Image-guided diagnostic block and radiofrequency ablation of the knee joint to manage pain require detailed understanding of joint innervation in relation to soft tissue and bony landmarks. In this article, the origin, course, and relationship to anatomic landmarks of articular nerves supplying the knee joint are discussed. The innervation pattern of the anterior and posterior aspects of the knee joint capsule is relatively consistent, with some variation in supply by the saphenous, anterior division of obturator, and common fibular nerves. To improve nerve capture rates for diagnostic block and radiofrequency ablation, multiple target sites could be beneficial.

Genicular nerve radiofrequency ablation has quickly become one of the most promising interventions for chronic knee pain secondary to osteoarthritis, with consistent improvements in pain and function. Although there are multiple techniques using slightly variable lesion locations, cannulas, lesion types, and imaging modalities, the clinical effectiveness targeting the anterior branches of the superior medial, superolateral, and inferior medial has reproducibly demonstrated clinically and statistically significant improvements up to 24 months after the procedure with minimal adverse events. This article summarizes the current knowledge of the sensory innervation of the knee joint, the principles of radiofrequency ablation, and the current literature on clinical outcomes.

In this article, the literature describing the origin, course, and termination of the nerves innervating the ankle joint is reviewed and discussed. The anterior aspect of the joint capsule receives innervation from articular branches from the saphenous, superficial, and deep fibular nerves; laterally from the sural and superficial fibular nerves; and medially and posteriorly from the saphenous and tibial nerves. Comprehensive mapping of the trajectory, spatial relationships, and termination of the articular branches innervating the ankle joint capsule will aid in developing new and improving existing image-guided nerve block and radiofrequency ablation protocols to treat chronic joint pain.

Ablation therapies in the foot and ankle are accessible adjuncts to surgery and comprehensive pain management in recalcitrant pain syndromes. Techniques are best applied to individual patient anatomy with strong advantages in a working knowledge of neuromuscular real-time imaging with ultrasound. Interventionists face the unique challenge in this region of preserving balance and proprioception as well as intrinsic muscle function, while optimizing pain relief. A decision-making approach emphasizing selectivity by using regional and target-specific ablations is optimal. This article reviews basic technique, approaches, potential complications, and ultrasound anatomy for a practical introduction to ablation options in the foot and ankle.

# PHYSICAL MEDICINE AND REHABILITATION CLINICS OF NORTH AMERICA

## SERIES OF RELATED INTEREST

*Orthopedic Clinics*
*https://www.orthopedic.theclinics.com/*
*Neurologic Clinics*
*https://www.neurologic.theclinics.com/*
*Clinics in Sports Medicine*
*https://www.sportsmed.theclinics.com/*

**VISIT THE CLINICS ONLINE!**
Access your subscription at:
www.theclinics.com

# Foreword

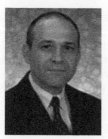

Santos F. Martinez, MD, MS
*Consulting Editor*

The techniques within the field of interventional pain management continues to expand and provide a critical resource for patients suffering from a wide range of conditions. The collaboration of Anaesthesiology and Physical Medicine and Rehabilitation has provided a rich diversity of viewpoints and orientation to further develop our options. Although the comprehensive pain management model with a multidisciplinary approach remains a gold standard, much of the emphasis noted in the ortho-neuro-logic setting, especially among Physical Medicine and Rehabilitation practitioners, has been directed towards the spine. Approaches such as diagnostic/therapeutic differential blocks became very useful for helping delineate and treat primary pain generators. There were instances where pain relief was transitory, leaving a niche of patients with unresolving pain and a great opportunity for expansion of the technology of ablation techniques. The success of more centrally utilized ablation modalities has evolved into peripheral radiofrequency ablation field which is growing. This may be partially related with the frequent integration of PMR and pain management practitioners with the Orthopaedic Surgical settings where there are a large number of patients that need pain management techniques not traditionally available. Likewise, these modalities have continued to expand with innovative research among Anesthesiologists dedicated to this population of patients. This edition discusses the anatomical considerations and approaches for primarily non-spine radiofrequency ablation techniques.

We are honored to have an exceptional panel of authors, which provide both anatomical and clinical guidance for peripheral ablation procedures.

Phys Med Rehabil Clin N Am 32 (2021) xiii–xiv
https://doi.org/10.1016/j.pmr.2021.07.001
1047-9651/21/© 2021 Published by Elsevier Inc.

This edition is dedicated to late Dr. Steven F. Brena, who was the director of the Emory Pain Control Center and served as a great mentor for many fellows and residents.

Santos F. Martinez, MD, MS
American Academy of Physical Medicine and Rehabilitation
Campbell Clinic Orthopaedics
Department of Orthopaedics
University of Tennessee
Memphis, TN 38104, USA

*E-mail address:*
smartinez@campbellclinic.com

# Radiofrequency Ablation for Craniofacial Pain Syndromes

Vwaire Orhurhu, MD, MPH[a,b], Shawn Sidharthan, MD[c], Jacob Roberts, MD[d],
Jay Karri, MD[e], Nelly Umukoro, MD[f], Jonathan M. Hagedorn, MD[g],
Charles A. Odonkor, MD, MA[h,i], Alaa Abd-Elsayed, MD, MPH[j],*

## KEYWORDS

- Headache • Facial pain • Chronic pain • Radiofrequency lesioning
- Radiofrequency ablation

## KEY POINTS

- Craniofacial pain syndrome, represented by headache disorders and trigeminal neuralgia, can significantly impact quality of life.
- Traditional management includes pharmacotherapy and supportive management, but can often fail to provide adequate pain relief.
- Radiofrequency ablation is often cited in publications as an effective and safe treatment option for craniofacial pain syndrome.
- Continuous radiofrequency and pulsed radiofrequency are the 2 types of radiofrequency ablation.
- Continuous radiofrequency overall has been shown to have minimal adverse effects in the use for craniofacial pain syndrome.

[a] Department of Anesthesia, Critical Care and Pain Medicine, Division of Pain, Massachusetts General Hospital, Harvard Medical School, Boston, MA, USA; [b] University of Pittsburgh Medical Center, 1100 Grampian Boulevard, Williamsport, PA 17701, USA; [c] Department of Neurology, Northwell Health–Northshore-LIJ, 300 Community Drive, Manhasset, NY 11030, USA; [d] Johns Hopkins School of Medicine, 733 N Broadway, Baltimore, MD 21205, USA; [e] Department of Physical Medicine and Rehabilitation, Baylor College of Medicine, 7200 Cambridge Street, Houston, TX 77030, USA; [f] Department of Anesthesia, Riley Hospital for Children, Indiana University Health, 705 Riley Hospital Drive, Indianapolis, IN 46202, USA; [g] Department of Anesthesiology and Perioperative Medicine, Division of Pain Medicine, Mayo Clinic, 200 First Street Southwest, Rochester, MN 55905, USA; [h] Department of Orthoapaedic Surgery, Division of Physical Medicine and Rehabilitation, Yale University School of Medicine, Yale New Haven Hospital, New Haven, CT, USA; [i] Yale University School of Medicine, 633 Middlesex Turnpike, Old Saybrook, CT 06475, USA; [j] Department of Anesthesiology, University of Wisconsin School of Medicine and Public Health, 600 Highland Avenue, B6/319 CSC, Madison, WI 53792-3272, USA
* Corresponding author.
E-mail address: alaaawny@hotmail.com

Phys Med Rehabil Clin N Am 32 (2021) 601–645
https://doi.org/10.1016/j.pmr.2021.05.003
1047-9651/21/© 2021 Elsevier Inc. All rights reserved.

## BACKGROUND

Headache subtypes include the following, but are not limited to, occipital neuralgia, cluster headache, cervicogenic headache, chronic migraine, and headaches associated with nasal congestion. Trigeminal neuralgia is another subtype of craniofacial pain syndrome that presents from mild to severe facial pain affecting the fifth cranial nerve. These pain syndromes are associated with significant detriment to well-being. Unfortunately, the effective management of these conditions can be challenging, often because of varying effectiveness and poor adverse effect profiles associated with oral and intravenous medications.

Radiofrequency ablation (RFA) has been increasingly used as a tool to treat resistant, chronic pain of both headache subtypes and trigeminal neuralgia. Multiple cases and trials have been reported that illustrate the efficacy of RFA in the treatment of these chronic pain conditions. RFA includes use of continuous radiofrequency (CRF) or pulsed radiofrequency (PRF) modalities, which are each associated with differing effectiveness and complication rates. CRF operates by producing coagulative tissue necrosis through use of high temperature (between 60 °and 80 °C) and high-frequency alternating currents. However, the high temperature used in CRF can lead to neural injury and result in key motor or sensory compromise. PRF uses short high-voltage bursts followed by a silent phase that allows for heat elimination and overall decreased heat exposure. Consequently, PRF is thought to be associated with both lower rates of procedure complications and success. The use of concomitant CRF and PRF modalities has shown favorable results. This narrative review aims to characterize and summarize the existing evidence, for RFA-associated pain reduction and complications in persons with headache disorders and trigeminal neuralgia.

## RADIOFREQUENCY ABLATION FOR HEADACHES
### Occipital Neuralgia and Headache

According to the International Headache Society, occipital neuralgia is defined as a sudden, stabbing pain in the posterior scalp region in the distribution of the greater occipital nerve, lesser occipital nerve, and/or third occipital nerve.[1] According to Huang and colleagues,[2] 85% of occipital neuralgias present in a unilateral fashion, with more prevalence of greater occipital nerve involvement over lesser occipital nerve involvement. This form of headache is idiopathic; however, it frequently occurs after some form of cranial trauma or whiplash.[1] Other causes include compression of the greater and/or lesser occipital nerve by long-term contracted muscles and spondylosis of the superior cervical spine.[2] Symptom response to occipital nerve block are hallmarks of this type of headache.[2] Currently, there is no universal standard for the treatment of occipital neuralgia, but overall includes steroid injections and/or PRF. Numerous studies have investigated the use of RFA for symptom improvement (**Table 1**). Cohen and colleagues in 2015[1] published a multicenter randomized double-blind comparative effectiveness study in 81 patients with occipital headaches. Inclusion criteria for the 81 patients were as follows: at least 18 years of age, diagnosis of occipital neuralgia based on the International Classification of Headache Disorders (ICHD), paroxysmal stabbing pain in the greater or lesser occipital nerve distribution, tenderness over the affected nerve(s), and relief of pain for at least 3 hours after local bupivacaine anesthetic block of the affected nerve(s), or ICHD-2 diagnosis of migraine with primarily occipital pain and nerve tenderness that responded to local anesthetic blockade; 4 or greater out of 10 pain; failure to respond to prior therapy to include nonopioid analgesics; and headache frequency for more than or equal to 10 days per month. Exclusion criteria were as follows: unstable medical or psychiatric condition, cardiac

**Table 1**
Characteristics of investigating the role of RFAs for headache disorders

| Author (Year) | Diagnosis | Study Design | Patient Population | Ablation Technique | Target Nerve | Duration of Pain Relief | Secondary Outcome | Conclusion | Side Effect |
|---|---|---|---|---|---|---|---|---|---|
| Cohen et al,[1] 2015 | Occipital neuralgia | Double blind comparative effectiveness study | Sample size: 81 Mean age: 41.6 Male (%): 52 | PRF 42 °C, 40–60V, 2 Hz, 20 ms pulses in 1 s cycle; 120 s duration per cycle. Control: sham PRF. | Greater occipital nerve | Patients who received PRF had better pain relief compared with patients who received steroids. PRF group had greater change from average occipital pain, and worst occipital pain. Difference in worst occipital pain stopped being significant for PRF at 6 mo. | Decrease in HA frequency did not reach significance at any time point between groups. Use of rescue medications for occipital neuralgia and migraines + occipital nerve tenderness did not differ at any follow-up. The PRF group had significant reduction in insomnia score. | PRF is superior to steroid injections for pain relief in occipital neuralgia but no difference for other outcomes. | PRF group: 1 report of worsening HA, 1 of swelling, and 1 of rash. |
| Huang et al,[2] 2012 | Occipital neuralgia | Retrospective study | Sample size: 102 Mean age: 51.2 Male (%): 26.5 | PRF: 42 °C plateau temps; 40–60 V, 2 Hz, 20 ms pulses in a 1-s cycle, 120 s duration per cycle | Greater and/or lesser occipital nerve | 51%[50] patients experienced ≥50% pain reduction after treatment for at least 3 mo. | Factors associated with procedural success: inciting event, presence of greater occipital neuralgia by itself, lower injectate volumes during diagnostic blocks, multiple cycles of PRF. | PRF may provide intermediate-term benefit in occipital neuralgia to a significant proportion of refractory cases. | 6 patients: temporary worsening pain, new painful sensation behind ear and cheek that resolved in 3 wk |

(continued on next page)

**Table 1**
*(continued)*

| Author (Year) | Diagnosis | Study Design | Patient Population | Ablation Technique | Target Nerve | Duration of Pain Relief | Secondary Outcome | Conclusion | Side Effect |
|---|---|---|---|---|---|---|---|---|---|
| Govind et al,[3] 2003 | Occipital headache | Prospective observational study | Sample size: 49 (51 nerves) Mean age: 43 Male (%): 42.9 | 80 °C for 90 s | Occipital nerve | 88%[41] of patients achieved >90 d of pain relief; 13%[6] patients did not achieve pain relief lasting >90 d, 6%[3] of patients had headache recurrence that were manageable by simple analgesics. Median duration of complete pain relief was 297 d, with 8 patients having ongoing relief. The median duration of complete pain relief with repeat neurotomy was 217 d, with 6 patients having ongoing relief. | N/A | RF neurotomy provides relief of occipital headache though the relief may be limited in duration and can require repeated procedures. | 97% numbness, 95% ataxia, 55% dysesthesia, 15% hypersensitivity, 10% itch |
| Salgado-Lopez et al,[4] 2019 | Chronic cluster headache | Prospective Observational Study | Sample size: PRF 24 RFA 13 Mean age: 40 Male (%): 78.4 | PRF: 80°C for 60 s; RFA: 42oC and 40V for 120s | Sphenopalatine Ganglion | A total of 5 patients (13.5%) experienced complete clinical headache relief of both pain and parasympathetic symptoms, 21 patients (56.7%) presented partial and transient relief, and 11 patients (29.7%) did not improve. | A total of 5 patients (13.5%) experienced complete clinical headache relief of both pain and parasympathetic symptoms, 21 patients (56.7%) presented partial and transient relief, and 11 patients (29.7%) did not improve. | There are no statistical differences between RFA and PRF. Because of the similarity in efficacy and the greater theoretic risk of thermal complications, we recommend the use of the PRF. | None reported |

| Study | Condition | Study Type | Sample | RF Parameters | Target | Outcomes | Notes | Conclusion | Adverse Events |
|---|---|---|---|---|---|---|---|---|---|
| Fang et al,[5] 2016 | Cluster headache | Prospective Observational Study | Sample size: 16 Mean age: 44.6 Male (%): 87.5 | Pulsed with max temp of 42°C for 120 | Sphenopalatine Ganglion | 85% (11/13) of episodic cluster headache cases showed positive treatment outcomes. 33% (1/3) of chronic cluster headache cases showed positive treatment outcomes. Mean remission before RFA was $8.7 \pm 2.9$ mo; mean remission after RFA was $16.6 \pm 5.2$ mo. Mean cluster duration pre-RFA was $2 \pm 0.9$ mo; mean cluster duration after RFA was $05 \pm 0.3$ mo. | 1 patient underwent 3 PRF treatments as symptoms recurred 3 times. 15%[2] episodic cluster headaches and 67%[2] patients with chronic cluster headaches did not respond to PRF treatment at 1-mo f/u. | RFA of sphenopalatine ganglion is effective and safe for relief of episodic cluster headaches. | N/A |
| Narouze et al,[6] 2009 | Chronic cluster headache | Prospective Observational Study | Sample size: 15 Mean age: N/A Male (%): N/A | Two 80°C RF lesions for 60s each | Sphenopalatine Ganglion | At 1 month after the operation, the mean attack intensity decreased from 8.6 (on a scale of 1–10) to 2.6 and the mean attack frequency improved from 17 attacks/wk to 5.4. | Precise needle placement with the use of real-time fluoroscopy and electrical stimulation prior to attempting RF lesioning may reduce the incidence of adverse events. | Percutaneous RF ablation of the sphenopalatine ganglion is an effective modality of treatment for patients with intractable chronic cluster headaches. | 50% (7/15) reported temporary paresthesia in the upper gums and cheek. One patient had a coin-like area of permanent anesthesia over his cheek. |

(continued on next page)

**Table 1**
*(continued)*

| Author (Year) | Diagnosis | Study Design | Patient Population | Ablation Technique | Target Nerve | Duration of Pain Relief | Secondary Outcome | Conclusion | Side Effect |
|---|---|---|---|---|---|---|---|---|---|
| Halim et al,[8] 2010 | Cervicogenic headache | Retrospective Study | Sample size: 86 Mean age: 50 Male (%): 37 | PRF: 45V, 2 Hz, 10 ms for 10 min | C1-C2 joint | 50%[41] patients had ≥50% relief at 2 mo 50%[41] patients had ≥50% relief at 6 mo 44.2%[37] patients had ≥50% relief at 1 y. Long-term pain relief (6 mo, 1 y) were reliably predicted by ≥ 50% relief at 2 mo. | Duration of pain preprocedure and baseline pain score were nonsignificant predictors of ≥50% pain relief at 2 mo, 6 mo, and 1 y. | PRF of lateral C1-2 facet joint is a safe technique in patients with cervicogenic headache. | 1 patient experienced increased severity of occipital headache lasting several hours. |
| Haspeslagh et al,[9] 2006 | Cervicogenic headache | Retrospective Study | Sample size: 30 (15 in RFA) Mean age: 48.3 Male (%): 26.7 | RFA of facet: 67°C for 60s; RFA of cervical segmental nerves: 50 Hz and 2 Hz threshold; RFA of cervical facet joint, followed by cervical dorsal root ganglion | Greater occipital nerve | Differences in VAS pain scores, effect scores, and quality of life scores between 2 groups were not statistically significant at any time point. After 16 wk, success rate of RFA was 66.7% vs 55.3% of the steroid group. | N/A | RFA of cervical facet joints and upper dorsal root ganglions is not a better treatment for trigeminal neuralgia than treatment of greater occipital nerve. | N/A |
| Lee et al,[10] 2007 | Cervicogenic headache | Prospective Observational Study | Sample size: 30 Mean age: 54 Male (%): 53.3 | 80°C for 90s | Occipital nerve | Number of patients who showed pain relief > 75% were 60% at 1 wk, 83.3% at 1 mo, 76.7% at 6 mo and 73.3% at 12 mo. The average number of headaches per week decreased from 6.2 to 2.8 after the operation. | There was a 70% reduction in analgesic intake/week. | RF neurotomy represents a moderate duration of pain relief without any serious side effects in the majority of these chronically disabling patients. | 12 patients complained of soreness on the posterior neck for 2–7 d following the procedures, all of which resolved within a week. |

| | | | Sample | | | | | | |
|---|---|---|---|---|---|---|---|---|---|
| Lang et al,[11] 2010 | Cervicogenic headache | Retrospective Study | Sample size: 31 Mean age: 46 Male (%): 61.3 | 80°C for 90s | Occipital nerve | The mean percentage of pain relief on the first day after the RF neurotomy was 91.64%. The median duration of pain relief until recurrence of 50% of the precoagulation pain was 125.11 d (minimum 6 d, maximum 732 d). | Eight patients worked full-time after successful coagulation, 5 of them underwent re-coagulation subsequent to headache recurrence. The 2 patients who remained unable to work were in the arthritis group. | Our results indicate that this therapy is effective in patients with underlying diseases of primarily degenerative origin. | All patients complained of numbness in the neck or the occipital region, which subsided without treatment. |
| Stovner et al,[12] 2004 | Cervicogenic headache | Randomized, Double Blind, Sham-controlled Study | Sample size: 12 Mean age: 48 Male (%): 50 | 3-4 lesions of 85°C for 60s | Greater occipital nerve | In month one both groups tend to be better, but in month 3 there seems to be a tendency that the RF-group is doing better than the sham group with regard to all variables except analgesics intake. In month 6 and later the 2 groups seem to be similar, but in month 24, the sham group is better on most variables. | All patients had at least a 50% effect on at least one of the blockades, but only 4 patients had more than 90% effect on at least one of the blockades. | We do not find much evidence that RF-treatment of facet joints C2-C6 is a promising procedure for most patients fulfilling purely clinical criteria for cervicogenic headache | More patients in the RF-group reported increased neck pain (4/6) than in the sham group (1/6) at discharge from the hospital 1-2 d after the procedure. |
| van Suijlekom et al,[13] 1998 | Cervicogenic headache | Prospective Observational Study | Sample size: 15 Mean age: N/A Male (%): N/A | N/A | N/A | There was a significant reduction in headache severity in 12 (80%) patients. Mean VAS decrease was 31.4 mm (P < .001) and 53.5 mm (P < .0001) respectively in 8 wk and 16.8 mo follow up. | The average mean number of headache days per week decreased from 5.8 d to 2.8 d (P = .001). | A definitive conclusion about the clinical efficacy of this treatment can only be drawn from a randomized controlled trial. | N/A |

(continued on next page)

**Table 1**
*(continued)*

| Author (Year) | Diagnosis | Study Design | Patient Population | Ablation Technique | Target Nerve | Duration of Pain Relief | Secondary Outcome | Conclusion | Side Effect |
|---|---|---|---|---|---|---|---|---|---|
| Yang et al,[14] 2015 | Chronic migraine | Randomized clinical trial | Sample size: 40 Mean age: 43.5 Male (%): 17.5 | 42°C for 120s twice | Occipital nerve | The mean decrease of headache duration in the treatment group was 8.9 d per month at the 6-mo follow-up. There was a significant difference in the decrease of headache duration between the treatment and the sham groups at the 1-mo (t = 8.14, $P < .001$), 2-mo (t = 7.93, $P < .001$), and 6-mo (t = 7.11, $P < .001$) follow-up time points | The VAS differed significantly between the treatment and the sham groups at the 1-mo (t = 4.08, $P < .001$), 2-mo (t = 4.86, $P < .001$), and 6-mo (t = 3.27, $P < .01$) follow-up periods | RF on the cervical 2–3 posterior medial branches could provide a satisfactory treatment that can reduce pain intensity, headache duration, and disability scores. The procedure was relatively easy to perform and resulted in few side effects. | One patient in the treatment group reported mild pain at the injection site and the pain subsided within 6 h without any treatment. |
| Shabat et al,[15] 2013 | Chronic headache | Retrospective Study | Sample size: 69 Mean age: 48 Male (%): 42 | 42°C for 120s | Suprascapular nerve | After 4 wk, 41 patients (59%) had improvement in their headache. After 3 mo, 38 (55%) of the patients reported significant pain relief. | 31 patients (45%) reported long-term pain relief for the headache (defined as reduction of VAS by at least 30%) | PRF for the suprascapular nerve is a safe and an effective procedure for patients who suffer from headache that is, attributed to the lower cervical nerve roots | No complications were found except for mild discomfort in the treated area which spontaneously resolved up to 3 wk after the procedure. |
| Celiker et al,[16] 2011 | Chronic nasal obstruction | Randomized Clinical Trial | Sample size: 84 Mean age: N/A Male (%): 60.7 | N/A | Inferior nasal concha | At 3 mo, RF turbinate reduction was superior to nasal steroids for nasal blockage, HA, and snoring. RF turbinate reduction + nasal steroids better for headaches vs RF turbinate reduction alone | RF turbinate reduction group had better nasal flow post treatment. | RF turbinate reduction is superior than nasal steroids for improving symptoms associated with nasal obstruction | N/A |

| Study | Condition | Study design | Sample | Parameters | Target nerve | Outcomes | Results | Conclusion | Complications |
|---|---|---|---|---|---|---|---|---|---|
| Bakshi et al,[17] 2017 | Nasal obstruction secondary to bilateral inferior turbinate hypertrophy | Randomized Clinical Trial | Sample size: RFA 44, TP 42; Mean age: RFA 33.8, TP: 35.6; Male (%): RFA 50, TP 43.2 | 350J delivered for 50–60s | Anterior, middle, and posterior end of turbinate | 75% of RFA and 87.1% of TP had improvement in HA by 1 y. Relief of HA in RFA was s significant by 3 mo. | N/A | RFA more effective than TP for treating nasal obstruction, equally effective in managing sneezing. Not significantly better for HA relief. | RFA: 9 patients had bloody nasal discharge; 5 patiers had persistent burning sensation of the nose |
| Abd-Elsayed et al,[18] 2019 | Neuralgia-associated headache conditions | Retrospective study | Sample size: 168, 244 ablations; Mean age: 43.6; Male (%): 24.4 | Continuous 80 °C for 180 s | Greater and lesser occipital nerve | Mean pain score before RFA = 5.69 ± 2.23, then significant reduction to 2.86 ± 2.29 after RFA. Mean duration of pain relief = 182.2 d ± 154.5 d | Mean % pain improvement = 62.6% ± 33.7. Maximum duration of pain relief was 831 d' 89.3% of RFAs led to some degree of improvement; remaining 10.7% had no improvement. | RFA is a safe and effective treatment for patients with chronic headache conditions associated with pericranial neuralgias. | 3 patients developed eyelid swelling after supraorbital + supratrochlear RFAs. 2 patients had worsening of HA-symptoms. 1 patient had superficial infection at procedure site, treated with antibiotics. |
| Hamer et al,[19] 2014 | Cervicogenic headache and/or occipital neuralgia | Retrospective study | Sample size: 40; Mean age: 46.9; Male (%): 11.4 | 80 °C for 90 s | C2 dorsal root ganglion, and/or third occipital nerve | 90%[35] of patients reported ≥50% pain reduction after treatment. 35% (14 patients) reported 100% pain relief, 70% (28 patients) reported ≥80% relief. 7.5%[3] of patients reported zero pain relief, 2.5%[1] of patients reported 30% relief. 48% (19 patients) reported 30% relief. 48% (19 patients) reported <6 mo of pain relief. 52%[21] patients reported >6 of pain relief. The mean duration of improvement was 22.35 wk; 24.16 wk if patients with no pain relief are excluded. | 90%[35] of patients reported ≥50% pain reduction after treatment. 35% (14 patients) reported 100% pain relief, 70% (28 patients) reported ≥80% relief. 7.5%[3] of patients reported no pain relief, 2.5%[1] of patients reported 30% pain relief. 48% (19 patients) reported <6 mo of pain relief. 52%[21] of patients reported >6 mo of pain relief. Mean duration of improvement was 22.35 wk; 24.16 wk if patients with no pain relief are excluded. | RFA of C2 dorsal root ganglion and/or third occipital nerve can provide many months of ≥50% pain relief in majority of recipients, with expected duration of symptom improvement of 5–6 mo. | 2.5% reported hyperesthesia along greater occipital and lower occipital nerves, lasting 1–6 mo and 1 patient reported occipital hyperesthesia that was worse than her headache after unsuccessful ablation. |

*Abbreviation:* HA, headache; N/A, not applicable; TP, turbinoplasty.

pacemaker or defibrillator, prior PRF intervention on any nerve, and nonoccipital neuralgia or nonmigrainous headache. Govind and colleagues[3] analyzed 49 patients in a double-blind controlled study of PRF specifically targeting only the third occipital nerve with a modified technique. The 49 patients were selected from a larger source population of 120 patients who were noting general headache symptoms associated with neck pain or history of neck injury. The selected 49 patients were diagnosed with occipital neuralgia based on symptom improvement from a first (lignocaine 2% or bupivacaine 0.5%) and second nerve (whichever local anesthetic not used in the first block) block of the third occipital nerve. The median age range for these patients was 45 years, with 21 males and 28 females. Huang and colleagues[2] published a multicenter retrospective data analysis of 102 patients. In this study, medical records were analyzed from 2004 to 2011 and patients with an *International Classification of Disease*, 9th edition, code of 723.8 corresponding with "other diseases affecting cervical region-subheading occipital neuralgia" and a Current Procedural Terminology code of 64,999 corresponding with "unlisted procedure, nervous system-subheading PRF." Overall, 102 patients were selected.

In Cohen and colleagues' study,[1] all patients in both cohorts were positioned prone with target sites identified via anatomic landmarks. For each nerve, a 20G radiofrequency needle with a 10-mm tip was inserted at a 25° to 45° angle toward the target. Electrical stimulation was elicited with corresponding symptoms in the occipital nerve(s) distribution. The mean voltage was approximately 0.3 or less. Once needle placement was confirmed, the 2 cohorts received 1 of 2 interventions. The first cohort received a 2.75 mL injection containing 1 mL 0.5% bupivacaine, 1 mL 2% lidocaine, and 0.75 mL normal saline at each targeted nerve region. PRF was started after 4 minutes with the following parameters: voltage output 40 to 60 V, 2 Hz frequency, 20 ms pulses for a 1-s cycle, 120 s duration per cycle, impedance range between 150 and 400 $\Omega$ and 42 °C plateau temperature. A total of 3 cycles were formed. The second group received the same 2.75 mL injection, but with 0.75 mL of 40 mg/mL depomethylprednisolone at each nerve, with the RF generator never being activated. For Govind and colleagues' study,[3] only the third occipital nerve was targeted using fluoroscopy. Specific RF parameters were not discussed in their study. Using a Ray electrode, 3 insertions at multiple levels were made at the superior articular process of the C3 vertebral body, so that the third occipital nerve did not escape coagulation, depending on its anatomic position. In Huang and colleagues' study,[2] each occipital nerve was targeted with a 20G radiofrequency needle placed at an oblique angle. Sensory stimulation was used to ensure proper electrode placement to maximize electrical stimulation at the lowest possible voltage. For this study, the radiofrequency generator used the following parameters: voltage output 40 to 60 V, 2 Hz frequency, 20 ms pulses in 1-s cycle, 120 s duration/cycle, impedance range between 150 and 500 $\Omega$, 42 °C temperature plateau.

The primary outcomes, in Cohen at al's study,[1] were defined by headache intensity after PRF. The PRF group, when compared with the steroid injection group, experienced an overall decrease in the primary outcome with average occipital pain at 6 weeks. Participants in the steroid injection group experienced worst occipital pain at 2 weeks and persisted through 6 months for average occipital pain. Nonpain secondary outcomes defined by the frequency of occipital pain, sleep quality, medication reduction, and depression score did not reach statistical difference between the 2 cohorts. Three complications in the PRF group were reported, which included worsening headache, rash, and swelling, each in 3 separate individuals. In the steroid group, adverse effects of dizziness, swelling at the injection site, and worsening of headache for only 6 individuals. In Govind and colleagues' study,[3] the primary outcome was defined as complete pain relief that did not require any medicinal treatment, and secondary outcomes were defined as resuming daily activities. Of the 49 patients, 43 (88%) achieved the designated primary outcome with an average relief duration of 297 days. Regarding adverse effects, mild ataxia, hypersensitivity, and dysesthesia occurred in the skin territory of the third occipital nerve, which subsided within 10 days. Huang and colleagues' study[2] defined the primary outcome as a more than 50% pain relief for at least 3 months, whereas the secondary outcome was described as procedural satisfaction. Fifty-two patients (51%) achieved the primary outcome. More clarity is needed as to what percentage of the study participants achieved the secondary outcomes.

## Cluster Headache

According to the third edition of the ICHD, cluster headaches are defined as an episodic unilateral attack, at least 5, that range primarily from 15 to 180 minutes, associated with at least 1 parasympathetic ipsilateral symptom.[4] Parasympathetic symptoms include conjunctival injection, nasal congestion and/or rhinorrhea, eyelid edema, or ptosis and/or miosis on the affected side. Individuals with cluster headaches have been refractory to pharmacologic and interventional nonpharmacologic treatments, resulting in variable effectiveness.[4] A prospective study by Salgado-Lopez and colleagues[4] investigated the usefulness of either RFA or PRF to help treat chronic refractory cluster headache. For the study population, the mean age was 40 years with a range of 26 to 59 years. Twenty-four patients received PRF and 13 patients received RFA, for a total of 37 patients. All 37 patients were diagnosed with cluster headaches according to the ICHD and met certain criteria for treatment refractoriness. In another study by Fang and colleagues,[5] 16 patients with diagnosed cluster headaches were evaluated to determine if computed tomography (CT)-guided sphenopalatine ganglion PRF ablation would provide symptom improvement. Of the 16 patients, 14 were males and 2 were females with a mean age of 44.6 years, ranging from 15 to 75 years of age. According to the classification system designated by the International Headache Society, 16 patients suffered from cluster headaches. Exclusion criteria for the study by Fang and colleagues included abnormal blood, urinalysis, kidney, liver, glucose results. Additional exclusion criteria were abnormal findings on radiographs, electrocardiograms, head MRI, and CT scans of the head. Psychological disorders or a history of narcotic abuse were other exclusion criteria. In a prospective observational study by Narouze and colleagues,[6] 15 patients with diagnosed intractable chronic cluster headache were evaluated for the efficacy of sphenopalatine ganglion RFA. No specific inclusion or exclusion criteria were outlined, except for the fact that participants had experienced partial relief with sphenopalatine ganglion nerve block. Medical records and headache diaries were reviewed.

In the study by Salgado-Lopez and colleagues,[4] either RFA or PRF techniques were used for the study. According to the analysis, no scientific literature exists that favors 1 radiofrequency over the other. A 22G needle a with 10 cm length with an active tip of 5 mm was used for skin entry. After insertion and under fluoroscopic guidance, with proper placement of the guide needle laterally to the nasal wall at the level of the middle turbinate, the guide needle is replaced by the electrode. After confirmation of proper electrode positioning, either RFA or PRF is done with the following parameters: RFA being 0.5 cm$^3$ of 0.2% ropivacaine injected first and a lesion being made at 80 °C for 60 seconds, or PRF being 42 °C and 40 V for 120 seconds. The study from Fang and colleagues[5] initially used a 21G needle with a 5 mm active tip to enter the skin and track to the pterygopalatine fossa, with the assistance of CT imaging. After the needle core is removed, a radiofrequency electrode, connected to a radiofrequency generator, is placed, which then induces 50-Hz electrical stimulation that would induce paresthesia of the nasal root, confirming location accuracy. Parameters for RFA in this study were as follows: manual mode radiofrequency with a maximum temperature of 42 °C with output voltage slowly increasing until pain tolerance was maximally reached by each patient. Participants were treated twice at 120 seconds each session. In Narouze and colleagues study,[6] a 22-gauge, 10 cm RFA needle with a 5-mm active tip was advanced to the pterygopalatine fossa under fluoroscopic guidance. Once placement is confirmed and an electrode is inserted to illicit the proper sensory stimulation, 2 radiofrequency lesions were performed at 80 °C for 60 seconds each.

According the study by Salgado-Lopez and colleagues,[4] 5 patients (13.5%) had clinical headache resolution of both general pain and ipsilateral parasympathetic symptoms. Twenty-one patients (56.7%) experienced partial and transient relief and 11 patients did not have symptoms improvement.[4] No complications were reported for any of the patients. When comparing PRF with RFA, patients receiving PRF had a higher rate of clinical improvement (70.8% vs 61.5%), however, not at a statistically significant level ($P = .48$). The study from Fang and colleagues[5] evaluated treatment at 3 levels: complete pain relief with drug treatment cessation, partial pain relief by at least 50% compared with the preoperative state, and no pain relief compared with the preoperative condition. Eleven of the 13 participants with episodic cluster headaches (85%) and 1 of 3 participants with chronic cluster headaches had complete relief within an average of 6.3 ± 6.0 days after intervention. Similar to the study by Salgado-Lopez and colleagues, no treatment-related adverse effects or complications were reported. Results for the study from Narouze and colleagues[6] were organized in to 3 subheadings: mean attack intensity, mean attack frequency, and pain disability index. The overall mean attack intensity, mean attack frequency, and pain disability index parameters saw improvement and can be referred to the article. Twenty percent of the patients (3/15) showed no change or increase in symptom intensity or frequency. Approximately 46.7% of participants reported improving symptoms with relapse to the episodic cluster headaches form. Unlike the studies by Salgago-Lopez and colleagues and Fang and colleagues, adverse effect of paresthesia in the cheek and upper gums were reported in 7 of the 15 patients. One patient had a permanent focal coinlike distribution of numbness on the cheek.

### Cervicogenic Headache

Unlike other types of headache disorders previously discussed, cervicogenic headaches are a referred pain originating from a cervical pathology. Etiologies may be muscular, neurogenic, osseous, articular, or vascular.[7] Diagnosis is often difficult owing to the considerable overlap of symptoms with migraines. Nonspecific symptoms of nausea, vomiting, and throbbing may or may not be present. The Cervicogenic Headache International Study Group designated the following diagnostic criteria for cervicogenic headaches: (1) unilateral pain (sometimes bilateral), (2) decreased range of motion by neck movement, (3) head pain by neck movement, (4) provocation of head pain by overlying pressure over the upper cervical or occipital region on the occipital side, (5) minimal ipsilateral nonradicular neck, shoulder, or arm pain, (6) confirmed local anesthetic blocks in the cervical region, (7) considerable response to pharmacologic treatments, and (8) posterior onset of head pain. A retrospective study, by Halim and colleagues[8] analyzed PRF treatment efficacy using an anterolateral approach into the lateral atlantoaxial (C1–C2) joint. Of the 86 patients selected, 32 were male and 54 were female, with a mean age of 50.0 ± 2.1 years and a mean duration of headache for 9.4 ± 1.1 years. Haspeslagh and colleagues[9] conducted a randomized controlled trial comparing radiofrequency treatment, designated group 1, to steroid and bupivacaine injection, designated group 2, for cervicogenic headaches. A total of 45 patients were analyzed in the study, with 30 patients in group 1 and 15 in group 2. Additional inclusion criteria included individuals aged between 20 and 65 years, cervicogenic headaches of at least 2 years duration, a visual analog scale (VAS) score of more than 50 mm during a pain episode, and considerable pain for at least 2 days per week. Exclusion criteria were as followed: patients with prior cervical spine procedures, coagulation anomalies, currently pregnant, or had severe cervical degenerative disease or whiplash syndrome. Lee and associates[10] evaluated the clinical efficacy of radiofrequency neurotomy at the cervical zygapophyseal joint in patients with cervicogenic headaches. A total of 40 patients were enrolled, with 16 being men and 14 being women, ranging in age from 35 to 67 years. The mean age was 54 years. Individuals requiring multilevel cervical blocks and/or involved in litigation or compensational programs were excluded. Lang and Buchfelder[11] conducted a prospective study on radiofrequency neurotomy for patients with headaches symptoms originating from the C2 to C3 and C3 to C4 joint levels. Of the 31 patients selected for the study, 19 were male and 12 were female with a mean age of 46 years. Inclusion criteria for these patients presented with one of the following: cervical fusion followed by postoperative pseudoarthrosis, traumatic cervical fractures without fusion, and arthritis. Stover and colleagues[12] in a randomized, double-blind, sham-controlled study examined the radiofrequency denervation of C2-C6 facet joints in patients with cervicogenic headaches. Patients were diagnosed based on the traditional criteria described initially in this section and aged between 34 and 64 years, with a mean age of 44.5 for radiofrequency group and 52.5 for the sham treatment group. Exclusion criteria included: cervical spine stenosis, prior neck surgery, malignant disease, disease necessitating analgesic intake, concomitant headache disorder, pending litigation or compensation secondary to trauma. Six patients were enrolled for the radiofrequency group, while 6 patients were enrolled for the sham treatment. Van Suijlekom at al.[13] published a prospective study of 15 patients with cervicogenic headaches who had undergone zygapophyseal joint neurotomy.

In Halim and colleagues' study,[8] a 22G 45 mm insulated radiofrequency needle with a 5 mm active tip was advanced, under fluoroscopic guidance, posterolaterally and then anteromedially at the C1 to C2 joint, with a characteristic pop heard. After sensory innervation at 50 Hz up to 1.0 V confirms positioning of the active tip, PRF activation was started with the following parameter: 45V, 2 Hz, and 10 ms for 10 minutes after positive sensory stimulation. Targeted lesions for radiofrequency in Haspeslagh and colleagues[9] study focused on the cervical facet and cervical segmental nerves at the following parameters respectively: 67 °C for 60 seconds, 50 Hz and 2 Hz threshold. RFA of the cervical facet was performed initially, followed by the cervical dorsal root ganglion. The greater occipital nerve was targeted. In Lee and colleagues'[10] observational study, a 22G, 10 cm needle with an expose tip of 5 mm was used to generate a final lesion at 80 °C for 90 seconds at the occipital nerve. For Lang and Buchfelder's study,[11] radiofrequency neurotomy, under fluoroscopy, was performed at the cervical dorsal rami of the C3 and C4 at 80 °C for 90 seconds. In Stovner and colleagues' study,[12] patients in the radiofrequency treatment group received 3 to 4 lesions at 85 °C for 60 seconds targeting the third occipital nerve. Patients in the sham procedure went to the same procedure with no lesions targeted. Both groups had procedures lasting approximately 90 minutes.

In a study by Halim and colleagues,[8] 43 patients (50%) experienced at least 50% pain relief at 2 and 6 months. Thirty-eight patients (44.2%) experienced at least

50% pain relief at 1 year. At 2 months, long-term pain relief at 6 months and 1 year were predicated reliably at a statistically significant rate ($P < .001$). As per the study's secondary outcome, pain duration, preradiofrequency neurotomy, and baseline pain were not significant predictors of at least 50% pain relief at the 2 months, 6 months, and 1 year. Overall, only 1 patient noted worsening of occipital headache of several hours duration. In the study by Haspeslagh and colleagues,9 VAS pain scores, effect scores, and quality of life scores presented no statistically significant differences between group 1 and group 2. After 16 weeks of treatment, RFA had a 66.7% success rate compared with the 55.3% success rate of the steroid group. No side effects or complications were recorded. A study by Lee and colleagues[10] reported more than 75% pain relief for 60% of the patients at week 1%, 83.3% of the patients at 1 month, and 76.7% at 6 months and 73.3% at 1 year. Postoperatively, the average frequency of headache symptoms decreased to 2.8 from 6.2. The secondary outcome for this study revealed a 70% decrease in analgesic usage per week. As per adverse effects, 12 patients noted posterior neck soreness for approximately 2 to 7 days that resolved within the week. No postoperative infections or other procedure-related complications occurred. The study by Lang and Buchfelder[11] showed that all patients in all 3 study groups experienced pain relief on the first day after neurotomy. Pain relief of at least 70% was noted in all procedures, and pain relief was 100% in 38 procedures. For the analysis by Stovner and colleagues,[12] pain relief was seen in both groups until month 3, where the radiofrequency group surpassed the sham group. When arriving to month 6, both groups seemed to have little to no difference in pain relief. At month 24, the sham group outperformed the radiofrequency group in all variables of pain relief. Results of the study by Van Suilekom and colleagues[13] showed a considerable decrease in the severity of cervicogenic headache in 12 of the 15 patients. The average VAS decrease was 31.4 mm at a statistically significant rate ($P < .001$) and 53.5 mm, also at a statistically significant rate at 8 weeks and 16 weeks of follow-up. Of note, a secondary outcome revealed in this study average number of headache days decreased to 2.8 from 5.8 ($P = .001$).

## Chronic Migraine

Chronic migraines are a debilitating headache condition affecting approximately 2% of the general population.[14] Individuals with chronic migraines have symptoms for at least 15 days per month, with at least 8 days of the month where the headache and associated symptoms meet the criteria for migraine diagnosis.[14] Characteristics and associated symptoms include the following: (1) unilateral, (2) throbbing pain, (3) exacerbation with physical activity, along with (a) nausea and/or vomiting and (b) photophobia and/or phonophobia. In current literature, very few studies evaluate the usefulness of PRF on helping to treat individuals with chronic migraines. Yang and colleagues[14] in a 2015 published study evaluated 40 patients to compare the efficacy of PRF with sham treatment. The number of men and women in the treatment group were 3 and 17, respectively, and the number of men and women in the sham treatment group were 4 and 16, respectively. The mean age for whole study was approximately 43.5 years, with a baseline VAS score of $7.75 \pm 0.96$ in the treatment group. Inclusion criteria were as follows: at least 18 years of age, chronic migraines diagnosed by the ICHD-III, at least 6 months duration of chronic migraines, and a 30% decrease in pain after occipital nerve block. Psychosis, an inability to adhere to physician advice, involvement in other trials, diagnosed pregnancy, or an inability to complete the study were exclusion criteria.

Under fluoroscopic guidance, Yang and colleagues[14] used a 21G needle with a 5 mm exposed tip to puncture at the C2 level. The needle was advanced until the tip reached the inferior articular process of the C2, resulting in alignment with the third occipital nerve. Sensation test mode was conducted at 50 Hz and 0.3 V. After confirmation of needle placement, the generator was turned on to the PRF mode with the following parameters: 42 °C, 120 seconds, performed twice for each level. The second entry point was at the C3 level to align with the C3 nerve medial branch, repeating the same steps for the C2 PRF.

Outcome measures in the report by Yang and colleagues[14] were measured by headache intensity, duration, analgesic dose, Migraine Disability Assessment Questionnaire score and reported adverse reactions. In the PRF group, mean VAS decreased by 2.52 points compared with a 0.55-point decrease in the sham group at the 6-month follow-up. The VAS scores also differed dramatically from the sham group at the 1-, 2-, and 6-month follow-up periods. Effective outcomes, with effective being defined as at least a 30% decrease in pain, were identified in the PRF group ($P < .05$). The mean decrease in headache duration at the 6-month follow-up was 8.9 days per month. Patients within the treatment cohort revealed considerably lower required aspirin doses at all follow-up periods. Significant differences between the 2 groups were evident in headache duration and aspirin dose for symptom relief. The Migraine Disability Assessment Questionnaire scores were decreased in the posttreatment phase compared with pretreatment. Of note, the Migraine Disability Assessment Questionnaire scores in the PRF group were lower, by 21.57 points, compared with the sham group. No patient experienced infection, increased bleeding, substantial pain, numbness, or postoperative paresthesia. Mild pain was noted at the second PRF cycle for 1 patient, which resolved within approximately 6 hours without treatment. Follow-up evaluations revealed no complications.

### Chronic Headache

Chronic headache is a generalized diagnosis of sharp or dull head pain defined by a duration of at least 15 days for at least 3 to 6 months. In the past, chronic headache etiologies stemmed from the upper cervical spine. However, investigators recently have suggested that the cervical spine nerve roots can also play a role in symptomology.[15] Shabat and colleagues[15] conducted a retrospective study that looked at PRF at the C5 and C6 nerve roots to determine efficacy for chronic headache symptom management. The C5 and C6 nerve roots give rise to the suprascapular nerve and thus have been targeted in the past for PRF to help improve shoulder pain. The retrospective study aimed to see if the same PRF techniques targeted at the same nerve roots, originally for shoulder pain treatment, also improved chronic headache symptoms. The study by Shabat and colleagues[15] examined 69 patients between 2005 and 2015 with both chronic shoulder pain and headache who underwent a PRF intervention at the suprascapular nerve. Twenty-nine of the patients were men and 40 were women, with a mean age of 48 years. The age range of the study population was 22 to 70 years.

For the 69 patients, sensory stimulation with 50 Hz and motor stimulation with 2 Hz was performed to confirm electrode placement. A core temperature of 42 °C around the electrode tip for 120 seconds. A Radionics RFG 3C generator was used.

The primary outcomes were evaluated via VAS scores for pain relief, which were separately scored for headache and shoulder pain. Follow-up evaluations were performed at 4 weeks, 3 and 6 months, and 1 year. A good result was defined by Shabat and colleagues[15] as at least 50% pain relief, and no effect was defined by less than 30% relief. A moderate result was identified as pain relief in the 30% to 50% range. At 4 weeks, 41 patients (59%) noted general improvement in headache. By 3 months after the PRF treatment, 38 patients (55%) reported headache relief in the pain free, good, or moderate designations. Similar trends were seen in the remaining 6-month and 1-year follow-up visits. Shabat and colleagues[15] also used the Owestry disability questionnaire to assess functional status. Individuals experienced average score improvements at a statistically significant rate; 76 points at preprocedure to 30 points (1 month) to 35 points (3 month) to 44 points (6 month) to 46 points (1 year). Nineteen patients experienced discomfort in the innervated region post PRF, which resolved within 3 weeks. Overall, no complications were reported for any study patients.

*Others*

RFA has been reported to have considerable efficacy in nasal obstruction conditions and other neuralgia-associated types of headache. Celiker and associates[16] in 2011 published a randomized clinical trial comparing RFA with steroid patch treatment for nasal congestion and concha hypertrophy. Nasal congestion and hypertrophic concha are commonly known to cause generalized headaches. The randomized control trial examined a total of 84 patients, with 51 being male and 33 being female. The age range was between 18 and 65 years. Of note, this study by Celiker and associatess[16] entailed the study participants switching treatment modalities at the 3-month timepoint, thus having all participants undertake both RFA and steroid patch placement by the end of the study. Baksha and colleagues[17] conducted another randomized clinical trial, consisting of 86 patients, comparing RFA with surgical turbinoplasty to relieve turbinate hypertrophy. Of the 86 patients, 40 were males and 46 were females, with 42 being assigned to the RFA group and the remaining 44 patients being assigned to surgical turbinoplasty. In a publication from Abd-Elsayed and colleagues,[18] a retrospective study was performed to evaluate the efficacy and safety of RFA treatment in 168 patients for headaches associated with precranial neuralgia. Of the 168 patients, 41 were male and 127 were female, with a mean age of 43.6 years and age range of 16 to 83 years. Hamer and Purath[19] published a single-center retrospective observational study looking at both occipital neuralgia and cervicogenic headache patients and their response to PRF to the C2 dorsal root ganglion and third occipital nerve, respectively. Forty patients with a mean age of 46.9 years were evaluated.

The study performed by Celiker and colleagues[16] inserted the RF probe specifically at 3 sites within the inferior concha for a treatment duration of 8 to 10 minutes. Specific settings for the RFA were not reported in the study. In a trial conducted by Baksha and colleagues,[17] a 10-mm active tip was used at 350 J for 50 to 60 seconds. Targeted regions were the anterior, middle, and posterior ends of the turbinate for 3 total applications, for an overall procedure time of less than 15 minutes. Overall, patients in the study conducted by Abd-Elsayed and colleagues[18] received RFA at 80 °C for 180 seconds with a 21G needle with a 4-mm active tip. A small percentage of the patients received RFA at 60 °C and 90 °C for durations ranging between 60 and 165 seconds. The greater and lesser occipital supraorbital and supratrochlear nerves were targeted for RFA. For the study by Hamer and Purath,[19] sensory testing at 50 Hz and motor testing at 2 Hz, along with radiographic imaging, was performed to confirm proper electrode placement. RFA was performed specifically at the third occipital nerve at 80 °C for 90 seconds.

The RF turbinate reduction group, in a study by Celiker and colleagues,[16] at 3 months had a statistically significant and more effective advantage compared with the nasal steroid patch group with regard to nasal blockage ($P < .01$) and headache ($P < .05$). In the study by Bakshi and colleagues,[17] 75% of the RF group experienced headache improvement by the third month until year end at a statistically significant level. As noted, relief in headache is likely caused by a decrease in nasal congestion secondary to decreased turbinate size or loss of septum and turbinate interface. No adverse reactions were noted in studies conducted by Bakshi and colleagues and Celiker and colleagues. In the analysis performed by Abd-Elsayed and colleagues,[18] the mean pain scores decreased from 5.69 ± 2.23 to 2.86 ± 2.29 in the post-RFA stage. Mean duration of pain relief was 182.2 ± 154.5 days. Overall, 89.3% of RFA patients reported symptom improvement and 10.7% reported otherwise. Three patients developed eyelid swelling after RFA to the supraorbital and supratrochlear nerves, for which resolution occurred within 1 week. One patient experienced superficial infection at the intervention site, which resolved with antibiotics. In the study from Hamer and Purath,[19] pain relief was reported, with 35% of the participants reporting 100% pain relief and 70% of the participants reporting at least 80% pain relief. Overall, the duration of pain relief ranged between 0 and 72 weeks, with the mean duration being 22.35 weeks. Approximately 12.5% of the patient reported hyperesthesia and 1 patient reported exacerbation of known dizziness.

### Trigeminal Neuralgia

Trigeminal neuralgia is a chronic neuropathic pain condition associated with severe pain that is described as excruciating and can cause serious impairments to daily functioning. The condition affects the fifth cranial nerve, one of the most widely distributed nerves in the head. The typical form of the disorder causes extreme, sporadic sudden burning or shock-like facial pain that lasts anywhere from a few seconds to as long as 2 minutes per episode. These attacks can occur in quick succession, in volleys lasting for up to 2 hours. The atypical form of the disorder is characterized by constant aching, burning, and stabbing pain of somewhat lower intensity than typical trigeminal neuralgia. Both forms of trigeminal neuralgia may occur in the same individual at the time. Rarely, both sides of the face may be affected at different times in an individual, or even more rarely at the same time in bilateral trigeminal neuralgia. Although pharmacologic treatment is often initiated for patients with trigeminal neuralgia, medical management eventually fails in most trigeminal neuralgia cases. For patients with persistent pain despite pharmacologic therapy or who are unable to tolerate the adverse effects of certain drugs, several alternative surgical modalities for trigeminal neuralgia have emerged.

### Randomized Controlled Studies

Several randomized controlled studies have investigated the use of surgical treatment for idiopathic trigeminal neuralgia. The average age of the study populations ranged from 48 to 60 years and the percentage of male patients in these studies ranged from 36.6% to 56.0% (Table 2). The sample size varied across studies, with smallest size (n = 40) being studied by Erdine and colleagues[20] and the largest (n = 1354) being studied by Yao and colleagues.[21]

Each of the randomized control studies assessed the use of surgical ablation techniques that targeted branches of the trigeminal nerve. Most studies assessed a broad distribution and targeted all 3 branches as affected within their patient populations, although Luo and colleagues[22] targeted largely the V2 distribution and Yao and colleagues[23] targeted the V1 distribution. The ablation techniques included PRF, conventional radiofrequency (CRF), percutaneous radiofrequency thermocoagulation (PRT or RFT), and nerve combing. These techniques were assessed with variations in ablation temperature, voltage differences, with or without CT guidance, combinations of therapies, and with comparisons between techniques.

Yao and colleagues[21] used a controlled study to assess differences in performance between RFT performed at 68 °C and 75 °C. Excellent pain relief was achieved equally

**Table 2**
Characteristics of randomized trials investigating the role of RFAs for the management of facial pain

| Author (Year) | Clinical Diagnosis | Study Design | Patient Population | Ablation Technique | Target Nerve | Duration of Pain Relief | Secondary Outcome | Conclusion | Side Effect |
|---|---|---|---|---|---|---|---|---|---|
| Yao et al,[21] 2016 | Idiopathic trigeminal neuralgia | Prospective randomized cohort study | Sample size (n): 81 Mean age (y): 41.6 Male (%): 52 | RFT performed at 68 °C and 75 °C | Trigeminal neuralgia | Excellent relief achieved at 75 °C in 99.2% of patients and in 98.2% of patients treated with 68 °C RFT at discharge, 95.1% and 93.5% at 1 y, 84.3% and 78.1% at 3 y, 80.7% and 74.4% at 5 y. | All patients were satisfied with bilateral RFT at discharge. At year 1, treatment was scored as satisfactory in 69.0% and 90.3% of patients (75 °C and 68 °C); at 5 y these rates decreased to 50.1% and 63.6% | Consistent pain relief was achieved after RFT at both 68 °C and 75 °C, but RFT at 68 °C was superior to RFT at 75 °C in terms of the rate and severity of complications and patient satisfaction. | Facial swelling, facial numbness, corneal hypoesthesia, masticatory atonia. Facial numbness persisted at discharge on the side undergoing 68 °C RFT (12.9%) less than often the side undergoing 75 °C RFT (79.0%), and all patients recovered within 1 y |
| Erdine et al,[20] 2007 | Idiopathic trigeminal neuralgia | Prospective randomized double-blinded | Sample size (n): 40 Mean age (y): 62.2 Male (%): 52.5 | PRF compared with CRF | Trigeminal neuralgia | VAS pain scores significantly decreased in CRF treatment patients 1 d after the procedure compared with baseline. Pain relief was not significantly achieved by PRF. VAS scores at 1 d, 3 mo, and 6 mo after CRF were significantly reduced compared with baseline. CRF applied to PRF patients at the end of 3 mo decreased VAS scores. All CRF patients maintained pain relief at 6 mo of follow-up. | Patient Satisfaction Scale scores significantly improved in CRF patients 1 d after procedure. No differences in Patient Satisfaction Scale values in the PRF group. All CRF patients were able to stop additional medical treatment. All PRF patients required further medical treatment at 3 mo. | Unlike CRF, PRF is not an effective method for the treatment of idiopathic trigeminal neuralgia. | Moderate headache reported in 25% of CRF patients after the procedure. 15% of PRF patients reported mild headache after the procedure. All CRF patients reported mild hypoesthesia and paresthesia after the procedure. PRF patients did not report paresthesia until the application of CRF at 3 mo. |
| Elawamy et al,[24] 2017 | Idiopathic trigeminal neuralgia | Prospective randomized double blinded | Sample size (n): 43 Mean age (y): 55.8 (PRF), | PRF at 42 °C for 10 min, CRF at 75 °C for 270 s, or PRF | Trigeminal neuralgia | Assessment of pain by VAS showed the most significant reductions in scores among the | Decreases in carbamazepine doses were observed in all groups. Patients in the | CCPRF results in excellent pain relief for patients maintained at 24 mo and decreases the | The CRF group had the most complications (45.5%), with the CCPRF group having the |

| Study | Condition | Study design | Sample size | Intervention | Pain condition | Results | Medication/satisfaction | Conclusions | Side effects/complications |
|---|---|---|---|---|---|---|---|---|---|
| | | | 56.0 (CRF), 52.6 (CCPRF) Male (%): 50.0 (PRF), 54.5 (CRF), 35.0 (CCPRF) | at 42 °C for 10 min followed by CRF at 60 °C for 270 s (CCPRF group) | | CCPRF group, followed by CRF, and then PRF group. All groups had significant pain reduction immediately after the intervention maintained at 1 wk, 1 mo, 6 mo, 12 mo, and 24 mo after the intervention. Excellent pain relief was achieved at 24 mo only with CCPRF (90%). | CCPRF group reported significantly higher satisfaction than other groups at 1 and 6 mo after the intervention. Satisfaction was maintained in all groups over 24 mo of follow-up. | consumption of analgesics by patients with idiopathic trigeminal neuralgia. CCPRF intervention also decreases complications compared with PRF and CRF. | lowest complications (20.0%). Numbness and weakness (18.2% among CRF) and paresthesia (10.0% among CCPRF) were most often reported. |
| Fang et al,[26] 2015 | Idiopathic trigeminal neuralgia | Prospective randomized double-blinded | Sample size (n): 60 Mean age (y): 63.5 (standard voltage), 60.5 (high-voltage) Male (%): 46.7 (standard voltage), 43.3 (high-voltage) | PRF, standard or high voltage | Trigeminal neuralgia | 41% of standard voltage patients had favorable outcomes at 6 mo as assessed by NRS scores. The effective rate at 1 y was only 19% for standard voltage treatment patients. Of these patients, 59% failed to respond to treatment 1-mo postoperatively. Those standard voltage patients who responded experienced the greatest pain relief 2 wk to 1 mo after intervention. Significant pain decreases were achieved in 69% of high-voltage patients at 6 mo and 1 y, and none of these patients experienced recurrence. | 41% of standard voltage patients stopped or greatly decreased carbamazepine treatment at 6 mo; 69% of high-voltage patients stopped or required only low doses of carbamazepine for pain control after treatment. The effective rates of the high-voltage group were higher at 1, 3, 6, and 12 mo after the operation compared with standard voltage treatment. | Although high-voltage PRFT is more effective than standard voltage PRFT without obvious side effects, the short-term effective rate is still lower than that of RFTC. The efficacy of high-voltage PRFT is still needed to be improved. | No side effects were experienced in patients who underwent PRFT. |

(continued on next page)

**Table 2**
*(continued)*

| Author (Year) | Clinical Diagnosis | Study Design | Patient Population | Target Nerve | Ablation Technique | Duration of Pain Relief | Secondary Outcome | Conclusion | Side Effect |
|---|---|---|---|---|---|---|---|---|---|
| Li et al,[25] 2012 | Idiopathic trigeminal neuralgia | Prospective randomized double blinded | Sample size (n): 60. Mean age (y): 54.4 (SCRF), 61.1 (LCRF), 55.6 (PCRF). Male (%): 40 (SCRF), 40 (LCRF), 35 (PCRF) | Trigeminal neuralgia | CRF at 75 °C for 120–180 s (SCRF), CRF at 75 °C for 240–300 s (LCRF), PRF at 42 °C for 10 min then CRF 75 °C for 120–180 s (PCRF) | After RF treatment, all patients had significant pain relief as assessed by NRS scores. After 12 mo, the rate of excellent pain relief exceeded 70% in all groups. There were no significant differences in the rate of excellent pain relief and mean NRS scores between groups. | After 6 and 12 mo, only 1 SCRF patient required low-dose carbamazepine to relieve pain. Within 12 mo, all patients reported significant improvement in QOL compared with baseline. | Although the combined treatment resulted in more severe dysesthesia immediately after the procedure, patients with this treatment achieved comparable efficacy and safety to treatment with CRF alone over a longer follow-up time. | All patients experienced facial dysesthesia 1 d after the procedure. The intensity of dysesthesia was most serious in the PCRF group and mildest in the SCRF group. Dysesthesia in the LCRF group was higher than in the PCRF group 12 mo after treatment; the degree of dysesthesia in the PCRF group decreased more rapidly with time. |
| Luo et al,[22] 2017 | Idiopathic trigeminal neuralgia | Prospective randomized double blinded | Sample size (n): 60. Mean age (y): 65 (standard voltage), 61 (high-voltage). Male (%): 46.6 (standard voltage), 36.6 (high-voltage) | Trigeminal neuralgia (V2) | PRF, standard or high voltage | 1-mo, 3-mo, 6-mo, and 1-y response rates were all 90% in the high-voltage group, which were significantly higher than in the standard voltage group (67%, 67%, 63%, and 60%, respectively), as measured by NRS scores. | 67% of standard voltage patients discontinued or required low-dose carbamazepine for pain relief during follow-up. 90% of patients in the high-voltage group discontinued or required only low-dose carbamazepine. | High-voltage PRF was effective and safe for patients with refractory neuralgia in the infraorbital nerve and could become a treatment option in patients who do not respond to conservative treatment. | 27% of patients in the high-voltage group and 13% of patients in the standard voltage group experienced minor transient numbness after PRF. |
| Xu et al,[27] 2006 | Idiopathic trigeminal neuralgia | Prospective randomized control | Sample size (n): 54. Mean age (y): 63 (navigation), 59 (control). Male (%): 53.8 (navigation), 46.4 (control) | Trigeminal neuralgia | PRT with or without neuronavigation | Immediate and complete pain relief was 100% in the navigation group and 95% in the control group. The proportion of sustained pain relief in the navigation group at 12, 24, and 36 mo after the | Recurrences in the control group were common than in the navigation group. Adverse effects were also more common in the control group. | Neuronavigator-guided PRT is a safe and promising method for the treatment of intractable trigeminal neuralgia with better short- and long-term outcomes and lower complication rates | No side effects or complications were noted in the navigation, except for minimal temporary facial hypoesthesia. In the control group, dysesthesia occurred in 2 patients, absent or |

| Study | Condition | Study design | Sample size / demographics | Intervention | Diagnosis | Results | Outcomes / QOL | Conclusions | Complications |
|---|---|---|---|---|---|---|---|---|---|
| | | | | | | operation was 85%, 77%, and 62%, respectively, whereas those in the control group were 54%, 40%, and 35%, respectively (significant difference at all time points). | | than PRT without neuronavigation. | diminished corneal reflex in 2 patients, corneal keratitis in 1, and masseter dysfunction in 1. |
| Yao et al,[21] 2016 | Idiopathic trigeminal neuralgia | Prospective randomized cohort study | Sample size (n): 1354 Mean age (y): 56.4 (62 °C), 61.1 (65 °C), 59.2 (68 °C) Male (%): 52.7 (62 °C), 48.6 (65 °C), 47.7 (68 °C) | CT-guided RFT, completed at 62 °C, 65 °C, or 68 °C | Trigeminal neuralgia | At discharge, pain relief was achieved in 94.2%, 98.3%, and 98.8% of the patients in the 62 °C, 65 °C, and 68 °C groups, respectively. At 1 year, these rates were 83.8%, 90.1%, and 91.4%. At 3 y, they were 66.7%, 80.5%, and 88.2%. At 5 y, they were 59.0%, 64.3%, and 77.2%. The 68 °C group was the only group to demonstrate >60% effectiveness with pain relief at 9 y. | The highest long-term health-related QOL scores were seen in the 68% group, followed by the 65 °C and then 62 °C groups. | 68 °C is effective for RFT of V2/V3 RFN. The alternative option of 62 °C or 65 °C for RFT minimizes the occurrence of complications but yields a higher recurrence rate. | The number of patients with facial numbness, masticatory atonia, or corneal hypoesthesia was increased with the elevation of temperature, but these complications were all mild. |
| Yao et al,[23] 2016 | Idiopathic trigeminal neuralgia | Prospective randomized cohort study | Sample size (n): 56 Mean age (y): 55.6 (CRF), 56.1 (CRF + PRF) Male (%): 42.9 (CRF), 46.4, (CRF + PRF) | CRF, CRF + PRF | Trigeminal neuralgia (V1) | At discharge, all patients in both groups had pain relief. At 1 y, pain relief as assessed by a BNI score of I was found in 81.6% of patients who underwent CRF and 92.0% of patients who underwent CRF + PRF. The rates of pain relief at 2 y were 68.4% and 92%, and rates at 3 y were 68.4% and 83.6%. | During follow-up, 32.1% of patients who received CRF developed recurrence, whereas only 7.2% of patients who underwent CRF + PRF developed recurrence. Patients in the CRF + PRF treatment group reported higher QOL scores during follow-up at 2 and 3 y. | CRF + PRF can decrease the recurrence rate of V1 trigeminal neuralgia, decrease the incidence rate and shorten the recovery time of corneal hypoesthesia, and lead to increased QOL scores after CRF. | Patients in both groups experienced postoperative corneal hypoesthesia, with shorter recovery times in the CRF + PRF treatment group. Facial numbness was also experienced in both groups but recovered by 6 mo. |

(continued on next page)

**Table 2**
*(continued)*

| Author (Year) | Clinical Diagnosis | Study Design | Patient Population | Ablation Technique | Target Nerve | Duration of Pain Relief | Secondary Outcome | Conclusion | Side Effect |
|---|---|---|---|---|---|---|---|---|---|
| Ding et al,[28] 2016 | Idiopathic trigeminal neuralgia | Prospective randomized study | Sample size (n): 108<br>Mean age (y): 57.9<br>Male (%): 38 | CT-guided RFT, access through either Hartel anterior approach (group H) or percutaneous puncture through mandibular angle (group G) | Trigeminal neuralgia | On day 1 after the procedure, 96.2% of group H patients and 98.0% of group G patients experienced initial pain relief. In group G patients, successful response was maintained in 89.8% of patients at 1 y, 85.7% at 2 y, and 81.6% at 3 y. In group H, success rates at 1, 2, and 3, y were 82.7%, 76.5%, and 60.8%, respectively. | In group H, the 24 and 36-mo recurrence rates were 23.5% and 39.2%, respectively. In group G, these recurrence rates were 12.2% and 16.3%. The mean QOL score at 36 mo for group G was higher than that for group H. | Compared with the Hartel approach of the Gasserian ganglion for RFT, the submandibular approach offers similar complication profiles but better long-term efficacy in terms of pain reduction. | Similar complications between the 2 groups included hematoma formation associated with needle entry, numbness, diminished corneal reflex, and masseter weakness. |
| Zhou et al,[29] 2016 | Idiopathic trigeminal neuralgia | Prospective randomized study | Sample size (n): 105<br>Mean age (y): 48.9 (nerve combing), 49.3 (RFT)<br>Male (%): 56 (nerve combing), 54.5 (RFT) | Nerve combing or RFT | Trigeminal neuralgia | At the end of follow-up, 82% of nerve combing treatment patients experienced pain relief. Initially, 90% of nerve combing treatment patients had experienced pain relief. In the RFT treatment group, 76.4% of patients reported satisfactory pain relief at the end of follow-up. Both procedures had similar efficacy. | 13 patients with recurrence in the nerve combing treatment group underwent a repeat procedure and experienced satisfactory pain relief. The recurrence rate in the nerve combing group was 10%, and the recurrence rate was 14.5% in the RFT group. | Nerve combing and RFT are both satisfactory treatment strategies for patients with idiopathic trigeminal neuralgia. Because of the higher risk of sensory morbidity and surgical risk as open surgery, RF is preferred as the recommended procedure for patients with idiopathic trigeminal neuralgia. | In the nerve combing group, postoperative morbidity included dysesthesia (16%), diplopia (2%), and partial nerve dysfunction (14%). In the RFT group, the most frequent complications were dysesthesia and tinnitus, which developed in 3.6% of patients. |

*Abbreviations:* BNI, Barrow neurological institute; CRF, conventional radiofrequency; NRS, numeric pain rating scale; PRT, percutaneous radiofrequency thermocoagulation; QIL quality of life.

at both temperatures with 99.2% of patients treated with RFT at 75 °C and 98.2% of patients treated with RFT at 68 °C having complete pain relief at discharge. Pain relief persisted, with 80.7% of patients treated at 75 °C and 74.4% of patients treated at 68 °C with RFT experiencing complete pain relief at 5 years of follow-up. Although these results were similar between the 2 groups, RFT at 68 °C was superior to RFT at 75 °C in terms of the rate and severity of complications and patient satisfaction. Patients in both treatment groups experienced transient facial swelling and numbness that recovered in all cases within 1 year.

Erdine and colleagues[20] compared PRF with CRF treatment and demonstrated the superiority of CRF for the treatment of idiopathic trigeminal neuralgia. All CRF patients in this study experienced pain relief immediately after the procedure; however, pain scores in the PRF group did not decrease from baseline at 1 day after the procedure. The decrease in pain scores was maintained by the CRF group at 3 months and 6 months after the procedure. Furthermore, all CRF patients were able to discontinue all medical treatment after the procedure, whereas all PRF patients required further medical treatment 3 months after the procedure. Fewer mild headaches were reported in the PRF group compared with CRF patients, and although only CRF patients experienced paresthesia, all patients undergoing either procedure reported mild transient hypoesthesia. Elawamy and colleagues[24] also compared PRF and CRF technique efficacy, although ablation temperature variations were also assessed in this study. All treatment groups in this study showed significant decreases in pain scores immediately after the procedure, with this pain relief maintained for up to 24 months after the intervention. Excellent pain relief was only achieved at 24 months by the group treated with PRF at 42 °C for 10 minutes followed by CRF at 60 °C for 270 seconds (CCPRF group). Decreases in medical treatment were seen in all groups, although the CCPRF treatment group reported the highest patient satisfaction rates at 1 and 6 months of follow-up. All groups maintained adequate satisfaction rates at 24 months of follow-up. The CCPRF group experienced the lowest rate of complications, with the most common complications being facial numbness, weakness, and transient paresthesia. Li and colleagues[25] also compared PRF and CRF treatment in combinations with varying ablation temperatures. All patients in this study had significant pain relief, with the rate of excellent pain relief exceeding 70% in all patient groups at 12 months after the procedure. All patients reported significant quality of life improvements, with only 1 patient requiring further low-dose medication to assist with relieving pain. All patients experienced facial dysesthesia 1 day after the procedure, although the intensity of dysesthesia was the most serious in the group treated with combined PRF and CRF. Yao and colleagues23 also compared CRF with combined CRF and PRF. All patients in this study experienced immediate pain relief after the procedure. Pain relief was sustained at 1 year of follow-up in 81.6% of patients who underwent isolated CRF, and pain relief was sustained in 92.0% of patients who underwent combined CRF and PRF. These rates at 2 years were 68.4% in the CRF group and 92.0% in the combined treatment group. Patients in the combined treatment group also reported higher quality of life scores at 2 to 3 years of follow-up. Patients in both groups experienced postoperative corneal hypoesthesia, although the recovery times were shorter in the combined treatment group. Facial numbness was also experienced in both groups, but resolved by 6 months.

Fang and colleagues[26] compared PRF application at standard with high-voltage pulses for the treatment of idiopathic trigeminal neuralgia, which showed that high-voltage PRF was more effective than standard voltage PRF for the treatment of idiopathic trigeminal neuralgia. Of all patients treated with high-voltage PRF, 69% achieved significant pain reductions at 6 months and 1 year. Standard voltage PRF only provided 41% of patients with favorable outcomes at 6 months. However, in comparing their results with previous literature, the authors noted that the positive results with PRF still presented lower effectiveness rates than treatment with RFT. No serious side effects were reported in this study. Luo and colleagues[22] also compared standard voltage PRF with high-voltage PRF. The 1-month, 3-month, and 6-month treatment response rates in the high-voltage group were all significantly higher than those seen in the standard voltage group. Furthermore, although 90% of patients treated with high-dose PRT were able to discontinue medical treatment during follow-up, only 67% of the patients receiving a standard voltage were able to discontinue this treatment. Minor transient facial numbness was experienced in both treatment groups, with higher rates of this complication seen in the high-voltage PRF group.

Among the studies investigating guided ablation techniques, Xu and colleagues[27] compared the effectiveness of PRT with or without the use of neuronavigation. This study found that all patients treated with guided PRT achieved immediate pain relief after the procedure, whereas 95% of patients treated with PRT without guidance experienced immediate relief. The proportion of sustained pain relief in the navigation-guided group was significantly higher at all time points up to 36 months after the procedure. Both pain recurrences and complications were more common in the control group than in the navigation group. Minimal transient hypoesthesia was the only complication experienced in the navigation-guided PRT group. Yao and colleagues[21] and colleagues used CT-guided RFT with varying ablation temperatures. The results of this study showed that the highest temperature used (68 °C) produced the highest treatment success rates at follow-up from 1 to 9 years after the procedure. Lower temperatures (62 °C and 65 °C) were associated with lower rates of complications, but also resulted in higher rates of recurrence. Only the highest ablation temperature group had an effective treatment rate of more than 60% at 9 years of follow-up, although all treatment groups had demonstrated an initial immediate response to the intervention. Complications included facial numbness, masticatory atonia, and corneal hypoesthesia, all of which increased in frequency with higher ablation temperatures. Ding and colleagues[28] examined differing approaches to CT-guided RFT, comparing effectiveness using the Hartel approach or puncture through the mandibular angle. Patients undergoing the procedure in which the mandibular angle approach was used experienced improved long-term pain relief compared with those who underwent the procedure when the Hartel approach was used. Patients in the mandibular angle approach group had lower rates of pain recurrence and reported higher quality of life scores than in the Hartel approach treatment group. Similar complication profiles were seen between the 2 groups, with hematoma formation, facial numbness, diminished corneal reflex, and masseter weakness.

Zhou and colleagues[29] compared the effectiveness of nerve combing and RFT for the treatment of idiopathic trigeminal neuralgia. Among those patients undergoing nerve combing, 82% experienced long-term pain relief. In the RFT treatment group, 76.4% had continued long-term pain relief. Pain relapse rates were 10.0% in the nerve combing treatment group and 14.5% in the RFT treatment group. Postoperative complications occurred at higher rates in the nerve combing treatment group, which included dysesthesia, diplopia, and partial nerve dysfunction.

### Observational Studies

The observational studies examining ablation techniques for the treatment of idiopathic trigeminal neuralgia assessed similar patient populations with the average patient age in these studies ranging from 53.8 to 78.0 years (**Table 3**). The percentage of

**Table 3**
Characteristics of observational studies investigating the role of RFAs for the management of facial pain

| Author (Year) | Clinical Diagnosis | Study Design | Patient Population | Ablation Technique | Target Nerve | Duration of Pain Relief | Secondary Outcome | Conclusion | Side Effect |
|---|---|---|---|---|---|---|---|---|---|
| Adler et al,[33] 2009 | Idiopathic trigeminal neuralgia | Prospective study | Sample size (n): 46 Mean age (y): 78 Male (%): 37 | Nonisocentric radiosurgical CyberKnife rhizotomy | Trigeminal neuralgia | 85% of patients experienced complete relief by 5.2 wk of follow-up. At 15 mo, 72% of patients graded their pain as excellent (pain free and off medication) and 24% (>90% improvement while still on medication) graded it as good. | No recurrences were experienced in patients after a pain-free interval of 7 mo 72% of patients required no medication by 15 mo of follow-up. | Nonisocentric radiosurgical rhizotomy demonstrates both high rates of pain relief and an acceptable incidence of facial numbness. | Facial numbness occurred in 15% of cases. |
| Chen et al,[34] 2019 | Idiopathic trigeminal neuralgia | Prospective study | Sample size (n): 37 Mean age (y): 59.8 Male (%): 35.1 | Radiofrequency rhizotomy | Trigeminal neuralgia | 67.5% of patients experienced pain relief at 1 y of follow-up, as assessed by VAS pain scores. | None assessed. | Conclusions discussed pathophysiology of pain resistant to treatment. | None discussed. |
| Xue et al,[32] 2015 | Idiopathic trigeminal neuralgia | Prospective study | Sample size (n): 25 Mean age (y): 64.4 Male (%): 48 | RFT through foramen rotundum | Trigeminal neuralgia (V2) | Complete or near pain relief was experienced by 92% of patients immediately after the initial procedure and in all patients after those not experiencing initial relief underwent a second procedure. Recurrence of pain occurred in 36% of patients during the 15-mo follow-up. | Total reoperation rate was 44%, with all patients experiencing complete pain relief after a second procedure. | Percutaneous RFT of the maxillary branch through the foramen rotundum under fluoroscopy is a safe and effective procedure for the treatment of isolate trigeminal neuralgia of the maxillary nerve. | Transient facial numbness occurred in 92% of patients. |

(continued on next page)

Table 3
(continued)

| Author (Year) | Clinical Diagnosis | Study Design | Patient Population | Ablation Technique | Target Nerve | Duration of Pain Relief | Secondary Outcome | Conclusion | Side Effect |
|---|---|---|---|---|---|---|---|---|---|
| Huang et al,[35] 2016 | Idiopathic trigeminal neuralgia | Prospective study | Sample size (n): 80 Mean age (y): not described; age range 27–88 Male (%): 32.5 | RFT | Trigeminal neuralgia | Excellent pain relief was achieved in 98.8% of patients after 1 wk, 1 mo, and 3 mo. | None assessed. | Temperature controlled TRF to V1 of the semilunar ganglion is effective and safe for trigeminal neuralgia treatment. | 97.5% of patients experienced tolerable facial numbness. 17.5% experienced a mild decrease in the corneal reflex. |
| Mathews et al,[36] 2000 | Idiopathic trigeminal neuralgia | Prospective study | Sample size (n): 258 Mean age (y): not described Male (%): not described | RTR | Trigeminal neuralgia | Pain relief was scored as excellent in 87% of patients within 6 mo of follow-up. At long-term follow-up beyond 6 mo, 83% of patients had excellent to good pain relief. | Long-term follow-up beyond 6 mo required reoperation in 12% of patients. | With the use of the specific diagnostic and management algorithm used in the study, patients with trigeminal neuralgia can be successfully treated with RTR. | Dysesthesia developed in 8% of patients and corneal analgesia developed in 3%. Anesthesia dolorosa developed in 2% of patients. |
| Meng et al,[40] 2009 | Idiopathic trigeminal neuralgia | Prospective study | Sample size (n): 26 Mean age (y): 61 Male (%): 34.6 | RFT assisted by virtual reality imaging with CT scan | Trigeminal neuralgia | Immediate pain relief was achieved in 100% of patients following the procedure. No recurrence of pain was reported in 96.2% of patients after 16 mo. | None assessed. | Virtual reality-assisted RFT represents a minimally invasive, low-risk technique with a higher efficacy compared with traditional RFT. | No permanent complications or mortality. |
| Telischak et al,[30] 2018 | Idiopathic trigeminal neuralgia, glossopharyngeal neuralgia, atypical facial pain | Prospective study | Sample size (n): 3 (idiopathic trigeminal neuralgia), 15 (atypical facial pain) Mean age (y): not described Male (%): not described | Percutaneous RFA using C-arm and CT guidance | Trigeminal neuralgia, glossopharyngeal neuralgia | All patients with trigeminal neuralgia/patients with glossopharyngeal neuralgia had both immediate and sustained pain relief at 1, 3, and 12 mo follow-up. Only 33% of patients with atypical facial patients had sustained pain relief. | None assessed. | RFA using this guided technique has a satisfying effect for trigeminal neuralgia patients but is less successful for patients with atypical facial. | Mild to moderate facial numbness occurred in most trigeminal neuralgia patients and some mild throat numbness occurred in patients with glossopharyngeal neuralgia. |

| Yang et al,[41] 2007 | Idiopathic trigeminal neuralgia | Prospective study | Sample size (n): 12 Mean age (y): 53.8 Male (%): 58.3 | Neuronavigation-assisted percutaneous RFT | Trigeminal neuralgia | Neuronavigation-assisted RFT resulted in immediate acute pain relief for all patients. During follow-up periods of 6–22 mo, trigeminal neuralgia symptoms recurred in 16.7% of patients. | None assessed. | Neuronavigation-assisted RFT successfully provided acute pain relief in all patients while avoiding major complications. | Facial hypoesthesia occurred in all patients, and transient masseter weakness occurred in 16.7% of patients. |
| Zakrzewska et al,[37] 1999 | Idiopathic trigeminal neuralgia, mixed trigeminal neuralgia | Prospective study | Sample size (n): 48 Mean age (y): not described Male (%): 39.6 | RFT | Trigeminal neuralgia, Gasserian ganglion | The mean time to recurrence of pain was 40 mo for the trigeminal neuralgia group and 36 mo for the mixed trigeminal neuralgia group. | Depression and anxiety dropped more in the trigeminal neuralgia group than the mixed trigeminal neuralgia group. The trigeminal neuralgia group also reported greater satisfaction with their outcome and experienced fewer complications. | Selection of patients for surgery for trigeminal neuralgia should involve object criteria because outcomes can vary by diagnosis. | More mixed trigeminal neuralgia patients experienced problems with eating than trigeminal neuralgia patients. Ophthalmic complications were also more common in the mixed trigeminal neuralgia group. |
| Hamid et al,[38] 1993 | Idiopathic trigeminal neuralgia | Prospective study | Sample size (n): 127 Mean age (y): age range 26–97 Male (%): 70.1 | PRF | Trigeminal neuralgia | Results of PRF were excellent in 67% of patients without any complications and good in 19% of patients with minor complications. | Recurrence was less frequent in patients that experienced a resulting deep sensory deficit. | Excellent to good results were obtained in most patients with limited complications. PRF has a high success rate as observed in this study. | Transient vision blurring, hearing disturbances, and diplopia were observed in some patients. Poor results were experienced in 14% of patients who experienced complications including masseter weakness or anesthesia dolorosa. |

(continued on next page)

**Table 3**
*(continued)*

| Author (Year) | Clinical Diagnosis | Study Design | Patient Population | Ablation Technique | Target Nerve | Duration of Pain Relief | Secondary Outcome | Conclusion | Side Effect |
|---|---|---|---|---|---|---|---|---|---|
| Kanpolat et al,[31] 2001 | Idiopathic trigeminal neuralgia | Prospective study | Sample size (n): 1600 Mean age (y): 56.8 Male (%): 47.9 | RFT | Trigeminal neuralgia | Acute pain relief was achieved in 97.6% of patients. Complete pain relief was maintained at 5 y in 57.7% of patients who underwent a single procedure. Pain relief was reported in 92% of patients with a single procedure or with multiple procedures 5 y after the first RFT was performed. At 10 y, 52.3% of the patients who underwent a single procedure and 94.2% of patients who underwent multiple procedures had experienced pain relief. Early pain recurrence (<6 mo) was experienced in 7.7% of patients. Late recurrence (>6 mo) occurred in 17.4% of patients. | 76% of patients were managed with a single treatment and 24% of patients were managed with multiple procedures. The overall pain recurrence was 25.1% during the total follow-up period. | Percutaneous RFT represents a minimally invasive, low-risk technique with a high rate of efficacy. The procedure may be safely repeated if pain recurs. | Complications included a diminished corneal reflex in 5.7% of patients, masseter weakness and paralysis in 4.4% of patients, dysesthesia in 1% of patients and anesthesia dolorosa in 0.8% of patients. |

| Liu et al,[42] 2005 | Idiopathic trigeminal neuralgia | Prospective study | Sample size (n): 18 Mean age (y): not described Male (%): not described | RFT with 3-dimensional CT guidance | Trigeminal neuralgia | Acute pain relief was achieved in 94.4% of patients after the procedure. Early (<6 mo) pain recurrence occurred in 11.1% of patients, whereas late (>6 mo) recurrence was reported in 16.7% of patients. Complete pain control was achieved in 72.2% of patients. | None assessed. | 3-dimensional CT foramen ovale locations can raise the successful rate of puncture, enhance the safety, and decrease the incident rate of complications. | No serious complications were reported. |
|---|---|---|---|---|---|---|---|---|---|
| Onofrio et al,[39] 1975 | Idiopathic trigeminal neuralgia | Prospective study | Sample size (n): 140 Mean age (y): not described Male (%): not described | PRF | Trigeminal neuralgia | Satisfactory analgesia was achieved in 86.9% of patients. | Sensation was preserved in the areas of surgically induced analgesia in 80% of patients. | PRF of the Gasserian ganglion and posterior root is a safe and effective mode of treatment for patients with severe trigeminal neuralgia. | Postoperative complications included V1 analgesia, transient sixth-nerve palsy, neuroparalytic keratitis, and anesthesia dolorosa. |
| Zheng et al,[43] 2015 | Idiopathic trigeminal neuralgia | Prospective study | Sample size (n): 27 Mean age (y): 56.3 Male (%): 29.6 | CT-guided RFT | Trigeminal neuralgia | The immediate success rate 3 d after the procedure was 100%, and pain-free status was observed in 92.6% of patients at 12 mo follow-up. | Masticatory dysfunction was significantly decreased in most patients between 3 d and 3 mo after the procedure but resolved by 12 mo postoperatively. | CT-guided PT-RFT is a safe and effective procedure for idiopathic trigeminal neuralgia, but there is a high rate of masticatory dysfunction during a short time after the procedure, appearing to be reversible within 12 mo. | Mild facial dysesthesia was experienced in all patients. Temporary masticatory dysfunction was often experienced patients but resolved within 12 mo. |

Abbreviation: RTR, radiofrequency thermal rhizotomy.

male patients in these studies ranged from 29.6% to 70.1%. The sample size of these studies varied, ranging from 3 patients in the report from Telischak and colleagues[30] to 1600 in the study conducted by Kanpolat and colleagues.[31] Each of the studies used ablation techniques that targeted the trigeminal nerve, with some studies targeting specific branches, including the study by Xue and colleagues[32] that directly targeted treatment in the distribution of V2. Ablation techniques that were assessed included nonisocentric radiosurgical CyberKnife rhizotomy, RFT, radiofrequency thermal rhizotomy, navigation-guided techniques, or PRF.

Adler and colleagues[33] examined the used of nonisocentric radiosurgical rhizotomy for the treatment of idiopathic trigeminal neuralgia. This study found that 85% of patients demonstrated pain relief at 5 weeks of follow-up. The complete pain reduction rate decreased to 72% at 15 months of follow-up, meaning that these patients required no further medical treatment. Furthermore, 24% of patients reported good pain relief, but still required medication treatment. Facial numbness was experienced in 15% of cases studied. Chen and colleagues[34] examined the use of radiofrequency rhizotomy and found that 67.5% of patients treated with this technique demonstrated pain relief 1 year after the procedure. Xue and colleagues in 2015[32] assessed RFT used with an approach through the foramen rotundum to examine the effectiveness of this technique in treating pain associated with a V2 distribution. This study showed that 92% of patients experienced pain relief immediately after the initial procedure and that all patients experienced complete relief if a second procedure was performed. The total reoperation rate was 44%, and transient facial numbness occurred in 92% of patients undergoing the procedure. Huang and colleagues 2016[35] also used RFT and achieved pain relief in 98.8% of patients up to 3 months after the procedure was performed. Almost all patients in this study experienced tolerable facial numbness as a side effect, and 17.5% of patients experienced a mild decrease in the corneal reflex. Mathews and Scrivani[36] assessed the use of radiofrequency thermal rhizotomy in treating idiopathic trigeminal neuralgia. This study demonstrated that 87% of patients had pain relief within the first 6 months of follow-up. At the long-term follow-up beyond 6 months, 83% of patients reported excellent to good pain relief. Minor side effects were mild dysesthesia in 8% of patients and corneal analgesia in 3% of patients. Zakrzewska and colleagues[37] used RFT and demonstrated long-term pain relief in patients undergoing the procedure. Secondarily, depression and anxiety decreased in patients undergoing RFT and minimal complications were reported. Hamid and colleagues[38] used PRF and found that 67% of patients experienced excellent pain relief without complications and 19% of patients experienced good pain relief with only minor associated complications. The authors noted that recurrence was less frequent in patients that experienced greater sensory deficits immediately after the procedure. Reported minor side effects included transient vision blurring, hearing disturbances, and diplopia. Poor results were experienced in 14% of patients who experienced complications, including masseter weakness or anesthesia dolorosa. Kanpolat and colleagues[31] also used RFT for the treatment of idiopathic trigeminal neuralgia and achieved acute pain relief in 97.6% of patients. Complete pain relief was maintained at a rate of 57.7% at 5 years of follow-up. Of the patients who underwent multiple procedures, 92% experienced sustained pain relief 5 years after the initial procedure. As a result, this study provides evidence that RFT may be repeated safely and effectively in pain recurrence. Complications in this study included diminished corneal reflex, masseter weakness, and dysesthesia in a limited number of patients. Onofrio and colleagues[39] in 1975 applied PRF for treating idiopathic trigeminal neuralgia and achieved satisfactory pain relief in 86.9% of patients. Postoperative complications in this study included V1 analgesia, transient sixth nerve palsy, neuroparalytic keratitis, and anesthesia dolorosa in a limited number of patients.

Several studies also examined guided ablation techniques for the treatment of idiopathic trigeminal neuralgia. Meng and colleagues in 2009[40] assessed the use of CT-guided RFT and reported immediate pain relief in 100% of patients after the procedure. No recurrence of pain was reported in 96.2% of patients after 16 months of follow-up. Telischak and colleagues[30] examined the use of CT-guided RFT in a limited sample and showed both immediate and sustained pain relief in all patients up 12 months after the procedure. Mild to moderate facial numbness was reported by most patients in this study. Yang and colleagues 2007[41] used neuronavigation-assisted RFT and demonstrated that all patients undergoing this procedure experienced immediate pain relief. During the follow-up, idiopathic trigeminal neuralgia symptoms occurred in only 16.7% of patients, with masseter weakness also occurring in these patients. All patients in this study reported transient facial hypoesthesia following the procedure. Liu and colleagues[42] used RFT with 3-dimensional CT guidance and achieved acute pain relief in 94.4% of patients. Early pain recurrence within 6 months of the procedure occurred in 11.1% of patients, and late pain recurrence after 6 months was reported in 16.7% of patients. Overall, complete pain control was achieved in 72.2% of patients, and no serious complications were reported. Zheng and colleagues[43] also used CT-guided RFT and achieved immediate pain relief in all patients by day 3 after the procedure. Pain-free status was also observed in 92.6% of patients at 12 months of follow-up. High rates of masticatory dysfunction were reported in these patients, although it resolved by 12 of months follow-up. Mild facial dysesthesia was also experienced by all patients in this study.

## Retrospective Studies

The retrospective studies examining ablation techniques for idiopathic trigeminal neuralgia treatment revealed the average age in these studies ranging from 50.0 to 69.4 years (**Table 4**). The percentage of male patients in these studies ranged from 26.1% to 47.1%. The sample size of these studies varied, ranging from 23 in a study by Abhinav and colleagues[44] to 1137 in the study by Tang and colleagues.[45] Each of these studies used ablation techniques that targeted specific distributions of the trigeminal nerve, from Fraioli and colleagues in 2009 (V3),[46] Kosugi and colleagues (V2, V3),[47] and Wang and colleagues in 2019 (V2).[48] Ablation techniques included RPR, neurovascular decompression, RFT, CRF, partial sensory rhizotomy, guided techniques, microvascular decompression, or radiosurgery.

Texeira and colleagues[49] compared the effectiveness of RPR and neurovascular decompression for the treatment of idiopathic trigeminal neuralgia. All patients experienced immediate pain relief with the use of both of these procedures. Pain relapse within 1 year occurred in 44% of RPR treatment patients, but data were not available for follow-up on patients who underwent neurovascular decompression. Reported complications resulting from RPR included transient trigeminal paresis, facial paresthesia, anesthesia dolorosa, and facial numbness. Neurovascular conflict occurred in all patients treated with neurovascular decompression. Tang and colleagues[50] used CT-guided RFT and achieved pain relief at rates of 88% at 1 year, 79% at 3 years, and 72% at 5 years. Long-term excellent pain relief was significantly increased in the V2 distribution compared with all other distributions, although high rates of long-term pain relief were achieved in all distributions. Most patients experienced side effects of facial numbness immediately after RFT, and a limited numbers of patients experienced masseter weakness, corneitis, and diplopia.

**Table 4**
Characteristics of retrospective studies investigating the role of RFAs for the management of facial pain

| Author (Year) | Clinical Diagnosis | Study Design | Patient Population | Ablation Technique | Target Nerve | Duration of Pain Relief | Secondary Outcome | Conclusion | Side Effects |
|---|---|---|---|---|---|---|---|---|---|
| Teixeira et al,[49] 2006 | Idiopathic trigeminal neuralgia, symptomatic facial pain, atypical facial pain, PHN | Retrospective study | Sample size (n): 290 (idiopathic trigeminal neuralgia), 52 (symptomatic facial pain), 16 (atypical facial pain), 9 (PHN) Mean age (y): 290 (idiopathic trigeminal neuralgia), 52 (symptomatic facial pain), 16 (atypical facial pain), 9 (PHN) Male (%): 42.7 (idiopathic trigeminal neuralgia), 75.8 (symptomatic facial pain), 50 (atypical facial pain), 55.6 (PHN) | RPR, neurovascular decompression (neurovascular decompression) | Trigeminal neuralgia | Complete pain relief immediately after the intervention in all idiopathic trigeminal neuralgia patients treated with RPR. All neurovascular decompression patients also experienced immediate complete pain relief. Pain relapse within 1 y in 44% of RPR patients. Recurrence rates were 9.6% in symptomatic facial pain patients undergoing RPR. Only 37.5% of patients with atypical facial undergoing RPR had pain relief. After RPR, 88.8% of PHN patients had pain relief. | None assessed. | Both RPR and neurovascular decompression provided immediate complete pain relief and were useful in the treatment of idiopathic trigeminal neuralgia. RPR was effective in treating symptomatic facial pain and PNH but was not effective in treating atypical facial pain and inflammatory pain (sinusitis). | Transient trigeminal paresis, facial paresthesia, anesthesia dolorosa, and numbness sensations in RPR patients. Neurovascular conflict in all neurovascular decompression patients. |
| Tang et al,[50] 2015 | Idiopathic trigeminal neuralgia | Retrospective study | Sample size (n): 1137 Mean age (y): 61.5 Male (%): 40.6 | CT-guided RFT | Trigeminal neuralgia | Pain relief was achieved 88% at 1 y, 79% at 3 y, 72% at 5 y, 65% at 7 y, 57% at 9 y, and 52% at 11 y. Long-term excellent pain relief of V2 was significantly increased compared with V3, V1 + V2, and V2 + V3. | Immediate pain relief outcomes were rated as excellent (no pain, no medications) by 98.4% of patients at the time of hospital discharge. | CT-guided RFT is a safe and effective procedure for idiopathic trigeminal neuralgia. All trigeminal branch divisions achieved comparable satisfactory curative effect. The highest rates of excellent pain relief were achieved in the V2 branch alone. | 84.7% of patients experienced degrees of facial numbness immediately after RFT; 67.3% of patients experienced numbness during follow-up. All patient reported gradual decreases in facial numbness after the procedure; masseter weakness (8%); corneitis (2.6%); diplopia (1.2%) |

| Ding et al,[51] 2018 | Idiopathic trigeminal neuralgia | Retrospective study | CT-guided CRF, PRF + CRF (PCRF) | Sample size (n): 80 Mean age (y): 56.4 (PRF), 55.8 (PCRF) Male (%): 37.5 (PRF), 35.0 (PCRF) | Trigeminal neuralgia | VAS scores were significantly lower in both groups compared with baseline. At 1 mo, VAS scores were lower in the PCRF group compared with CRF. By 6 mo, VAS scores increased in the CRF group, while the duration of pain relief was longer in the PCRF group. VAS score in the PCRF group was significantly lower than that of the CRF group in the later stages of follow-up and remained lower at each time point from 1 mo to 2 y. | Pain relief observed immediately in both groups, 1 day after surgery, with significant pain relief after 1 wk. Postoperative recurrence rates in the CRF and PCRF groups within 2 y were 20% and 5%. | CT-guided PCRF for treating idiopathic trigeminal neuralgia can effectively relieve pain, increase the pain remission rate in the late stage, reduce complications, and reduce recurrence rates. | Facial numbness, weakness of masticatory muscles, and weakened corneal reflex were the most reported side effects. Numbness gradually reduced or recovered within 1 y. Recovery times from side effects were shorter in the PCRF group compared with RPF. |
| Abhinav et al,[44] 2012 | Idiopathic trigeminal neuralgia | Retrospective study | Partial sensory rhizotomy | Sample size (n): 23 (MS), 47 (non-MS) Mean age (y): 50 (MS), 50.3 (non-MS) Male (%): 26.1 (MS), 38.3 (non-MS) | Trigeminal neuralgia | Long-term pain relief was achieved in 87% of MS patients and 93.6% of non-MS patients had mild or no pain at last follow-up. | Patient satisfaction was achieved in 82.6% of MS patients and 80.9% of non-MS patients. Recurrent trigeminal neuralgia was more common in patients with a compressing vessel. | Demyelination in the inferior part of the trigeminal nerve root entry zone may contribute to trigeminal neuralgia in most patients with MS and in idiopathic trigeminal neuralgia associated with vascular compression of the nerve root. The outcome after partial sensory rhizotomy was largely successful in both groups of patients. | Both MS and non-MS patients reported facial numbness in the affected trigeminal nerve distribution. Patients also experience reduced corneal reflex. |

(continued on next page)

**Table 4**
*(continued)*

| Author (Year) | Clinical Diagnosis | Study Design | Patient Population | Ablation Technique | Target Nerve | Duration of Pain Relief | Secondary Outcome | Conclusion | Side Effects |
|---|---|---|---|---|---|---|---|---|---|
| Fraioli et al,[46] 2009 | Idiopathic trigeminal neuralgia | Retrospective study | Sample size (n): 158 Mean age (y): age range 52–93 Male (%): not described | CT- or non-CT-guided RFT | Trigeminal neuralgia (V3) | Complete pain relief was achieved immediately after the procedure in all patients. Recurrences were observed in 7.8% of patients followed for a median duration of 11.6 y. | None assessed. | RFT is easily performed under CT-guided control and results in limited complications. It is immediately effective with a low rate of pain recurrence. | A limited number of patients experienced hypoesthesia. |
| Koning et al,[52] 2014 | Idiopathic trigeminal neuralgia | Retrospective study | Sample size (n): 28 Mean age (y): 68 Male (%): 53 | RFT | Trigeminal neuralgia | Acute pain relief was achieved in 89% of patients, with pain relief sustained in 60% of patients at the 12-mo follow-up. | A lower sensory stimulation threshold during treatment was associated with better patient satisfaction, improved pain relief, and trended toward greater hypoesthesia. | This study supported the high efficacy of RF treatment, but there was a high rate of associated side effects. | Complications included hypoesthesia (56%), dry eye (20%), and masseter muscle weakness (12%). |
| Kosugi et al,[47] 2015 | Idiopathic trigeminal neuralgia | Retrospective study | Sample size (n): 89 Mean age (y): 69.4 Male (%): 33.7 | RFT | Trigeminal neuralgia (V2, V3) | Immediate success rates of PRT for V2 trigeminal neuralgia, V2 + V3 trigeminal neuralgia, and V3 trigeminal neuralgia were 100%, 86.6%, and 100%, respectively. The durations pain-free for V2 trigeminal neuralgia and V2 + V3 trigeminal neuralgia were significantly shorter than that for V3 trigeminal neuralgia. The | For V2 trigeminal neuralgia and V2 + V3 trigeminal neuralgia, median pain-free durations were 18 mo in patients with anesthesia, 15 mo in patients with severe hypesthesia, and 9 mo in patients with mild hypesthesia. Similar pain-free durations were seen in V3 trigeminal neuralgia patients with anesthesia and hypoesthesia. | For V2 trigeminal neuralgia and multiple-division trigeminal neuralgia, less long-term pain relief after PRT of the Gasserian ganglion can be expected compared with that for isolated V3 trigeminal neuralgia, even if immediate pain relief is achieved. The recurrence of pain can be treated safely and effectively by repeated RFT. | Complications included severe and mild hypoesthesia. |

| | | | | | | | | |
|---|---|---|---|---|---|---|---|---|
| Liu et al,[53] 2016 | Idiopathic trigeminal neuralgia | Retrospective study | Sample size (n): 84 Mean age (y): 66.1 Male (%): 35.7 | RFT | probabilities of pain relief of V3 being maintained were 80.2% at 12 mo and 54.9% at 24 mo. Those of V2 trigeminal neuralgia and V2 + V3 trigeminal neuralgia were 40.5% and 49.3% at 12 mo, and 19.6% and 17.1% at 24 mo, respectively. | Immediate pain relief was 98%. Sustained pain relief without medications at 1, 2, and 3 y after RFT were 85%, 68%, and 54%, respectively, with an overall 80% effective rate for pain control during the study period. | Of those patients that underwent a second RFT, 95% benefited from multiple RFT procedures and were satisfied with their pain relief. | Percutaneous RFT is a safe and effective treatment for patients with persistent or recurrent trigeminal neuralgia after surgery. | All patients experienced numbness of varying degrees. The complication rate was 15%, with side effects including masseter weakness, impaired taste acuity, absent or decreased corneal reflex, and oculomotor paralysis. |
| Luo et al,[54] 2013 | Idiopathic trigeminal neuralgia | Retrospective study | Sample size (n): 28 Mean age (y): not described Male (%): not described | CT-guided PRF | A ≥50 decrease in NRS pain score 2 wk postoperatively was described as effective treatment. Only 39.3% of patients experienced effective treatment. These patients had satisfactory outcome up to 6 mo after the procedure. Pain relapse at 7–11 mo occurred in 54.5% of patients that had experienced an effective pain relief response. | Intraoperative PRF output voltage and electric field intensity were both significantly lower in the ineffective group compared with the effective treatment response group. | Intraoperative PRF output voltage and electrical field intensity was higher in the group that received effective treatment compared with the group in which treatment was ineffective. | No serious complications were reported. |

(continued on next page)

**Table 4**
*(continued)*

| Author (Year) | Clinical Diagnosis | Study Design | Patient Population | Ablation Technique | Target Nerve | Duration of Pain Relief | Secondary Outcome | Conclusion | Side Effects |
|---|---|---|---|---|---|---|---|---|---|
| Sanchez-Mejia et al,[55] 2005 | Idiopathic trigeminal neuralgia | Retrospective study | Sample size (n): 209 for initial treatment, 32 for retreatment<br>Mean age (y): 69.1 (retreatment patients)<br>Male (%): 40.6 (retreatment patients) | Assessed retreatment after microvascular decompression, RFT, or radiosurgery | Trigeminal neuralgia | After retreatment, the majority of patients attained complete or very good pain relief. Of the 209 patients that underwent treatment, 15.3% required retreatment. | The initial treatment for the 209 patients was microvascular decompression with or without rhizotomy in 93 patients, RFA in 12, and radiosurgery in 104. The mean time between the initial and second treatment was 13 mo. No patient required more than 2 retreatments per affected side. | The number of patients requiring retreatment is not negligible. Lower retreatment rates were seen in patients undergoing radiosurgery, compared with those that underwent microvascular decompression or RFT. Radiosurgery was more likely to be the final treatment for recurrent trigeminal neuralgia regardless of the initial treatment. Pain relief after retreatment correlated with postoperative facial numbness. | Facial numbness was experienced with all procedures. |
| Tang et al,[50] 2014 | Idiopathic trigeminal neuralgia | Retrospective study | Sample size (n): 146 for initial PRT, 33 for retreatment<br>Mean age (y): 64.1 (retreatment patients)<br>Male (%): 36.4 (retreatment patients) | PRT | Trigeminal neuralgia | Of all patients undergoing PRT, 22.6% required retreatment. Pain relief was immediate in 90.9% of patients following a second PRT procedure. The percentage of patients who remained in an excellent or good pain relief condition after the second PRT was 75% at 1 y, 68% at 2 y, and 68% at 5 y. | The median time after initial PRT to recurrence was 79.3 mo. 54.5% of patients remained satisfied with their pain relief during the follow-up period after the retreatment. | Repeated PRT provides long-term pain relief benefits to patients with recurrent trigeminal neuralgia and should be considered as treatment for recurrent trigeminal neuralgia. | Postoperative complications included masseter weakness. |

| | | | Sample size | Intervention | Indication | Results | Conclusion | Postoperative complications |
|---|---|---|---|---|---|---|---|---|
| Tronnier et al,[56] 2001 | Idiopathic trigeminal neuralgia | Retrospective comparative study | Sample size (n): 225 (microvascular decompression), 206 (PRT) Mean age (y): not described Male (%): not described | PRF or microvascular decompression | Trigeminal neuralgia | There was a 50% risk for pain recurrence 2 y after PRF. This rate rose to 75% after 4.5 y. Of patients undergoing microvascular decompression, 76.4% were pain free after 2 y, 65% after 10 y, and 63% after 20 y. | Patients without sensory impairment after microvascular decompression were pain free significantly longer than patients who experienced postoperative hypoesthesia or partial rhizotomy. | Microvascular decompression proved to be a more effective and longer lasting procedure for patients with idiopathic trigeminal neuralgia than PRF. Patients without postoperative sensory deficit remained pain free significantly longer, providing evidence against the trauma hypothesis of the procedure. | Postoperative complications included varying degrees of hypoesthesia. |
| Wang et al,[48] 2019 | Idiopathic trigeminal neuralgia | Retrospective case control | Sample size (n): 38 Mean age (y): 67.7 (experimental), 65.8 (control) Male (%): 47.1 (experimental), 57.1 (control) | PRT with or without CT guidance | Trigeminal neuralgia (V2) | All patients experienced good pain remission postoperatively. At follow-up points of 1 wk, 3 mo, 6 mo, and 12 mo after operation, there was no significant difference in good pain relief between the 2 groups. Good pain relief rates in the experimental group at 7 d, 3 mo, 6 mo, and 12 mo were 100%, 100%, 94.1%, and 88.2%, respectively. Rates of good pain relief at each follow-up time point in the control group were 100%, 100%, 90.5%, and 85.7%, respectively. | The rate of 1-time successful puncture was higher in the CT-guided PRT group than in the control group were CT guidance was not used. | CT template-guided PRT is a safe and precise navigation instrument for treatment of isolated V2 trigeminal neuralgia. | No significant difference in complications was found between the 2 groups. All patients experienced mild facial numbness in V2 immediately after the surgery, and this symptom gradually subsided within 1–3 mo. There were 5 case of facial hematomas in the control group and 1 case in the experimental group. |

(continued on next page)

**Table 4**
*(continued)*

| Author (Year) | Clinical Diagnosis | Study Design | Patient Population | Ablation Technique | Target Nerve | Duration of Pain Relief | Secondary Outcome | Conclusion | Side Effects |
|---|---|---|---|---|---|---|---|---|---|
| Zhang et al,[57] 2011 | Idiopathic trigeminal neuralgia, recurrent after microvascular decompression | Retrospective study | Sample size (n): 62 Mean age (y): 54 Male (%): 40.3 | RTR, with (group B) or without virtual reality imaging guidance (group A) | Trigeminal neuralgia | All patients in both groups attained immediate pain relief after RTR. Group A had pain relief rates of 82.6% and 69.6% at year 1 and year 2 and group B had corresponding rates of 92.3% and 84.6%. The difference in rates became significant after 2 y. With virtual reality-guided RTR, group B demonstrated higher rates of pain relief than group A. The proportions of pain relief in group B at 3, 4, and 5 y were 82.5%, 76.2%, 68.8%, whereas those in the control group were 57.2%, 49.6%, and 36.4%, respectively. | All patients with pain relief required no further medications. | RTR provided both immediate and short-term pain relief in all patients. In addition, the long-term pain relief rate of RTR for trigeminal neuralgia under virtual reality guidance was comparable with microvascular decompression. RTR without guidance has a higher pain recurrence rate. | Facial hypoesthesia occurred in all patients immediately after operation. Transient masseter weakness, cornea insensitivity, and transient keratitis were experienced in a limited number of patients. |

*Abbreviations:* LCRF, long radiofrequency ablation; NRS, numeric pain rating scale; PCRF, power-controlled radiofrequency ablation; PHN, postherpetic neuralgia; QOL, quality of life; RFT, radiofrequency thermocoagulation; RPR, Radiofrequency percutaneous rhizotomy; SCRF, short radiofrequency ablation.

Ding and colleagues[51] similarly used CT-guided PRF, but compared effectiveness between CRF alone and CRF combined with PRF. Acute pain relief was achieved by both procedures, but sustained pain relief for up 2 years of follow-up was improved among patients undergoing the combined procedure. Recurrence rates in the combined procedure group were 5% at 2 years, whereas they were 20% when only CRF was used. Reported side effects included facial numbness, weakness of the masticatory muscles, and weakened corneal reflex. Most cases of numbness resolved within 1 year, and recovery times from side effects were decreased in the combined procedure group. Abhinav and colleagues[44] used partial sensory rhizotomy and achieved long-term pain relief in 87% of patients who had trigeminal neuralgia associated with multiple sclerosis (MS). Non-MS patients had long-term relief rates of 93.6%. High patient satisfaction was reported in both groups of patients. The authors noted that recurrent trigeminal neuralgia occurred more often in patients with structural associations including a compressed vessel. Both MS and non-MS patients in this study reported side effects of facial numbness and reduced corneal reflex. Fraioli and colleagues [46] compared treatment effectiveness between CT or non–CT-guided RFT. This study showed that complete pain relief was achieved immediately after both procedures, and recurrence rates with CT-guided RFT were just 7.8% in patients followed for a median duration of 11.6 years. A limited number of patients in this study reported experiencing mild hypoesthesia. Koning and colleagues[52] also studied RFT use and found that patients undergoing this procedure had 60% response rates with pain relief maintained at 12 months of follow-up. Side effects were reported in this study, including hypoesthesia (56%), dry eye (20%), and masseter muscle weakness (12%).

Kosugi and colleagues[47] examined the use of RFT for idiopathic trigeminal neuralgia and assessed its effectiveness in different distributions. This study demonstrated that RFT for V2 idiopathic trigeminal neuralgia and multiple-division idiopathic trigeminal neuralgia produces lower response rates than RFT for V3 VTN. Patients in this study were effectively treated with repeat RFT, with complications including mild to severe hypoesthesia. Liu and colleagues[53] also assessed the effectiveness of RFT for idiopathic trigeminal neuralgia. Immediate pain relief was achieved in 98% of patients, and sustained relief without medications at 1, 2, and 3 years after RFT were 85%, 68%, and 54%, respectively. Of patients undergoing a second RFT, 95% experienced long-term pain relief after the repeat procedure. Facial numbness was experienced by all patients in this study, with further complications including masseter weakness, impaired taste acuity, absent or decreased corneal reflex, and oculomotor paralysis. Luo and colleagues[54] provided a retrospective study examining CT-guided PRF and found that only 39.3% of the patients their study population experienced effective treatment as determined during the first 2 weeks of follow-up. Pain relapse rates were high in this study, with 54.5% of the patients who had responded initially experiencing pain relapses within 7 to 11 months of follow-up. The authors of this study noted that voltage and electric field intensity were both significantly lower in the patients who experienced ineffective treatment. Sanchez-Mejia and colleagues[55] assessed retreatment responses after failed response to microvascular decompression, RFT, or radiosurgery. This study demonstrated that, after retreatment, the majority of patients attained complete or very good retreatment. Retreatment occurred in 15.3% of patients who had undergone an initial procedure. Lower rates of retreatment were observed in patients undergoing radiosurgery compared with those who underwent microvascular decompression or RFT. Radiosurgery was also more likely to be used as the final treatment for recurrent idiopathic trigeminal neuralgia regardless of the initial treatment. The authors also noted that pain relief after retreatment correlated with postoperative facial numbness, a side effect that was experienced in all procedures. Tang and colleagues[45] examined PRT for idiopathic trigeminal neuralgia and found that, out of all the patients undergoing PRT in their study population, 22.6% required retreatment and 90.0% experienced immediate pain relief after a second procedure. The percentage of patients who remained in an excellent or good pain relief condition after the second PRT was 75% at 1 year, 68% at 2 years, and 68% at 5 years. Postoperative complications in this study included masseter weakness occurring in a limited number of patients. Tronnier and colleagues[56] compared PRF and microvascular decompression treatment. This study found that patients undergoing microvascular decompression experienced pain-free conditions significantly longer than patients undergoing PRF. Both procedures were associated with side effects, including varying degrees of hypoesthesia. Wang and colleagues[48] retrospectively assessed the effectiveness PRT with and without CT guidance for V2 idiopathic trigeminal neuralgia in their patients. Short- and long-term pain relief rates were similar in both treatment groups, with no differences in complications observed between them. All patients experienced mild facial numbness immediately after the procedure, which resolved within 1 to 3 months. Higher rates of facial hematoma complications were observed in the group treated without CT guidance. Zhang and colleagues[57] also compared radiofrequency thermal rhizotomy treatment with and without image guidance. Patients undergoing procedures with image guidance demonstrated significantly higher rates of long-term pain relief than patients undergoing the procedure without image guidance. The use of radiofrequency thermal rhizotomy without the image guidance resulted in much higher rates of pain recurrence. Facial hypoesthesia occurred in all patients immediately after the operation, with transient masseter weakness, cornea insensitivity, and transient keratitis seen as less common complications.

### Other Facial Pain Conditions

Other chronic facial pain conditions have also been targeted by ablation techniques. These conditions include atypical facial pain, symptomatic facial pain associated with another condition, postherpetic neuralgia (PHN), cluster headache with facial symptoms, glossopharyngeal neuralgia, mixed trigeminal neuralgia, chronic facial and head pain, and cervicogenic headache. Types of ablation techniques include RPR, neurovascular decompression, percutaneous stereotactic radiofrequency rhizotomy, RFT, and PRF, which are highlighted in the following studies (see **Table 4**).

Teixeira and colleagues[49] retrospectively assessed the use of RPR for the treatment of symptomatic facial pain, atypical facial pain, and PHN. Although the sample size varied among these groups of patients, this study demonstrated low pain recurrence rates among symptomatic facial pain and PHN patients undergoing RPR. Among the 16 symptomatic facial pain patients undergoing RPR, only 9.6% experienced pain recurrence after the procedure. Among the 9 PHN patients undergoing RPR, 88.8% experienced persistent pain relief. Although RPR was effective in treating SPF and PHN, it was not effective in treating atypical facial pain, because only 37.5% of these patients experienced pain relief. Across all patient groups, transient facial numbness was experienced along with limited cases of trigeminal paresis. Telischak and colleagues[30] also examined ablation for the treatment of atypical facial pain, using a prospective study to assess the effectiveness of CT-guided RFT for the treatment of both atypical facial pain and glossopharyngeal neuralgia. All patients with glossopharyngeal neuralgia in this study had both immediate and sustained pain relief at 1, 3, and 12 months of follow-up. However, only 33% of patients with atypical facial experienced pain relief. Therefore, both Teixeira and colleagues[49] and Telischak and colleagues[30] demonstrated a limited use for RFA procedures in treating atypical facial pain. Telischak and colleagues[30] further reported mild to moderate facial numbness occurring in most patients along with mild throat numbness in patients with glossopharyngeal neuralgia. Zakrzewska and colleagues[37] used a prospective study to examine RFT for the treatment of mixed trigeminal neuralgia. Patients in this study experienced immediate pain relief and had a mean time of 36 months for pain recurrence. Associated side effects included masticatory dysfunction and ophthalmic complications after the RFT procedure.

Ablation techniques have also been studied for headache disorders associated with facial pain symptoms. Taha and Tew[58] conducted a retrospective study to analyze the use of percutaneous stereotactic radiofrequency rhizotomy for the treatment of cluster headaches with facial pain symptoms. The study found that all patients undergoing the radiofrequency rhizotomy procedure experienced immediate pain relief after surgery. The long-term effects of treatment were somewhat maintained, with 28.6% of patients remaining pain free from 7 to 20 years after the procedure. Of all patients treated, 42.9% had mild pain recurrence that was well-controlled with medication 6 to 12 months after the procedure. Major pain recurrences occurred in 28.6% of patients within the first 2 months after the procedure. Overall, some patients with chronic cluster headaches achieved long-term pain relief, although surgery on the trigeminal neuralgia system alone may not completely eliminate pain symptoms localized to other areas. No adverse effects were discussed in this study. Zhang and colleagues[57] further examined the possible use of ablation for headache disorders and assessed the use of PRF for cervicogenic headaches. Using PRF of C2, the 2 patients in this small sample case report study experienced 100% pain relief lasting for 6 months after the procedure. Therefore, the limited sample size and positive response to PRF in this study provide potential evidence that PRF may be effective in treating cervicogenic headache. No serious complications were reported among the patients in this case report.

## SUMMARY

Numerous headache disorders and trigeminal neuralgia can significantly impact quality of life and cause significant distress for patients. RFA has gained popularity in the treatment of these chronic pain conditions refractory to traditional pharmacologic therapies. The studies presented in this extensive review were either prospective clinical studies or retrospective reviews. Overall, symptom improvement with the use of RFA has shown to reveal promising results for conditions responsible for craniofacial pain. Furthermore, minor adverse effects were reported, many of which that self-resolved. The current consensus in this comprehensive review supports the use of RFA for the treatment of various craniofacial syndromes.

## CLINICS CARE POINTS

- Craniofacial pain syndromes encompasses trigeminal neuralgia and a wide array of headache disorders that affect each individual's quality of life in varying degrees
- The focal origin of craniofacial syndrome subtypes makes them particularly susceptible to targeted RF interventions
- Further studies focusing on possible long-term effects of RFA should be considered

## REFERENCES

1. Cohen SP, et al. Randomized, double-blind, comparative-effectiveness study comparing pulsed radiofrequency to steroid injections for occipital neuralgia or migraine with occipital nerve tenderness. Pain 2015;156(12):2585–94.
2. Huang JH, et al. Occipital nerve pulsed radiofrequency treatment: a multi-center study evaluating predictors of outcome. Pain Med 2012;13(4):489–97.
3. Govind J, et al. Radiofrequency neurotomy for the treatment of third occipital headache. J Neurol Neurosurg Psychiatry 2003;74(1):88–93.
4. Salgado-Lopez L, et al. Efficacy of Sphenopalatine Ganglion Radiofrequency in Refractory Chronic Cluster Headache. World Neurosurg 2019;122:e262–9.
5. Fang L, et al. Computerized tomography-guided sphenopalatine ganglion pulsed radiofrequency treatment in 16 patients with refractory cluster headaches: twelve- to 30-month follow-up evaluations. Cephalalgia 2016;36(2):106–12.
6. Narouze S, et al. Sphenopalatine ganglion radiofrequency ablation for the management of chronic cluster headache. Headache 2009;49(4):571–7.
7. Grandhi RK, Kaye AD, Abd-Elsayed A. Systematic Review of Radiofrequency Ablation and Pulsed Radiofrequency for Management of Cervicogenic Headaches. Curr Pain Headache Rep 2018;22(3):18.
8. Halim W, Chua NH, Vissers KC. Long-term pain relief in patients with cervicogenic headaches after pulsed radiofrequency application into the lateral atlantoaxial (C1-2) joint using an anterolateral approach. Pain Pract 2010;10(4):267–71.
9. Haspeslagh SR, et al. Randomised controlled trial of cervical radiofrequency lesions as a treatment for cervicogenic headache [ISRCTN07444684]. BMC Anesthesiol 2006;6:1.
10. Lee JB, et al. Clinical efficacy of radiofrequency cervical zygapophyseal neurotomy in patients with chronic cervicogenic headache. J Korean Med Sci 2007;22(2):326–9.
11. Lang JK, Buchfelder M. Radiofrequency neurotomy for headache stemming from the zygapophysial joints C2/3 and C3/4. Cent Eur Neurosurg 2010;71(2):75–9.
12. Stovner, L.J., F. Kolstad, and G. Helde, Radiofrequency denervation of facet joints C2-C6 in cervicogenic headache: a randomized, double-blind, sham-controlled study.
13. van Suijlekom HA, et al. Radiofrequency cervical zygapophyseal joint neurotomy for cervicogenic headache: a prospective study of 15 patients. Funct Neurol 1998;13(4):297–303.
14. Yang Y, et al. Efficacy of pulsed radiofrequency on cervical 2-3 posterior medial branches in treating chronic migraine: a randomized, controlled, and double-blind trial. Evid Based Complement Alternat Med 2015;2015:690856.
15. Shabat S, Leitner J, Folman Y. Pulsed radiofrequency for the suprascapular nerve for patients with chronic headache. J Neurosurg Anesthesiol 2013;25(3):340–3.
16. Celiker S, Rosenblad A, Wilhelmsson B. A radiofrequency vs topical steroid treatment of chronic nasal obstruction: a prospective randomized study of 84 cases. Acta Otolaryngol 2011;131(1):79–83.
17. Bakshi SS, Shankar Manoharan K, Gopalakrishnan S. Comparison of the long term efficacy of radiofrequency ablation and surgical turbinoplasty in inferior turbinate hypertrophy: a randomized clinical study. Acta Otolaryngol 2017;137(8):856–61.
18. Abd-Elsayed A, Nguyen S, Fiala K. Radiofrequency Ablation for Treating Headache. Curr Pain Headache Rep 2019;23(3):18.

19. Hamer JF, Purath TA. Response of cervicogenic headaches and occipital neuralgia to radiofrequency ablation of the C2 dorsal root ganglion and/or third occipital nerve. Headache 2014;54(3):500–10.
20. Erdine S, Ozyalcin NS, Cimen A, et al. Comparison of pulsed radiofrequency with conventional radiofrequency in the treatment of idiopathic trigeminal neuralgia. Eur J Pain 2007;11(3):309–13.
21. Yao P, Hong T, Wang Z Bin, et al. Treatment of bilateral idiopathic trigeminal neuralgia by radiofrequency thermocoagulation at different temperatures. Med (United States) 2016;95(29). https://doi.org/10.1097/MD.0000000000004274.
22. Luo F, Wang T, Shen Y, et al. High voltage pulsed radiofrequency for the treatment of refractory neuralgia of the infraorbital nerve: a prospective double-blinded randomized controlled study. Pain Physician 2017;20(4):271–9.
23. Yao P, Hong T, Zhu YQ, et al. Efficacy and safety of continuous radiofrequency thermocoagulation plus pulsed radiofrequency for treatment of V1 trigeminal neuralgia A prospective cohort study. Med (United States). 2016;95(44). https://doi.org/10.1097/MD.0000000000005247.
24. Elawamy A, Abdalla EE, Shehata GA. Effects of pulsed versus conventional versus combined radiofrequency for the treatment of trigeminal neuralgia: a prospective study. Pain Physician 2017;20(6):E873–81.
25. Li X, Ni J, Yang L, et al. A prospective study of Gasserian ganglion pulsed radiofrequency combined with continuous radiofrequency for the treatment of trigeminal neuralgia. J Clin Neurosci 2012;19(6):824–8.
26. Fang L, Tao W, Jingjing L, et al. Comparison of High-voltage- with Standard-voltage Pulsed Radiofrequency of Gasserian Ganglion in the Treatment of Idiopathic Trigeminal Neuralgia. Pain Pract 2015;15(7):595–603.
27. Xu SJ, Zhang WH, Chen T, et al. Neuronavigator-guided percutaneous radiofrequency thermocoagulation in the treatment of intractable trigeminal neuralgia. Chin Med J (Engl) 2006;119(18):1528–35.
28. Ding W, Chen S, Wang R, et al. Percutaneous radiofrequency thermocoagulation for trigeminal neuralgia using neuronavigation-guided puncture from a mandibular angle. Medicine (Baltimore) 2016;95(40):e4940.
29. Zhou X, Liu Y, Yue Z, et al. Comparison of nerve combing and percutaneous radiofrequency thermocoagulation in the treatment for idiopathic trigeminal neuralgia. Braz J Otorhinolaryngol 2016;82(5):574–9.
30. Telischak NA, Heit JJ, Campos LW, et al. Fluoroscopic C-Arm and CT-Guided Selective Radiofrequency Ablation for Trigeminal and Glossopharyngeal Facial Pain Syndromes. Pain Med 2018;19(1):130–41.
31. Kanpolat Y, Savas A, Bekar A, et al. Percutaneous controlled radiofrequency trigeminal rhizotomy for the treatment of idiopathic trigeminal neuralgia: 25-year experience with 1600 patients. Neurosurgery 2001;48(3):524–34.
32. Xue T, Yang W, Guo Y, et al. 3D image-guided percutaneous radiofrequency thermocoagulation of the maxillary branch of the trigeminal nerve through foramen rotundum for the treatment of trigeminal neuralgia. Medicine (Baltimore) 2015;94(45):e1954.
33. Adler JR, Bower R, Gupta G, et al. Nonisocentric radiosurgical rhizotomy for trigeminal neuralgia. Neurosurgery 2009;64(2 Suppl):A84–90.
34. Chen S-T, Yang J-T, Weng H-H, et al. Diffusion tensor imaging for assessment of microstructural changes associate with treatment outcome at one-year after radiofrequency Rhizotomy in trigeminal neuralgia. BMC Neurol 2019;19(1):62.
35. Huang QD, Liu XM, Chen JS, et al. The effectiveness and safety of thermocoagulation radiofrequency treatment of the ophthalmic division (V1) and/or maxillary

(V2) and mandibular (V3) division in idiopathic trigeminal neuralgia: an observational study. Pain Physician 2016;19(7):E1041–7.

36. Mathews ES, Scrivani SJ. Percutaneous stereotactic radiofrequency thermal rhizotomy for the treatment of trigeminal neuralgia. Mt Sinai J Med 2000;67(4): 288–99.

37. Zakrzewska JM, Jassim S, Bulman JS. A prospective, longitudinal study on patients with trigeminal neuralgia who underwent radiofrequency thermocoagulation of the Gasserian ganglion. Pain 1999;79(1):51–8.

38. Hamid AI, Qureshi AA, Bhatti IH. Percutaneous radiofrequency retrogasserian rhizotomy for trigeminal neuralgia. J Pak Med Assoc 1993;43(7):132–3.

39. Onofrio BM. Radiofrequency percutaneous Gasserian ganglion lesions. Results in 140 patients with trigeminal pain. J Neurosurg 1975;42(2):132–9.

40. Meng F-G, Wu C-Y, Liu Y-G, et al. Virtual reality imaging technique in percutaneous radiofrequency rhizotomy for intractable trigeminal neuralgia. J Clin Neurosci 2009;16(3):449–51.

41. Yang Y, Shao Y, Wang H, et al. Neuronavigation-assisted percutaneous radiofrequency thermocoagulation therapy in trigeminal neuralgia. Clin J Pain 2007; 23(2):159–64.

42. Liu M, Wu C-Y, Liu Y-G, et al. Three-dimensional computed tomography-guided radiofrequency trigeminal rhizotomy for treatment of idiopathic trigeminal neuralgia. Chin Med Sci J 2005;20(3):206–9.

43. Zheng S, Wu B, Zhao Y, et al. Masticatory muscles dysfunction after CT-guided percutaneous trigeminal radiofrequency thermocoagulation for trigeminal neuralgia: a detailed analysis. Pain Pract 2015;15(8):712–9.

44. Abhinav K, Love S, Kalantzis G, et al. Clinicopathological review of patients with and without multiple sclerosis treated by partial sensory rhizotomy for medically refractory trigeminal neuralgia: a 12-year retrospective study. Clin Neurol Neurosurg 2012;114(4):361–5.

45. Tang Y-Z, Wu B-S, Yang L-Q, et al. The long-term effective rate of different branches of idiopathic trigeminal neuralgia after single radiofrequency thermocoagulation: a cohort study. Medicine (Baltimore) 2015;94(45):e1994.

46. Fraioli MF, Cristino B, Moschettoni L, et al. Validity of percutaneous controlled radiofrequency thermocoagulation in the treatment of isolated third division trigeminal neuralgia. Surg Neurol 2009;71(2):180–3.

47. Kosugi S, Shiotani M, Otsuka Y, et al. Long-Term Outcomes of Percutaneous Radiofrequency Thermocoagulation of Gasserian Ganglion for 2nd- and Multiple-Division Trigeminal Neuralgia. Pain Pract 2015;15(3):223–8.

48. Wang R, Han Y, Lu L. Computer-assisted design template guided percutaneous radiofrequency thermocoagulation through foramen rotundum for treatment of isolated V2 trigeminal neuralgia: a retrospective case-control study. Pain Res Manag 2019;9784020.

49. Teixeira MJ, Siqueira SRDT, Almeida GM. Percutaneous radiofrequency rhizotomy and neurovascular decompression of the trigeminal nerve for the treatment of facial pain. Arq Neuropsiquiatr 2006;64(4):983–9.

50. Tang Y-Z, Jin D, Li X-Y, et al. Repeated CT-guided percutaneous radiofrequency thermocoagulation for recurrent trigeminal neuralgia. Eur Neurol 2014;72(1–2):54–9.

51. Ding Y, Li H, Hong T, et al. Combination of pulsed radiofrequency with continuous radiofrequency thermocoagulation at low temperature improves efficacy and safety in V2/V3 primary trigeminal neuralgia. Pain Physician 2018;21(5):E545–53.

52. Koning MV, Koning NJ, Koning HM, et al. Relationship between sensory stimulation and side effects in percutaneous radiofrequency treatment of the trigeminal ganglion. Pain Pract 2014;14(7):581–7.
53. Liu P, Zhong W, Liao C, et al. The role of percutaneous radiofrequency thermocoagulation for persistent or recurrent trigeminal neuralgia after surgery. J Craniofac Surg 2016;27(8):e752–5.
54. Luo F, Meng L, Wang T, et al. Pulsed radiofrequency treatment for idiopathic trigeminal neuralgia: a retrospective analysis of the causes for ineffective pain relief. Eur J Pain 2013;17(8):1189–92.
55. Sanchez-Mejia RO, Limbo M, Cheng JS, et al. Recurrent or refractory trigeminal neuralgia after microvascular decompression, radiofrequency ablation, or radiosurgery. Neurosurg Focus 2005;18(5):e12.
56. Tronnier VM, Rasche D, Hamer J, et al. Treatment of idiopathic trigeminal neuralgia: comparison of long-term outcome after radiofrequency rhizotomy and microvascular decompression. Neurosurgery 2001;48(6):1261–7.
57. Zhang J, Shi DS, Wang R. Pulsed radiofrequency of the second cervical ganglion (C2) for the treatment of cervicogenic headache. J Headache Pain 2011;12(5): 569–71.
58. Taha JM, Tew JM. Long-term results of radiofrequency rhizotomy in the treatment of cluster headache. Headache 1995;35(4):193–6.

# Radiofrequency Ablation for Thoracic and Abdominal Chronic Pain Syndromes

Mani Singh, MD[a], Jay Karri, MD, MPH[b], Vwaire Orhurhu, MD, MPH[c],
Laura Lachman, MD[b], Alaa Abd-Elsayed, MD, MPH[d],*

## KEYWORDS

- Thoracic pain • Abdominal pain • Chronic pain • Radiofrequency ablation
- Neuroablation

## KEY POINTS

- Chronic thoracic pain and abdominal pain syndromes are common conditions that can significantly affect quality of life.
- Traditional management includes pharmacotherapy and supportive management but often fails to provide adequate pain relief.
- Radiofrequency ablation is often cited in publications as an effective and safe treatment option for chronic and resistant thoracic and abdominal pain.

## BACKGROUND

Thoracic and abdominal pain syndromes are chronic pain conditions that often arise secondarily to tumor infiltration, visceral organ involvement, operative interventions, and focal neuralgias. These pain syndromes are associated with significant detriment to quality of life and well-being. However, effective management of these conditions can be challenging, often because of varying effectiveness and poor adverse effect profiles associated with enteral medications that include standard neuropathic pain agents and opiates. On the contrary, the focal nature of tumor burden and other underlying disorders makes these pain syndromes particularly susceptible to targeted interventions.

Radiofrequency ablation (RFA) has increasingly been used as a tool to treat resistant, chronic pain of both thoracic and abdominal origins. Multiple cases and trials

a Department of Rehabilitation Medicine, Weill Cornell Medical Center, 180 Fort Washington Avenue, Harkness Pavilion First Floor, RM 168, New York, NY 10032, USA; b Department of Physical Medicine and Rehabilitation, Baylor College of Medicine, 7200 Cambridge Street, Houston, TX 77030, USA; c Department of Anesthesia, Critical Care and Pain Medicine, Division of Pain, Massachusetts General Hospital, Harvard Medical School, 55 Fruit Street, GRB 444, Boston, MA 02114, USA; d Department of Anesthesia, Division of Pain Medicine, University of Wisconsin School of Medicine and Public Health, 1102 S Park Street, Madison, WI 53715, USA
* Corresponding author.
E-mail address: alaaawny@hotmail.com

Phys Med Rehabil Clin N Am 32 (2021) 647–666
https://doi.org/10.1016/j.pmr.2021.05.004
1047-9651/21/© 2021 Elsevier Inc. All rights reserved.
pmr.theclinics.com

have been reported that show the efficacy of RFA in the treatment of these chronic pain conditions. RFA includes use of continuous radiofrequency (CRF) or pulsed radiofrequency (PRF) modalities, which are each associated with differing effectiveness and complication rates. CRF operates by producing coagulative tissue necrosis through use of high temperature (between 60° and 80°C) and high-frequency alternating currents. However, the high temperature used in CRF can lead to neural injury and result in key motor or sensory compromise. PRF uses short high-voltage bursts followed by a silent phase, which allows heat elimination and overall reduced heat exposure. Consequently, PRF is thought to be associated with both lower rates of procedure complications and success. The use of concomitant CRF and PRF modalities has shown promising results. This article characterizes and summarizes the existing evidence for RFA-associated pain reduction and associated complications in persons with thoracic and abdominal pain syndromes.

## THORACIC PAIN SYNDROMES

RFA has been shown to play a role in the management of a variety of thoracic pain syndromes. These syndromes include cancer pain, intercostal neuralgia (ICN), chronic postsurgical thoracic pain (CPTS), postthoracotomy pain syndrome (PTPS), and post–thoracic trauma pain (PTTP).

### Thoracic Cancer Pain

Primary malignancies, such as breast or lung cancer, as well as metastatic disease from extrathoracic cancer foci, can result in chronic thoracic pain syndromes. Common causes of thoracic metastasis include colon and prostate cancer. Despite the precise cause, thoracic malignancy can invade surrounding structures such as the chest wall, pleura, visceral organs, or intercostal nerves. Invasion of these structures can cause intractable thoracic pain that can be complex nociceptive and neuropathic, constant, and poorly localized. The pain can greatly affect quality of life, causing respiratory compromise, decreased ambulation, worsening immobility, and decreased function and independence. Because of the prevalence of these cancers, there has been increased research into the most effective ways to manage thoracic cancer pain.

Uchida[1] presented a case series of 3 patients using CRF of the T2 to T6 thoracic paravertebral nerves for neuropathic pain following modified radical mastectomy for breast cancer. Patients showed improvement in quality of life (measured by Short Form 36 [SF-36] questionnaire) and reported decreased visual analog scale (VAS) pain scores after 6 to 12 months. In Oh and colleagues,[2] a retrospective cohort of 100 patients received CRF of the thoracic nerve roots from T2 to T12. One week after CRF, this study found a modest decreased morphine equivalent daily dose (MEDD) reduction from 200 mg to 180 mg and decreased pain after 6 weeks measured by numerical rating scale (NRS). Reyad and colleagues,[3] was a single-blinded, parallel group, randomized clinical trial in 78 patients with lung cancer, mesothelioma, or secondary metastases to the chest. These patients received thermal RFA of T2 to T8 dorsal root ganglia (DRG); these patients had decreased VAS scores at 12 weeks as well as decreased use of oxycodone and pregabalin over a 12-week follow-up. Gulati and colleagues[4] was a retrospective review of 146 patients who received PRF ablation of the thoracic nerve roots of T3, T8, and T9.

In the Uchida[1] study, the patients were pretreated with betamethasone, making it difficult to conclude whether the pain improvement was related to the betamethasone or RFA individually or whether the improvement was related to both. In the Oh and colleagues[2] study, many patients died before the 1-month and 6-month follow-ups, suggesting that these patients had higher NRS scores that were excluded from the final results. Also, NRS scores may not represent only thoracic pain; they could represent overall pain. This study also failed to measure the effect on quality of life. The investigators also suggest that CRF may be more efficacious than PRF. The Reyad and colleagues[3] study compared RFA guided by standard fluoroscopy (N = 38) versus RFA guided by Xper computed tomography (CT) and fluoroscopy (N = 40) without another control group. No comparisons were made with pharmacologically treated patients or placebo. The CT-guided group had decreased VAS scores and fewer adverse events compared with the standard fluoroscopy group. Gulati and colleagues[4] used other therapies, not just RFA, including intercostal nerve blocks, paravertebral nerve blocks, intrathecal pumps, and neurosurgical options. The investigators recommended that pharmacologic treatment remains first line when treating thoracic chest wall cancer pain. The investigators recommended RFA specifically for posterior chest wall tumors or paravertebral tumors that were encroaching on the thoracic nerve roots. This study was observational and many recommendations were based on expert opinion rather than analyzed data.

This article summarizes 1 primary report on RFA treatment of thoracic cancer pain, 1 case series, and 2 review articles. Despite the varying types of treatment, targeted structures, and methods used to measure effectiveness, the overall conclusion of these studies is that RFA is an effective way to treat thoracic cancer pain and reduce the use of pain medication. Whether used in conjunction with other therapy modalities or used only in specific forms of cancer, RFA could help decrease pain and improve quality of life in these patients. More research is needed regarding the most effective target structures, type of treatments (CRF vs PRF or in conjunction with steroid injections, nerve blocks, and so forth), long-term effectiveness, and impact on quality of life. However, it can be concluded that RFA will play an increasingly important role in the treatment of thoracic cancer pain in the future.

### Intercostal Neuralgia

ICN can be seen after surgery, trauma, herpes zoster infections, iatrogenic neuromas, or nerve entrapment. It is sharp, shooting, burning pain in the distribution of an intercostal nerve that follows specific dermatomal patterns. It typically starts in the posterior axillary line and radiates anteriorly. This pain can be reproduced with deep inspiration or other chest movement. It is a complex condition and difficult to treat. Typical pharmacologic treatment includes tricyclic antidepressants or antiseizure medications. Nerve blocks can also be used but must be done carefully because of the proximity to the pleural space. Because this condition is difficult to treat, RFA has emerged as an intervention for resistant intercostal neuropathic pain.

Abd-Elsayed and colleagues[5] presented a case series of 2 patients who underwent thermal RFA of the intercostal nerves (T4–T7 and T9–T12) to treat intractable ICN. Both patients reported significant pain relief between 2 months and 1 year. Similarly, Engel[6] presented a case series of 6 patients with ICN following blunt trauma. These patients were effectively treated with intercostal CRF ablation at various levels between T4 and T12. Of these 6 patients, 5 reported immediate pain relief after RFA. Two of the 6 patients reported their pain returned between 6 and 10 months, but noted overall decreased pain compared with baseline and did not require additional interventional treatment.

In 1994, Stolker and colleagues[7] performed an observational study analyzing the efficacy of radiofrequency rhizotomy (CRF) of the thoracic dorsal ganglion, in the management of 4 patients with ICN. One patient reported complete relief, 1 reported greater than 50% relief, and 2 patients reported less than 50% relief. This study also analyzed the efficacy of CRF in the management of other thoracic pain syndromes (N = 41). Overall, the study showed that 66.7% of patients (N = 33) were pain free at 2 months following RFA, 24.4% (N = 11) reported 50% improvement, and 4 patients (8.9%) reported no improvement.

In a double-blinded, randomized control trial by Ke and colleagues,[8] 96 patients with thoracic postherpetic neuralgia (PHN) were treated with PRF. Patients underwent PRF of the intercostal nerves at, above, and below the affected dermatome levels (eg, for T2 pain, T1–T3 were treated). VAS scores and the SF-36 quality-of-life questionnaire were administered on day 3, day 7, day 14, month 1, month 2, month 3, and month 6 after the procedure. The investigators determined that postprocedure VAS scores were significantly lower compared with the placebo group, and SF-36 scores were improved in the treatment group versus the placebo group. The investigators also found that tramadol administration in the first month was lower in the treatment group compared with the control group.

In a retrospective study of 15 patients by Yang and colleagues,[9] 5 patients with PHN were treated with CT-guided coblation (PRF) of the thoracic paravertebral nerves. Four of these patients reported a significant decrease of pain symptoms following ablation, whereas 1 patient reported no change.

Of the 5 studies reviewed, 2 were case studies, 1 was observational, 1 was retrospective, and 1 was a randomized controlled trial (RCT). The overall study sizes were very small and the anatomic targets differed in each study. The causes of ICN also varied; in the Abd-Elsayed and colleagues[5] study, ICN was secondary to cancer surgery (breast, esophageal, non–small cell lung cancer), whereas in Engel[6] the cause was trauma. These studies also did not comment on the use of or the difference between CRF versus PRF. The follow-up time in Stolker and colleagues[7] was very short (only 2 months). In the Stolker and colleagues[7] study, 8 patients (17.7%) reported complications of transient burning pain and sensory loss. Despite the limitations of the Stolker and colleagues'[7] article, the investigators concluded that RFA was a safe and effective treatment of chronic thoracic pain when conservative treatment failed. In order to make that conclusion, there needs to be more research specifically regarding ICN with larger populations; that is, not just case studies or observational studies. These studies would also benefit from comparing the efficacy of RFA treatment in the different causes of ICN as well as including longer follow-up time. Although RFA does look promising in the treatment of ICN, only with stronger data can it be recommended.

### Chronic Postsurgical Thoracic Pain and Postthoracotomy Pain Syndrome

CPTS pain refers to persistent pain following thoracic surgery. Similar to CPTS, PTPS defines a more specific pain syndrome following thoracotomy. Although there is still ongoing debate regarding when acute pain transitions to chronic pain temporally, consensus defines CPTS/PTPS as pain persisting beyond the normal and expected time of healing. The sources causing postsurgical thoracic pain include large incisions through skin and multiple layers of muscle, retraction, possible rib fractures or dislocation of costovertebral joints, intercostal nerve damage, and pleural irritation from chest tubes. This pain can be neuropathic, such as burning or stabbing pain. Postsurgical thoracic pain can greatly affect respiratory function and ambulation. The inability to properly clear secretions by effective coughing can lead to pneumonia in these patients. Medical management of CPTS pain can include narcotics, nonsteroidal antiinflammatory drugs (NSAIDs), epidurals, and nerve blocks. RFA can possibly play a role in the treatment of CPTS pain. Cohen and colleagues[10] was a retrospective study of 49 patients treated with PRF for chronic pain following thoracic surgery. Of these 49 patients, 31 had thoracotomies, 5 had sternotomies, 9 had mastectomies, and 4 had other thoracic surgeries. This study compared pulsed RFA of the DRG and RFA of the intercostal nerves with traditional pharmacotherapy and conservative management. At 6 weeks of follow-up, 27.3% of the medically managed patients reported pain relief, 21.4% of ICN RFA patients reported pain relief, and 61.5% of DRG RFA patients reported pain relief. Similarly, at 3 months follow-up, 19.9% of medically managed patients reported pain relief, 6.7% of ICN RFA patients reported relief, and 53.8% of DRG RFA patients reported relief.

In a case series of 26 patients, Nash[11] also reviewed the efficacy of RFA of the DRG for treatment of thoracic pain. Fourteen patients underwent CRF ablation of thoracic DRG with 5 patients experiencing specifically postsurgical pain and 1 postthoracotomy scar pain. Of these 5 patients, 3 patients reported no response to treatment, 1 patient reported good response (reduced rate of analgesic consumption), and 1 patient reported an excellent response (virtually pain free). The patient with postthoracotomy scar pain did not experience any benefit from RFA treatment.

In a case report from Ladenhauf and colleagues,[12] a patient with CPTS following pectus excavatum repair was successfully treated with paravertebral CRF ablation of the T9 segment bilaterally. RFA provided the patient with up to 3 years of pain relief without any complications.

In a retrospective study of 15 patients by Yang and colleagues,[9] CT-guided ablation (PRF) of the thoracic paravertebral nerves was used to treat thoracic neuropathic pain. However, only 6 of the 15 patients had PTPS. Patients were selected following good response to paravertebral nerve blocks. Overall, 80% of the 15 patients achieved greater than 50% pain relief following ablation, with a decrease in VAS scores from 7.42 to 2.17 at 1 week and 1.58 at 6 months. Five of the 6 patients with PTPS reported excellent response to treatment and did not require any further postoperative medications, whereas 1 patient had some benefit following ablation but continued to require gabapentin for pain control. Many patients reported transient numbness following treatment that resolved within a few days to weeks without intervention.

Stolker and colleagues'[7] study of 45 patients who received CRF of the thoracic DRG for chronic thoracic pain included 9 patients with PTPS. Of these patients, 5 reported excellent pain relief, 3 reported greater than 50% pain relief, and 1 patient was lost to follow-up (died).

The evidence from these 5 articles was overall limited in strength, design, and variability in outcome measures reported. None of these articles were RCTs; 2 were retrospective studies, 1 observational study, 1 case series, and 1 case report. Also, the population size of these studies was very small. The Cohen study,[10] which had the largest population size, recommended that, although medical management should remain first-line therapy for CPTS, RFA of the DRG is safe and effective for refractory pain and superior to RFA of ICN. However, of note, 2 patients included in the study had pneumothoraxes caused by the intervention. One patient required a chest tube for symptomatic treatment, whereas another pneumothorax was an incidental finding. In the Yang and colleagues[9] study, most of patients reported transient numbness. Although RFA of thoracic DRG may be an effective treatment of chronic post–thoracic surgery pain, more evidence is required to conclude that the benefits outweigh the associated risks/complications.

### Other Thoracic Pain Syndromes

Yang and colleagues[9] similarly included patients with PTTP in their retrospective review. Of their 15 patients, 4 patients underwent thoracic paravertebral nerve ablation for PTTP. Three of the 4 patients reported a good response to treatment.

In a study by Pevsner and colleagues,[13] 122 patients were retrospectively reviewed after treatment of spinal mechanical pain with CRF ablation of the medial branch of the dorsal ramus. Patients with cervical and lumbar pain were included in the study as well. Thoracic pain was not separately analyzed. Limited data were provided on the patients selected and the cause of their pain. The investigators reported that 75% of patients reported pain relief at 1 month following RFA, and 63% of patients reported continued relief at 1 year with an average reduction in VAS scores of 4.3 points at this time. Importantly, all patients were treated with 4 to 6 weeks of NSAIDs and 1 month of physiotherapy following RFA as well. A high postprocedural complication rate was reported, although most patients reported spontaneous resolution of adverse symptoms within 1 month. However, because of the multiple additional treatments the patients received, it is difficult to determine which individual treatment was most effective. Also, because thoracic pain was not individually analyzed, RFA treatment of thoracic spinal mechanical pain cannot be fully recommended.

Stolker and colleagues[14] performed a more specific observational study for patients with chronic thoracic pain related to thoracic facet syndrome. Forty patients underwent percutaneous facet denervation (PFD) via radiofrequency lesioning (CRF) of the medial branch of the DRG at various thoracic levels. Patients were followed for 2 months after the procedure, at which time 51% of patients were pain free, 33% of patients reported greater than 50% pain reduction, and 16% reported no improvement. Long-term follow-up (31 months on average) revealed similar levels of pain control, with 44% of patients still reporting excellent pain control and 39% of patients reporting moderate pain control. Of note, 4 patients required multiple treatments, after which a transient neuritislike syndrome occurred but spontaneously resolved. Despite needing more research, CRF of thoracic DRG could possibly be used to treat chronic thoracic pain caused by thoracic facet syndrome.

Two additional studies investigated the utility of RFA in the treatment of chronic thoracic pain caused by multiple disorders. In a case series by Nash,[11] 26 patients with cervical, lumbar, and thoracic pain were treated with RFA of the DRG. Fourteen patients with thoracic pain were included. The disorders of these 14 patients included postradiation osteitis, failed laminectomy, postsurgical scar pain, carcinoma of the lung, posttraumatic neuralgia, and unspecified neuralgia. Four patients reported excellent pain response, 4 patients reported good response, and 6 patients reported no response to the RFA. No specific follow-up period was noted. No objective pain measurements were included. An observational study by Van Kleef and colleagues[15] also reviewed the efficacy of CRF ablation of DRG at variable thoracic levels for thoracic segmental pain. Forty-three patients with 6 months of unilateral thoracic segmental pain (unresponsive to conservative therapy) were selected. Clinical diagnoses for the thoracic pain included slipping rib syndrome, twelfth rib syndrome, PTTP, vertebral collapse, and segmental peripheral neuralgia (unspecified). The investigators reported that 67% of patients had good pain relief following RFA at 8 weeks and 52% of patients had good pain relief after 36 weeks. However, if patients had symptoms involving 2 or more thoracic segmental levels, RFA was less effective, with 62% of patients reporting no short-term benefits following RFA. In this study, the pain relief measures were all subjective; good was 50% or more reduction in pain, moderate was 30% to 50% reduction, no effect was less than 30% pain relief. In addition, the investigators recommended peripheral nerve blocks rather than spinal nerve blocks as part of the screening process for patients to include in future studies. RFA may be an effective treatment of chronic thoracic pain caused by multiple disorders. However, overall, much more research is needed in order for RFA to become a recommended treatment.

| Pain Condition | Nerve Targets | Highest Level of Evidence | Consensus for RFA Treatment | Comments |
|---|---|---|---|---|
| Refractory thoracic cancer chest wall pain<br>Oh et al,[2] 2018 | • Thoracic nerve root RFA<br>• T2 to T12 thoracic nerve roots<br>• CRF | • 2018 study<br>• N = 100<br>• Retrospective review | • Decrease in NRS when comparing pre-RFA pain with postprocedure pain at 1 wk, 1 mo, 6 mo<br>• Decrease MEDD 1 wk postprocedure but no difference at 1 or 6 mo | • Many patients died before the 1-mo and 6-mo analysis and likely had higher NRS scores<br>• NRS scores may represent overall pain and not just thoracic pain<br>• Quality of life was not measured |
| Refractory thoracic cancer chest wall pain<br>Reyad et al,[3] 2019 | • Thoracic DRG<br>• T2–T8 DRG<br>• CRF | • 2019 study<br>• N = 78<br>• Single-blinded, parallel-group, randomized clinical trial | • Decreased VAS scores in both groups, lower VAS scores in CT-guided group compared with standard group at weeks 4, 8, and 12<br>• Both groups had decreased VAS scores at 12 wk, decreased oxycodone and pregabalin consumption | • No comparison with pain control modalities apart from RFA<br>• Decreased adverse events in CT-guided group compared with standard group |
| Refractory thoracic cancer chest wall pain<br>Gulati et al,[4] 2015 | • Thoracic nerve root<br>• T3, T8, T9<br>• PRF | • 2015 study<br>• N = 146<br>• Retrospective review | • Recommend RFA if pharmacologic therapies fail, if lesion is in posterior chest wall, or is a paravertebral tumor, and if tumor is encroaching thoracic nerve root | • If no response to intercostal nerve blocks or paravertebral nerve blocks, then proceed to RFA |
| CPTP<br>Cohen et al,[10] 2006 | • Intercostal nerves and DRG at variable levels<br>• PRF | • 2006 study<br>• N = 49<br>• Retrospective review | • 6 wk: pain relief in 27.3% of patients in medical management group, 21.4% in ICN RFA group, 61.5% in DRG RFA group<br>• 3 mo: pain relief in 19.9% of medical management group, 6.7% in ICN RFA group, 53.8% in DRG RFA group | • Comparison between pharmacotherapy, pulsed RFA of intercostal nerves, and pulsed RFA of dorsal root ganglia in CPTP<br>• Pulsed RFA of DRG is superior to pharmacotherapy and RFA of ICN in patients with CPTP |

(continued on next page)

**(continued)**

| Pain Condition | Nerve Targets | Highest Level of Evidence | Consensus for RFA Treatment | Comments |
|---|---|---|---|---|
| Mechanical pain of spinal origin<br>Pevsner et al,[13] 2003 | • Medial branch of the dorsal ramus (levels varied depending on the patient, not mentioned specifically)<br>• CRF | • 2003 study<br>• N = 122<br>• Retrospective review | • 75% of patients reported pain relief at 1 mo following RFA<br>• 63% of patients reported continued pain relief at 12 mo following RFA<br>• Average reduction in VAS was 4.3 points after 12 mo compared with scores before RFA | • Thoracic pain was not separately categorized, but thoracolumbar pain was treated |
| PTPS, postherpetic neuralgia, post–thoracic trauma pain<br>Yang et al,[9] 2017 | • CT-guided coblation of thoracic paravertebral nerve<br>• Targeted regions included T1 to T11, patients had 2–5 nerves treated<br>• PRF | • 2016 study<br>• N = 15<br>• Retrospective review | • 80% of patients achieved >50% pain relief following ablation with a decrease in VAS scores from 7.42 to 2.17 at week 1<br>• At 6 mo, VAS scores remained low at 1.58 | • Most patients reported transient numbness following treatment |
| ICN, PTPS, pain following mastectomy, spinal pain, others<br>Stolker et al,[7] 1994 | - Intercostal nerve at variety of thoracic levels (T1–T12)<br>• Percutaneous partial rhizotomy suspected to target DRG<br>• CRF | • 1994 study<br>• N = 45<br>• Observational study | • 33 patients (66.7%) were pain free at 2 mo, 11 (24.4%) reported 50% improvement, 4 (8.9%) reported no improvement | • Success rates are higher compared with surgical rhizotomy<br>• Burning pain/sensory loss was transient and reported in 8 patients (17.7%) |
| Postherpetic neuralgia<br>Ke et al,[8] 2013 | • Thoracic intercostal nerves were selected and expanded 1 up and down (T2–T11)<br>• Eg, T3 pain treated at T2, T3, T4<br>• PRF | • 2013 study<br>• N = 96<br>• Double-blinded RCT | • Postprocedure VAS scores in pulsed RF group was significantly lower than placebo group<br>• SF-36 scores improved in treatment vs control group | • End points analyzed by intention-to-treat analysis<br>• Measured VAS scores and SF-36 questionnaire and side effects on day 3, 7, 14 and months 1, 2, 3, 6 |

| | | | | |
|---|---|---|---|---|
| Facet syndrome Stolker et al,[14] 1993 | • PFD, or radiofrequency lesioning used on the DRG (medial branch) • Levels included T1–T12 • CRF | • 1993 study • N = 40 • Observational study | • Patients followed 2 mo postprocedure; 51% of patients were pain free, 33% reported >50% pain reduction, 16% reported no improvement • Long-term follow-up (average 31 mo): excellent response in 44%, good response in 39%, and poor result in 17% | • Patients with negative response to facet nerve blocks excluded • 4 patients had multiple treatments, after which a transient neuritislike syndrome occurred that spontaneously resolved |
| Posttrauma thoracic pain, thoracic segmental pain, segmental peripheral neuralgia, slipping rib syndrome, 12th rib syndrome Van Kleef et al,[15] 1995 | • Radiofrequency of DRG at variable thoracic levels • CRF | • 1995 study • N = 43 • Observational study | • Pain limited to segmental distribution: 67% had short-term (8 wk) relief of pain; 52% had long-term relief • Pain involving >2 thoracic segments: 12% were pain free at short-term and long-term follow-up; 62% reported no short-term effects and 68% reported no long-term effects | • Pain relief measures were subjective; good = 50% or more reduction in pain, moderate = 30%–50% reduction, no effect ≤30% pain relief • Recommend peripheral nerve blocks rather than spinal nerve blocks when evaluating patients for RFA |

## ABDOMINAL PAIN SYNDROMES

RFA has become more popular in the treatment of abdominal pain syndromes. These pain syndromes include abdominal cancer pain, loin pain hematuria syndrome (LPHS), chronic pancreatitis, anterior cutaneous nerve entrapment syndrome (ACNES), and abdominal myofascial pain syndrome (AMPS).

### Abdominal Cancer Pain

Chronic abdominal pain can be caused by cancer. These types of cancer include pancreatic, gallbladder, hepatocellular, stomach, and colon. The pain can be a mixture of somatic, visceral, and neuropathic pain. Somatic pain refers to well-localized pain, whereas visceral pain is poorly localized. The causes of abdominal cancer pain include compression, inflammation, ischemia, and hemorrhage. Traditional management includes the use of opioids and other pharmacologic therapies, such as antidepressants, antiepileptics, and steroids. However, these therapies are often limited by side effects and lack of efficacy, especially in palliative cases. Because of the difficulty of managing cancer pain, other methods besides medical management are being studied. RFA, particularly of the celiac or splanchnic nerves, has gained more traction as an effective alternative to traditional therapies.

Two RCTs studying the effect of RFA on abdominal cancer pain caused by cancer were reviewed for this article. Bang and colleagues[16] studied the utility of endoscopic ultrasonography-guided RFA (EUS-RFA) of the celiac plexus. In their 2019 RCT, they compared EUS-RFA (CRF) with celiac plexus neurolysis (CPN). Compared with EUS-CPN patients (N = 14), patients who underwent EUS-RFA (N = 12) showed decreased pain scores and increased quality of life at 4 weeks with similar use of opioid analgesia. No adverse effects were seen other than transient gastrointestinal symptoms, and patients in the RFA group had fewer side effects. In Amr and colleagues,[17] patients were split into 2 groups and underwent bilateral splanchnic nerve block (T10 to T11) using CRF ablation (N = 30) or alcohol (N = 30). The investigators determined RFA to be more effective than alcohol, with larger reduction of mean VAS scores and improvement of global perceived effect satisfaction (GPES) scores. RFA acted more rapidly, provided longer duration of analgesia, and had a better safety profile compared with alcohol.

Two retrospective studies were reviewed. Papadopoulos and colleagues[18] performed a retrospective review of 35 patients with pancreatic cancer pain. These patients underwent radiofrequency thermocoagulation (CRF) of both splanchnic nerves, under fluoroscopic guidance, at the T11 to T12 levels. Patients reported a decrease in mean NRS scores from 8.9 to 3.6 5 months after RFA treatment. Similarly, patients reported improvement in quality-of-life scores from 1.05 to 8 at 1 month post-RFA. Raj and colleagues[19] also studied CRF ablation of the splanchnic nerves (T11 and T12 levels). In their study, 107 patients with chronic abdominal pain (secondary to pancreatitis, pancreatic cancer, liver cancer, or postsurgical pain) underwent RFA of the splanchnic nerves. Only 73 patients were followed prospectively and analyzed. At 6-month follow-up, 40% of patients reported VAS pain scores that decreased by 50% or more compared with baseline. The investigators concluded that RFA was more efficacious and had a lower side effect profile than chemical neurolysis of the celiac plexus.

There are many case reports that highlight the possible efficacy of RFA in the treatment of chronic abdominal cancer pain. In the case report by Jin and colleagues,[20] a 57-year-old man with pancreatic cancer pain with liver metastases underwent EUS-RFA (CRF) of the celiac ganglion. The patient had a subsequent decrease in his VAS score from baseline of 8 to 2, 3 days after RFA. At 2 weeks, the patient reported a VAS score of 4 and no longer required opioid analgesia. Miceli and colleagues[21] presented the case of a 55-year old woman who underwent PRF ablation of the left-sided iliohypogastric and ilioinguinal nerves for abdominal pain secondary to colorectal cancer metastasis. At 12 weeks after RFA, the patient's NRS score was 4 compared with a baseline of 9. Similarly, Evrard[22] reported a case of a 55-year-old woman who underwent left-sided splanchnic nerve RFA for pancreatic cancer with liver metastases. In this case, CRF ablation was performed as part of an exploratory laparotomy using anatomic landmarks. The patient reported being pain free at 1-month and 4-month follow-up visits.

Although RFA may play a future role in treating chronic abdominal pain related to abdominal cancer, the data are promising but limited. In 2 of the studies, by Bang and colleagues[16] and Papadopoulos and colleagues,[18] patients were receiving other pharmacologic treatments such as chemotherapy, radiation, opioids, steroids, antidepressants, and antiepileptics. Because the patients were receiving these other treatments, it is difficult to analyze the effect of RFA in the pain of these patients. In the Raj and colleagues[19] study, 40% of patients underwent repeat splanchnic RFA because of return of intolerable pain around 3 months. Also in this study, there were limited data because of attrition, and pain caused by cancer was unable to be analyzed individually. In the Jin and colleagues[20] study, it was the patient's second RFA procedure; his first was 2 months before this case report and offered limited benefit. Papadopoulos and colleagues[18] and Amr and colleagues[17] discussed side effects such as temporary paresthesia, diarrhea, and colic; in the Amr and colleagues[17] study, the group receiving the alcohol nerve block reported more side effects. Before recommending an interventional treatment such as RFA for chronic abdominal pain caused by cancer, there needs to be more focused research in this area. Topics could include the type of cancer in which RFA is most efficacious and side effects.

### Loin Pain Hematuria Syndrome

LPHS refers to severe bilateral or unilateral renal, flank, or abdominal pain associated with gross or microscopic hematuria. This diagnosis is one of exclusion; all glomerular and nonglomerular causes must be excluded. The cause of LPHS in unclear and it is often resistant to treatment. Traditional treatment includes an interdisciplinary approach: opioids, NSAIDs, muscle relaxants, antidepressants, behavior and psychological therapy, and nephrectomy as a last resort. In order to help the population with LPHS, RFA has been studied as a possible treatment.

Two case reports were reviewed for this article. Gambaro and colleagues[23] reported the case of a 40-year-old woman with LPHS poorly controlled with pharmacologic therapy. She underwent percutaneous renal sympathetic nerve continuous RFA, applied in the vicinity of the right renal artery. The patient reported a VAS pain score of 1 at 6-month follow-up. Similarly, Moeschler and colleagues[24] reported the case of a 50-year-old woman with chronic flank pain secondary to LPHS and chronic nephrolithiasis. She initially underwent bilateral splanchnic nerve blocks with short-lived pain relief. She then underwent pulsed RFA of the splanchnic nerves (bilateral T12–L1 levels). Before RFA, she reported a VAS score between 5 and 10. Six months after RFA, the patient reported near-complete resolution of her right-sided abdominal and flank pain but her left-sided pain remained unchanged These 2 case reports show the possible efficacy of RFA treatment of LPHS, but more research is needed in order to make this recommendation.

### Chronic Pancreatitis

Chronic pancreatitis can cause chronic abdominal pain that can be visceral, somatic, and neuropathic. It is usually refractory to treatment. The pain commonly starts in the epigastric area and radiates to the back. The pain is often worse after eating and is associated with postprandial nausea and vomiting. Causes of chronic pancreatitis include alcoholism, hypertriglyceridemia, cystic fibrosis, smoking, and gallstones. The pain can be so severe that it warrants hospital admission. Management of chronic pancreatitis pain includes NSAIDs, opioids, antidepressants, gabapentin, and N-methyl-D-aspartate (NMDA) receptor antagonists such as ketamine. Because chronic pancreatitis pain is often refractory to medical management, other forms of treatment are being studied, including RFA. Garcea and colleagues[25] performed a retrospective, observational study in patients with chronic pancreatitis and abdominal pain. Ten patients (8 with chronic pancreatitis, 2 with unknown cause of abdominal pain) underwent percutaneous RFA of the splanchnic nerve. Following CRF ablation, patients had decreased VAS scores, decreased opiate analgesia use, improved anxiety levels, improved daily activity levels, improved mood, and improved general perceptions of their health. One patient reported transient diarrhea, but otherwise no complications were reported. Verhaegh and colleagues[26] also performed a retrospective observational study in patients with chronic pancreatitis. Eleven patients underwent diagnostic bupivacaine blocks, followed by percutaneous RFA (CRF) of the splanchnic nerves with fluoroscopic guidance (at T11–12, both unilateral and bilateral). Mean NRS pain scores decreased from 7.7 to 2.8 following RFA, with a median duration of 45 weeks of pain relief (no formal follow-up period). Of note, 5 patients underwent a second RFA procedure and 2 patients underwent a third RFA procedure in order to sustain pain relief. In total, 18 RFA procedures were performed. Excellent pain response (>75% reduction in pain) was seen after 6 procedures, and good pain response was obtained in 14 procedures (>50% pain relief). One patient had transient hypoesthesia of the flank following RFA.

Brennan and colleagues[27] reported on 2 patients that underwent bilateral PRF lesioning of the splanchnic nerves (T12) to treat chronic pancreatitis pain. The first was a 48-year-old man with poorly controlled pain. Following RFA, his NRS pain score decreased from 10 to 2 and he required fewer oral pain medications. The second was a 63-year-old woman. Following RFA, her NRS score decreased from 8 to 4 and was sustained for at least 6 months. Three other patients were reviewed, but they did not respond to PRF lesioning No adverse effects were reported.

Because chronic pancreatitis pain is commonly refractory and often requires hospitalization, it is imperative to find other pain relief methods. RFA shows promise with minimal complications, but overall the data are limited. It is important to understand how many RFA treatments provide the most relief and to analyze the efficacy in different causes of chronic pancreatitis and the side effects. Although observational studies and case reports can provide some evidence, larger studies, particularly RCTs, need to be performed. Only with more evidence can RFA for chronic pancreatitis pain become standard practice.

### Anterior Cutaneous Nerve Entrapment Syndrome/Lateral Cutaneous Nerve Entrapment Syndrome

The anterior and lateral cutaneous nerves contribute to the sensory innervation of the abdominal wall in a dermatomal pattern. These nerves can become trapped in the rectus abdominis muscles, leading to chronic abdominal pain. These nerves can become trapped in scars, adhesions from surgery, and hernias. The pain is usually well localized and can be described as dull, sharp, and burning, and can cause significant distress. When the anterior cutaneous nerve is trapped, this is referred to as ACNES. In a similar pattern, when the lateral cutaneous nerve is involved, it is known as lateral cutaneous nerve entrapment syndrome (LACNES).

Maatman and colleagues[28] performed a RCT comparing pulsed RFA with anterior neurectomy in the management of ACNES. Sixty patients underwent either PRF or neurectomy of the anterior cutaneous nerve (varying between T7 and T12 levels) by targeting the anterior fascia of the rectus abdominis muscle. At 8-week follow-up, 61% of patients in the neurectomy group reported greater than 50% pain reduction, compared with only 38% of patients in the PRF group. Maatman and colleagues[29] also performed a retrospective observation study in patients with ACNES. Twenty-six patients were asked to locate points of maximal pain and underwent PRF targeted to those areas and the underlying fascia of the rectus abdominis muscles. At 6-week follow-up, NRS scores decreased from 6.7 to 3.8 with mean patient global impression of change scores of 4.9. In addition, 50% of patients reported short-term success (defined as >50% reduction in NRS scores) at 6 to 8 weeks, whereas 8% of patients reported being pain free for longer (median 15 months). The same group (Maatman and colleagues[30]) also completed an observational study of 30 patients with LACNES. Patients who did not respond initially or after to diagnostic/therapeutic repeat lidocaine injections underwent medical management or pulsed RFA (N = 6). However, limited data are available on the specific nature of the procedures performed, as well as how individual patients responded. Presumably, 2 of the 6 patients responded to radiofrequency therapy.

Two case reports have been published regarding the use of RFA in ACNES as well. Birthi and colleagues[31] reported the case of a 33-year-old woman who was diagnosed with ACNES and underwent pulsed RFA of the thoracic DRG (T10–T11). Her VAS score decreased from a 6 to a 1 for up to 10 months. Villaios and colleagues[32] presented a case of ACNES poorly controlled by oral medications. The patient underwent pulsed RFA of the abdominal cutaneous nerve near the left iliac fossa (T11–T12 intercostal level). Fifteen days after the procedure, the patient was able to return to work and reported continued pain relief for as long as 6 months postprocedure.

These studies show that RFA may have a role in ACNES/LACNES that is refractory to other treatments. However, before making that conclusion, it is important to look at the limitations of the studies presented earlier. In Maatman and colleagues,[28] the study was nonblinded and there was overlap between lidocaine administration and the PRF procedure. Both groups reported improved quality of life and minimal adverse events. Patients were also allowed to cross over from PRF to neurectomy if they did not have satisfactory results after 8 weeks, but only 1 patient made this switch. Because of the overlap between lidocaine administration and PRF treatment, this study cannot fully conclude that it was RFA treatment that improved pain scores and quality of life. In Maatman and colleagues,[29] many patients received corticosteroids after PRF, which again may have contributed to symptom improvement. Of note, in this study the investigators noted that there seemed to be a steep loss of analgesic effect observed 2 to 5 months after treatment. Therefore, there needs to be more research into RFA treatment of ACNES/LACNES and length of analgesic effect. Although data are limited, this study shows that RFA may have a role in LACNES refractory to other therapies.

### Abdominal Myofascial Pain Syndrome

AMPS describes musculoskeletal pain that arises from trigger points, or areas of discrete and sensitive muscle in the abdominal musculature. It is theorized that these trigger points can arise with stress or trauma to the muscle. These irritable points can cause significant discomfort and pain. The pain can be a constant dull pain with sharp flare ups, and is often relieved by curling up in a ball. In order to make the diagnosis of AMPS, it is necessary to exclude other disorders or inflammatory processes in the abdomen and pelvis. RFA may be a possible treatment of AMPS.

Niraj and colleagues[33] published an observational study analyzing the utility of a treatment protocol plan in AMPS and ACNES. In this 2018 study, patients were first treated with a local anesthetic and then underwent trigger point injection with steroids if they had less than 30% pain relief. If trigger point injections failed, then patients underwent PRF treatment of various abdominal trigger points. Of the 120 included patients, 18 were diagnosed with ACNES (none underwent RFA) and 102 patients were diagnosed with AMPS. Of these 102 patients diagnosed with AMPS, 43 patients required PRF to myofascial trigger points. Sixty percent of patients in this group reported pain relief lasting more than 6 months, whereas 12 patients reported minimal pain relief. On average, NRS pain scores decreased from 8.2 to 5.9 at 6-month follow-up. Tamimi and colleagues[34] reported a case series of 9 patients with abdominal myofascial trigger points. Of their 9 subjects, 1 patient with AMPS underwent pulsed RFA (twice) of the iliohypogastric region for chronic abdominal pain. They reported 50% pain relief for more than 6 months without any complications. Niraj and colleagues[35] also reported a series of patients that underwent ultrasonography-guided pulsed RFA of various abdominal and cervicothoracic trigger points. Of the 12 patients included, 8 patients underwent RFA for AMPS. Patients were followed at 1 month and 6 months postprocedure. NRS pain scores decreased from a baseline of 7.75 to 3.5 at 6-month follow-up.

Note that, in Niraj and colleagues,[33] 9 patients had side effects of pain flares after radiofrequency treatment that lasted greater than 1 week. Many patients also underwent multiple treatment options, including medical management and acupuncture, before PRF treatment. Obviously, these additional treatments could have influenced the results. Because of the limitations to their study, Niraj and colleagues[33] recommended that radiofrequency treatment should only be considered for AMPS if initial anesthetic injections or trigger point injections do not provide adequate and sustained pain relief. Although the studies discussed here show that RFA could play a role in the treatment of AMPS, there are still limited data regarding greater efficacy of RFA compared with anesthetic or steroid trigger point injections.

### Other Abdominal Pain Syndromes

Postsurgical abdominal pain has also been a target of RFA. Zaky and colleagues[36] presented the case of a 50-year old woman with resistant abdominal pain for more than 2 years following a cholecystectomy. She first underwent bilateral splanchnic nerve blockade with steroid injection and had 80% improvement in symptoms that lasted up to 3 weeks. She then underwent bilateral splanchnic nerve RFA (CRF) and reported 50% reduction in pain that persisted for up to 5 months.

An observational study by Niraj and colleagues[37] analyzed the utility of RFA in chronic abdominal pain stemming from a variety of causes, including AMPS, pancreatitis, appendicitis, gastritis, and biliary inflammation. The goal of their 2018 study was to establish a treatment pathway for chronic abdominal pain. Initially, patients were offered ultrasonography-guided trigger point injections and steroids. Thirty-five (out of 36) patients reported greater than 50% pain response with this initial treatment. However, patients who had less than 3 months of pain relief were offered radiofrequency therapy. Sixteen patients continued to the radiofrequency (PRF) treatment arm. Eleven patients (69%) reported greater than 50% pain relief with RFA, whereas the remaining 5 patients reported less than 50% pain relief at their 3-month follow-up. Three patients in the radiofrequency arm had transient postprocedure pain. No control group was present. The investigators determined that radiofrequency therapy was an appropriate treatment in patients that had less than 3 months of pain relief with trigger point injections.

| Pain Condition | Nerve Targets | Highest Level of Evidence | Consensus for RFA Treatment | Comments |
|---|---|---|---|---|
| Pancreatic cancer pain Papadopoulos et al,[18] 2013 | • Radiofrequency thermocoagulation of both splanchnic nerves under fluoroscopic guidance<br>• T11–T12<br>• CRF | • 2013 study<br>• N = 35<br>• Retrospective observational design | • Mean NRS before RFA was 8.9; NRS 3.6 at 5 mo<br>• Reduced pain, reduced consumption of systemic opioids, and improved quality of life | — |
| Abdominal cancer pain (pancreatic, gall bladder, hepatocellular, stomach, others) Amr et al,[17] 2018 | • Group 1: 30, bilateral splanchnic RFA at T10–T11<br>• Group 2: 30, bilateral splanchnic alcohol nerve block at T11<br>• CRF | • 2018 study<br>• N = 60<br>• RCT | • Significant reduction of VAS and GPES scores observed in both groups, with group 1 having a larger reduction | • More patients in group 2 complained of temporary paresthesia, colic, diarrhea; no major complications recorded |
| Pancreatic cancer pain Bang et al,[16] 2019 | • Group 1: 14 patients underwent EUS-CPN<br>• Group 2: 12 patients underwent EUS-RFA of celiac plexus<br>• CRF | • 2019 study<br>• N = 26<br>• RCT | • At 4 wk: pain scores (using PAN26, BPI, VAS scores) lower in RFA group compared with CPN group<br>• Quality-of-life scores (PAN26) better in RFA group compared with CPN group | • Many patients undergoing chemotherapy and radiation therapy at that time<br>• Opioid managed by primary oncologist and thus not regimented or controlled in study |
| Chronic pancreatitis and abdominal pain Garcea et al,[25] 2005 | • Percutaneous RFA of splanchnic nerve<br>• T12 level<br>• CRF | • 2005 study<br>• N = 10<br>• Retrospective observational study | • Splanchnic nerve RFA led to decreased pain scores, decreased opiate analgesia use; improved anxiety levels; improved daily activity, mood, and general perception of health | • No complications apart from 1 patient complaining of self-resolving diarrhea<br>• Decreased number of hospital admissions for pain |
| Chronic abdominal pain secondary to ACNES Maatman et al,[28] 2019 | • RFA of anterior cutaneous nerve (T7–T12, variable)<br>• RFA administered underneath anterior fascia of rectus abdominis<br>• PRF | • 2019 study<br>• N = 60<br>• RCT (multicenter, nonblinded) | • Neurectomy group showed greater pain reduction at 8-wk follow-up<br>• Treatment success reached in 38% of PRF patients and 61% of neurectomy group | • Comparison between pulsed RFA and anterior neurectomy<br>• Quality-of-life scores improved in both groups; neurectomy group reported higher patient satisfaction |

(continued on next page)

*(continued)*

| Pain Condition | Nerve Targets | Highest Level of Evidence | Consensus for RFA Treatment | Comments |
|---|---|---|---|---|
| Chronic abdominal pain (chronic pancreatitis, pancreatic cancer, liver cancer, postsurgical pain) Raj et al,[19] 2002 | • RFA of splanchnic nerves at the T11-T12 levels • CRF | • 2002 study • N = 107 but 73 followed closely • Retrospective observational study | • At 6-mo follow-up, 40% of patients reported VAS pain scores decreased by 50% or more • Poor results (VAS scale decreased by 10% or less) were seen in 15% | • 40% of patients underwent repeat splanchnic RFA because of return of intolerable pain around 3 mo • Investigators concluded RF to be better than chemical neurolysis of celiac plexus given fewer side effects |
| Chronic pancreatitis Verhaegh et al,[26] 2013 | • Percutaneous RFA of splanchnic nerves at T11-T12 levels with fluoroscopic guidance • Diagnostic test block performed at T11 with bupivacaine • CRF | • 2013 study • N = 11 • Retrospective observational study | • Mean NRS pain score decreased from 7.7 to 2.8 • Median period of pain relief was 45 wk • Excellent pain response seen in 6 procedures • Good pain response seen in 14 procedures | • 1 patient had transient hypoesthesia of the flank, no other complications reported • 4 patients reported significantly decreased analgesic use, 4 patients reported no analgesic use |
| ACNES Maatman et al,[29] 2018 | • Targeted point of maximal tenderness • Located underlying fascia of rectus abdominis and this area is anesthetized and then treated with RFA • PRF | • 2018 study • N = 26 • Retrospective observational study | • NRS decreased from 6.7 to 3.8 on average (at 6 wk) • 50% of patients reported short-term treatment success (6-8 wk) • 8% were pain free longer (median 15 mo) • Median effect duration was 4 mo (2-26 mo) | • No short-term neurologic complications seen • May patients received corticosteroids after PRF; may have played a small role in study results • Steep loss of analgesic effect observed between 2 and 5 mo after treatment |

| | | | |
|---|---|---|---|
| Chronic abdominal pain (AMPS secondary to pancreatitis, appendicitis, gastritis, biliary inflammation) Niraj & Chaudhri,[37] 2018 | • RFA performed at various locations based on trigger point locations in patients (limited location details provided) <br> • PRF | • 2018 study <br> • N = 43 <br> • Observational study, case series | • 35 of the 36 that were followed further had >50% pain response following trigger point injections <br> • Of these, 16 continued to PRF treatment <br> • 11 of the 16 patients (69%) reported >50% pain relief after procedure | • Limited specific data in PRF subset of patients <br> • 3 patients in PRF arm had transient postprocedure pain <br> • Used PRF for AMPS when patients did not have >3 mo of pain control with trigger point injection |
| AMPS, ACNES Niraj,[33] 2018 | • RFA of variable trigger point locations in abdomen <br> • Possible sites include rectus abdominis, oblique muscles, transversus abdominis, quadratus lumborum <br> • PRF | • 2018 study <br> • N = 120 <br> • 18 patients with ACNES; none underwent PRF <br> • 102 patients with AMPS <br> • Observational study | • 43 patients received PRF <br> • 26 patients (60%) reported sustained pain relief lasting >6 mo; 12 had minimal relief (28%) <br> • NRS pain scores of 8.2 at baseline with a mean score of 5.9 at 6-mo follow-up <br> • For AMPS: if patients fail initial anesthetic injection, use trigger point injection with steroids <br> • PRF is lower on the pathway if patients do not respond to injections | • Patients went through a protocol outlining when they would receive PRF treatment: patients were first treated with local anesthetic; if pain relief <30%, underwent trigger point injection with steroids; if pain relief <30%, underwent PRF treatment <br> • 9 patients reported pain flare after PRF that continued >1 wk |

## SUMMARY

Chronic thoracic and abdominal pain conditions can significantly affect quality of life and cause significant distress for patients. RFA has gained popularity in the treatment of chronic pain conditions refractory to traditional pharmacologic therapies, such as chronic cancer pain, ICN, chronic pancreatitis, and posttraumatic or postprocedural pain. Many of the studies currently published are case series, observational studies, or retrospective reviews, limited by small sample sizes. There is a lack of sizable and well-designed studies exploring the effectiveness of RFA relative to other to treatment strategies. Furthermore, there is a lack of uniform outcome measures and time points for comparing the effectiveness of RFA. Despite a shortage of high-level evidence, multiple trials have shown the efficacy and safety of RFA in the treatment of these conditions, particularly when other treatments fail. The current consensus in the literature supports the use of RFA for the treatment of various chronic thoracic and abdominal pain syndromes. Areas of investigation for future studies should include DRG RFA versus ICN RFA versus placebo, PRF versus CRF, quality-of-life and functional measures, reduction in the use of opiates and other pharmacotherapies, and the utility of diagnostic nerve blocks in the selection of patients to undergo RFA treatment.

## CLINICS CARE POINTS

- Many thoracic and abdominal pain syndromes often arise secondarily to tumor infiltration, visceral organ involvement, operative interventions, and focal neuralgias.
- The focal nature of localized tumor burden and other underlying pain disorders makes them particularly susceptible to targeted interventions.
- Further study exploring the safety and effectiveness of PRF versus CRF for various conditions is needed.

## REFERENCES

1. Uchida KI. Radiofrequency treatment of the thoracic paravertebral nerve combined with glucocorticoid for refractory neuropathic pain following breast cancer surgery. Pain Physician 2009;12:277–83.
2. Oh TK, Kim NW, Yim J, et al. Effect of radiofrequency thermocoagulation of thoracic nerve roots in patients with cancer and intractable chest wall pain. Pain Physician 2018;21:323–9.
3. Reyad RM, Ghobrial HZ, Shaker EH, et al. Modified technique for thermal radiofrequency ablation of thoracic dorsal root ganglia under combined fluoroscopy and CT guidance: a randomized clinical trial. BMC Anesthesiol 2019;19:234.
4. Gulati A, Shah R, Puttanniah V, et al. A retrospective review and treatment paradigm of interventional therapies for patients suffering from intractable thoracic chest wall pain in the oncologic population. Pain Med 2015;(16):802–10.
5. Abd-Elsayed A, Lee S, Jackson M. Radiofrequency ablation for treating resistant intercostal neuralgia. Ochsner J 2018;18(1):91–3.
6. Engel AJ. Utility of intercostal nerve conventional thermal radiofrequency ablations in the injured worker after blunt trauma. Pain Physician 2012;15:711–8.
7. Stolker RJ, Vervest ACM, Groen GJ. The treatment of chronic thoracic segmental pain by radiofrequency percutaneous partial rhizotomy. J Neurosurg 1994;80:986–92.

8. Ke M, Yinghui F, Yi J, et al. Efficacy of pulsed radiofrequency in the treatment of thoracic postherpetic neuralgia from the angulus costae: a randomized, double-blinded, controlled trial. Pain Physician 2013;16:15–25.

9. Yang LQ, Gong WY, Wang XP, et al. Computed tomography-guided percutaneously controlled ablation of the thoracic paravertebral nerve due to thoracic neuropathic pain. Pain Pract 2017;17(6):792–9.

10. Cohen SP, Sireci A, Wu CL, et al. Pulsed radiofrequency of the dorsal root ganglia is superior to pharmacotherapy or pulsed radiofrequency of the intercostal nerves in the treatment of chronic postsurgical thoracic pain. Pain Physician 2006;9:227–36.

11. Nash TP. Percutaneous radiofrequency lesioning of dorsal root ganglia for intractable pain. Pain 1986;24:67–73.

12. Ladenhauf HN, Stundner O, Likar R, et al. Successful treatment of persistent pain after pectus excavatum repair using paravertebral nerve radiofrequency thermoablation. AA Case Rep 2017;8(1):18–20.

13. Pevsner Y, Shabat S, Catz A, et al. The role of radiofrequency in the treatment of mechanical pain of spinal origin. Eur Spine J 2003;12:602–5.

14. Stolker RJ, Vervest ACM, Groen GJ. Percutaneous facet denervation in chronic thoracic spinal pain. Acta Neurochir 1993;122:82–90.

15. van Kleef M, Barendse GAM, Dingemans WAAM, et al. Effects of producing a radiofrequency lesion adjacent to the dorsal root ganglion in patients with thoracic segmental pain. Clin J Pain 1995;11:325–32.

16. Bang JY, Sutton B, Hawes RH, et al. EUS-guided celiac ganglion radiofrequency ablation versus celiac plexus neurolysis for palliation of pain in pancreatic cancer: a randomized controlled trial. Gastrointest Endosc 2019;89(1):58–66.

17. Amr SA, Reyad RM, Othman AH, et al. Comparison between radiofrequency ablation and chemical neurolysis of thoracic splanchnic nerves for the management of abdominal cancer pain, randomized trial. Eur J Pain 2018;22:1782–90.

18. Papadopoulos D, Kostopanagiotou G, Batistaki C. Bilateral thoracic splanchnic nerve radiofrequency thermocoagulation for the management of end-stage pancreatic abdominal cancer pain. Pain Physician 2013;16:125–33.

19. Raj PP, Sahinler B, Lowe M. Radiofrequency Lesioning of Splanchnic Nerves. Pain Pract 2002;2(3):241–7.

20. Jin ZD, Wang L, Li Z. Endoscopic ultrasound-guided celiac ganglion radiofrequency ablation for pain control in pancreatic carcinoma. Dig Endosc 2015;27(1):163–4.

21. Miceli L, Bednarova R. Pulsed radiofrequency analgesia in a patient with abdominal wall metastasis from colorectal cancer: a case report. Neuromodulation 2020;23(8):1220–1.

22. Evrard S. Surgical lesioning of splanchnic nerves using wet needle radiofrequency thermoablation. J Surg Oncol 2002;80:171–2.

23. Gambaro G, Fulignati P, Spinelli A, et al. Percutaneous renal sympathetic nerve ablation for loin pain haematuria syndrome. Nephrol Dial Transplant 2013;28(9):2393–5.

24. Moeschler SM, Hoelzer BC, Eldrige JS. Patient with loin hematuria syndrome and chronic flank pain treated with pulsed radiofrequency of the splanchnic nerves. The Clin J Pain 2013;29(11):26–9.

25. Garcea G, Thomasset S, Berry DP, et al. Percutaneous splanchnic nerve radiofrequency ablation for chronic abdominal pain. ANZ J Surg 2005;75(8):640–4.

26. Verhaegh BPM, van Kleef M, Geurts JW, et al. Percutaneous radiofrequency ablation of the splanchnic nerves in patients with chronic pancreatitis: results of single and repeated procedures in 11 patients. Pain Pract 2013;13(8):621–6.

27. Brennan L, Fitzgerald J, McCrory C. The use of pulsed radiofrequency treatment for chronic benign pancreatitis pain. Pain Pract 2009;9(2):135–40.

28. Maatman RC, Kuijk SMJ, Steegers MAH, et al. A randomized controlled trial to evaluate the effect of pulsed radiofrequency as a treatment for anterior cutaneous nerve entrapment syndrome in comparison to anterior neurectomy. Pain Pract 2019;19(7):751–61.

29. Maatman RC, Steegers MAH, Kallewaard JW, et al. Pulsed radiofrequency as a minimally invasive treatment option in anterior cutaneous nerve entrapment syndrome: a retrospective analysis of 26 patients. J Clin Med Res 2018;10(6): 508–15.

30. Maatman RC, Papen-Botterhuis NE, Scheltinga MRM, et al. Lateral Cutaneous Nerve Entrapment Syndrome (LACNES): a previously unrecognized cause of intractable flank pain. Scand J Pain 2017;17:211–7.

31. Birthi P, Calhoun D, Grider JS. Pulsed radiofrequency for chronic abdominal pain. Pain Physician 2013;16(4):443–5.

32. Villajos LT, Olmedillo BH, Vicente VM, et al. Pulsed radiofrequency in the treatment of abdominal cutaneous nerve entrapment syndrome. Gastroenterol Hepatol 2015;38(1):14–6.

33. Niraj G. Pathophysiology and management of abdominal myofascial pain syndrome (AMPS): a three-year prospective audit of a management pathway in 120 patients. Pain Med 2018;19(11):2256–66.

34. Tamimi MA, McCeney MH, Krutsch J. A case series of pulsed radiofrequency treatment of myofascial trigger points and scar neuromas. Pain Med 2009; 10(6):1140–3.

35. Niraj G. Ultrasound-guided pulsed radiofrequency treatment of myofascial pain syndrome: a case series. Br J Anesth 2012;109(4):645–6.

36. Zaky S, Abd-Elsayed A. Splanchnic nerve radiofrequency ablation for treating resistant abdominal pain. Saudi J Anesth 2017;11(4):504.

37. Niraj G, Chaudhri S. Prospective audit of a pathway for in-patient pain management of chronic abdominal pain: a novel and cost-effective strategy. Pain Med 2018;19(3):589–97.

# Overview of Innervation of Shoulder and Acromioclavicular Joints

John Tran, HBSc, PhD[a],*,
Sharon Switzer-McIntyre, BPE, BScPT, MEd, PhD[b],
Anne M.R. Agur, BSc(OT), MSc, PhD[a]

## KEYWORDS

- Shoulder joint • Innervation • Anatomy • Denervation

## KEY POINTS

- The shoulder joint was found to receive innervation from articular branches of the suprascapular, axillary, subscapular, and lateral pectoral nerves, with less frequent supply from the radial and musculocutaneous nerves.
- The acromioclavicular joint was reported to receive innervation from the suprascapular and lateral pectoral nerves.
- The consistent relationship of articular branches to anatomic landmarks provides the basis for specific image-guided targeting.
- In order to capture articular branches from all of these nerves, multiple target sites could be used to enhance nerve capture rates.
- Further clinical studies are required to determine the feasibility and analgesic implications.

## INTRODUCTION

Image-guided radiofrequency ablation (RFA) has emerged as an alternative intervention for the management of chronic shoulder pain. The detailed understanding of the course and location of articular nerves innervating the shoulder (glenohumeral) joint is paramount to the successful utilization of RFA. This article reviews the nerve supply to the glenohumeral joint (GHJ) and acromioclavicular joint (ACJ) to describe the origin and course of articular nerves and identify bony and soft tissue landmarks, visible with image-guidance, that can be used to target the articular nerves. Dissections documenting the innervation of the GHJ and ACJ in this article were carried out in the authors' laboratory.

---

[a] Division of Anatomy, Department of Surgery, Temerty Faculty of Medicine, University of Toronto, 1 King's College Circle, Room 1158, Toronto, Ontario M5S 1A8, Canada; [b] Department of Physical Therapy, Temerty Faculty of Medicine, University of Toronto, 500 University Avenue, Room 160, Toronto, Ontario M5G 1V7, Canada
* Corresponding author.
*E-mail address:* johnjt.tran@utoronto.ca

Phys Med Rehabil Clin N Am 32 (2021) 667–674
https://doi.org/10.1016/j.pmr.2021.05.005
1047-9651/21/© 2021 Elsevier Inc. All rights reserved.

## INNERVATION OF GLENOHUMERAL JOINT CAPSULE

Previous cadaveric studies that have reported the nerve supply to the GHJ are summarized in **Table 1**. The articular branches innervating the GHJ have been described to originate from the suprascapular, lateral pectoral, subscapular, and axillary nerves. The course of each articular nerve and its relationship to bony and soft tissue landmarks, visible with image-guidance, will be described.

### Suprascapular Nerve

Of the 12 cadaveric studies found investigating the nerve supply to the GHJ, 8 reported suprascapular nerve (SSN) innervation (**Table 1**). The articular nerves were described to terminate in the superior, posterior, and/or inferior regions of the capsule.

In 4 of the 8 studies, the SSN was found to terminate in the superior region of the GHJ capsule.[1–5] The articular branches of SSN were described as coursing posterior to the coracoid process, either at the margin of supraspinatus[3] or deep to the supraspinatus in the supraspinous fossa[1,2,4,5] to supply the superior capsule. In addition, Tran and colleagues[4] found superior articular branches that originated from the lateral trunk of SSN that coursed within the supraspinous fossa, deep to the supraspinatus (**Figs. 1A and 2**).

The posterior region of the GHJ capsule was found to receive innervation from SSN in all 8 studies (see **Table 1**). As the SSN courses along the floor of the supraspinous

**Table 1**
**Previous cadaveric studies of the innervation of the glenohumeral joint capsule**

| | Suprascapular Nerve | Axillary Nerve | Subscapular Nerve | Lateral Pectoral Nerve[a] |
|---|---|---|---|---|
| Gardner,[1] 1948 | Y | Ant: Y<br>Post: Y | Y | Y |
| Wrete,[2] 1949 | Y | Ant: 5/5<br>Post: 5/5 | Y | X |
| Aszmann et al,[3] 1996 | Y | Ant: Y<br>Post: Y | Y[b] | X |
| Akita et al,[12] 2002 | - | - | - | 2/125 |
| Gelber et al,[10] 2006 | - | Ant: 18/61<br>Post: 40/61 | - | - |
| Vorster et al,[5] 2008 | 27/31 | - | - | - |
| Ebraheim et al,[6] 2011 | Y | | | |
| Nasu et al,[9] 2015 | - | Inf: 16/20[c]<br>Post: 3/20 | - | - |
| Nam et al,[11] 2016 | - | - | - | 29/43 |
| Eckmann et al,[8] 2017 | 16/16 | Ant: -Post: 16/16 | - | 12/14 |
| Tran et al,[4] 2019 | 15/15 | Ant: 15/15<br>Post: 15/15 | 14/15 | 1/15 |
| Laumonerie et al,[7] 2019 | 15/15 | - | - | - |

*Abbreviations:* -, not investigated; Ant, anterior capsule; Inf, inferior capsule; Post, posterior capsule; X, not found; Y, found.
[a] Gardner referred to this nerve as the anterior thoracic nerve.
[b] Supplied subcoracoid bursa.
[c] Supplied subacromial bursa and humerus

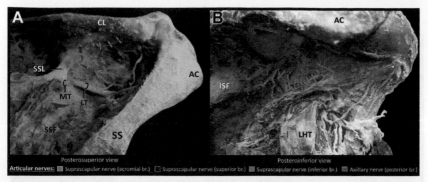

**Fig. 1.** Innervation of the superior and posterior shoulder joint capsule. (*A*) Articular branches of suprascapular nerve (acromial and superior branches). (*B*) Articular branches of suprascapular (inferior branch) and axillary (posterior branch) nerves. AC, acromion; CL, clavicle; ISF, infraspinous fossa; LHT, long head of triceps; LT, lateral trunk of suprascapular nerve; MT, medial trunk of suprascapular nerve; SS, spine of scapula; SSF, supraspinous fossa; SSL, suprascapular ligament. (*From* Philip Peng Educational Series; with permission.)

fossa to the spinoglenoid notch, it enters the infraspinous fossa deep to the infraspinatus. The articular branches supplying the posterior region of the capsule have been described as originating from the SSN prior to entry into the infraspinous fossa,[1,4,6,7] at the level of the spine of the scapula,[3,4] or just inferior to the spinoglenoid notch.[4,8] Eckmann and colleagues[8] further described these articular branches as supplying the posterior inferior GHJ capsule and head of the humerus.

The consistent descriptions of the course of articular branches of SSN in relationship to anatomic landmarks make these branches targetable with image guidance. The articular branches supplying the superior GHJ capsule can be localized using the posterior surface of the coracoid process and/or the floor of the supraspinous fossa (see **Fig. 1**A). When targeting the articular branches supplying the posterior and inferior GHJ capsule, the spinoglenoid notch can be used as a landmark (see **Fig. 1**B).

### Axillary Nerve

Six previous studies have reported articular branches of the axillary nerve (AN) innervating the anterior, posterior, and inferior regions of the GHJ capsule (see **Table 1**). The posterior capsule was found to be innervated by AN in all 6 studies, 4 of which localized innervation to the inferior portion.[1–4] The inferior aspect of the anterior capsule was described as receiving innervation from the AN in 4 studies.[1–4] Additional innervation to the anterior capsule has been reported from the musculocutaneous nerve[2] and posterior cord of the brachial plexus.[4] Furthermore, the inferior capsule[1,9] and inferior glenohumeral ligament[10] were found to receive innervation from the AN.

In 4 studies, the AN before entering the quadrangular space was found to give off articular branches that coursed around the inferior margin of the subscapularis to supply the inferior region of the anterior capsule.[1–4] The AN after passing through the quadrangular space was reported to give off additional articular branches to the posterior inferior capsule in all studies. More specifically, these branches were found to emerge from the posterior division of the AN[4] or from the branch to teres minor.[3,9] The inferior margin of the subscapularis can be used as an anatomic landmark for image guidance to localize the articular branches of AN that supply the inferior region of the anterior GHJ capsule (**Fig. 3**). To landmark the articular branches that supply the inferior region of the posterior GHJ capsule the plane deep to the tendon of the teres minor could be used (see **Figs. 1**B and **2**).

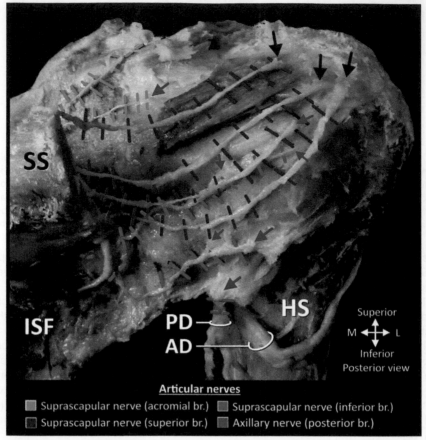

**Articular nerves**
🟥 Suprascapular nerve (acromial br.)    🟩 Suprascapular nerve (inferior br.)
⬜ Suprascapular nerve (superior br.)    ⬛ Axillary nerve (posterior br.)

**Fig. 2.** Overview of innervation of the superior and posterior shoulder joint capsule with the acromion process excised. AD, anterior division of axillary nerve; Black arrows, termination in subacromial bursa; br., branch; HS, humeral shaft; ISF, infraspinous fossa; PD, posterior division of axillary nerve; Red arrow, termination in GHJ capsule; SS, spine of scapula. (*From* Philip Peng Educational Series; with permission.)

### Nerves to Subscapularis

The nerves to subscapularis (NS) from the posterior cord of the brachial plexus were reported to provide innervation to the anterior/anterosuperior GHJ capsule in 4 previous studies (see **Table 1**). The articular branches from NS were found to pierce the subscapularis tendon,[1] course through the belly of subscapularis,[2] or course along the superior border of the subscapularis and then pass deep to its tendon to supply the anterior/anterosuperior GHJ capsule.[3,4] The articular branches of NS can be targeted at the junction of the superior border of the subscapularis and the inferior border of the coracoid process (see **Fig. 3**).

### Lateral Pectoral Nerve

The GHJ was reported to be innervated by articular branches originating from the lateral pectoral nerve (LPN) in 5 of 7 studies (see **Table 1**). Eckmann and colleagues[8] and Nam and colleagues[11] found LPN innervation in 86% and 67% of specimens, respectively, whereas Tran and colleagues[4] and Akita and colleagues[12] reported

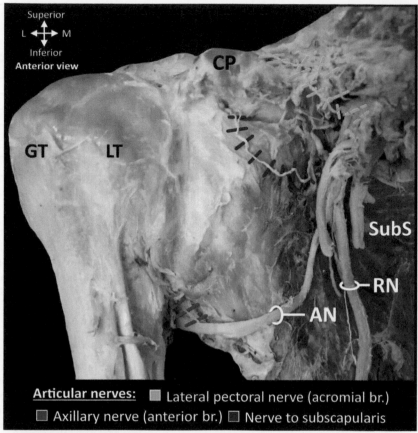

**Fig. 3.** Innervation of the anterior shoulder joint capsule. AN, axillary nerve; br., branch; CP, coracoid process; GT, greater tubercle; LT, lesser tubercle; RN, radial nerve; SubS, subscapularis. (*From* Philip Peng Educational Series; with permission.)

scarce innervation of 7% and 2%, respectively. In all studies, the articular branches from LPN were described as coursing superior to the coracoid process and coracoacromial ligament to supply the GHJ capsule. Further, Nam and colleagues[11] and Eckmann and colleagues[8] described the articular branch to pierce the coracoacromial ligament to supply the shoulder joint. The superior surface of the coracoid process can be used as an anatomic landmark to target the articular branches of LPN (see **Fig. 3**).

## INNERVATION OF ACROMIOCLAVICULAR JOINT CAPSULE

Previous cadaveric studies have reported articular branches from the SSN and LPN innervating the ACJ capsule. Articular branches terminating in the ACJ capsule were found to originate from the SSN in 6 studies and from the LPN in 3 studies (**Table 2**).

### Suprascapular Nerve

Of the 6 studies that found innervation of the ACJ capsule by articular branches of the SSN, only 4 reported the frequency of innervation. Innervation by SSN was found in all

**Table 2**
**Previous dissection studies of the innervation of acromioclavicular joint capsule**

|  | Suprascapular Nerve | Lateral Pectoral Nerve[a] |
|---|---|---|
| Gardner,[1] 1948 | Y | Y |
| Aszmann et al,[3] 1996 | Y | Y |
| Akita et al,[12] 2002 | 2/125 | - |
| Ebraheim et al,[6] 2011 | 12/12 | - |
| Tran et al,[4] 2019 | 15/15 | 15/15 |
| Borbas et al,[13] 2019 | 27/27 | - |

*Abbreviations:* Y indicates found; -, not investigated.
   [a] Gardner referred to this nerve as the anterior thoracic nerve.

specimens in 3 studies[4,6,13] and in 2% of specimens in 1 study.[12] The course of the articular branch of SSN supplying the ACJ capsule was similarly described in relation to anatomic landmarks, including the base/posterior surface of the coracoid process,[4,6] the supraspinatus muscle/tendon,[1,12] or both the coracoid process and supraspinatus muscle.[3,13] Dissections demonstrating articular branches from the acromial branch of SSN coursing along the posterior surface of the coracoid process and anterior margin of the supraspinatus are included in **Figures. 1A and 4.**

*Lateral Pectoral Nerve*

In 3 studies, the LPN was found to supply articular branches to the ACJ capsule. In all studies, the articular branches were reported to course superior to the coracoid process prior to terminating in the ACJ. In addition, the articular branches were described in relation to anatomic landmarks, including the acromial branch of the thoracoacromial artery[1,4] and the coracoclavicular and coracoacromial ligaments.[3] The superior surface of the coracoid process, the acromial branch of the thoracoacromial artery, and the coracoacromial and coracoclavicular ligaments can be used to target the articular branches of LPN before their termination in the ACJ capsule (**Fig. 5**).

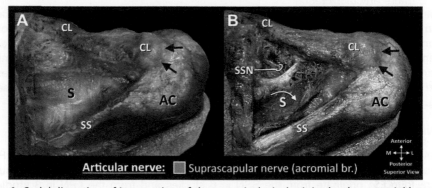

**Articular nerve:** ☐ Suprascapular nerve (acromial br.)

**Fig. 4.** Serial dissection of innervation of the acromioclavicular joint by the acromial branch of suprascapular nerve. (*A*) Superficial dissection with trapezius removed to show supraspinatus. (*B*) Deep dissection with supraspinatus reflected posteriorly to show the acromial branch of suprascapular nerve. AC, acromion; blue arrow, acromioclavicular joint; br., branch; CL, clavicle; S, supraspinatus; SS, spine of scapula; SSN, suprascapular nerve. (*From Philip Peng Educational Series; with permission.*)

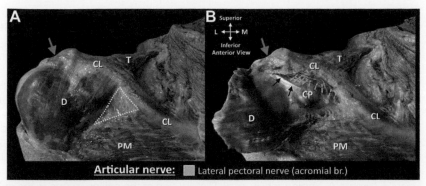

**Fig. 5.** Serial dissection of innervation of the acromioclavicular joint by the acromial branch of lateral pectoral nerve. (*A*) Superficial dissection. (*B*) Deep dissection with deltoid reflected to show the acromial branch of lateral pectoral nerve. Black arrow, coracoacromial ligament; Blue arrow, acromioclavicular joint; CL, clavicle; CP, coracoid process; D, deltoid; PM, pectoralis major; T, trapezius; white dotted line; outline of deltopectoral triangle. (*From* Philip Peng Educational Series; with permission.)

## SUMMARY

In the literature, the innervation of the shoulder and acromioclavicular joint capsules was consistent. The shoulder joint was found to receive innervation from articular branches of the suprascapular, axillary, subscapular, and lateral pectoral nerves, with less frequent supply from the radial and musculocutaneous nerves. Articular branches of the suprascapular and lateral pectoral nerves were reported to innervate the acromioclavicular joint capsule.

## CLINICAL PEARLS

In the context of radiofrequency ablation, the consistent relationship of articular branches of the suprascapular, axillary, subscapular, and lateral pectoral nerves to anatomic landmarks provides the basis for specific image-guided targeting. In order to capture articular branches from all of these nerves, multiple target sites could be used to enhance nerve capture rates. Further clinical studies are required to determine the feasibility and analgesic implications.

## DISCLOSURE

Anne Agur is an anatomy faculty member with Allergan Academy of Excellence.

## ACKNOWLEDGMENT

The authors wish to acknowledge the individuals who donated their bodies and tissue for the advancement of education and research.

## REFERENCES

1. Gardner E. The innervation of the shoulder joint. Anat Rec 1948;102(1):1–18.
2. Wrete M. The innervation of the shoulder-joint in man. Acta Anat 1949;7:173–90.
3. Aszmann O, Lee Dellon A, Birely B, et al. Innervation of the human shoulder joint and its implications for surgery. Clin Orthop Relat Res 1996;330:202–7.

4. Tran J, Peng P, Agur A. Anatomical study of the innervation of glenohumeral and acromioclavicular joint capsules: implications for image-guided intervention. Reg Anesth Pain Med 2019;44(4):452–8.
5. Vorster W, Lange C, Briët R, et al. The sensory branch distribution of the suprascapular nerve: an anatomic study. J Shoulder Elb Surg 2008;17(3):500–2.
6. Ebraheim N, Whitehead J, Alla S, et al. The suprascapular nerve and its articular branch to the acromioclavicular joint: an anatomic study. J Shoulder Elbow Surg 2011;20(2):e13–7.
7. Laumonerie P, Blasco L, Tibbo M, et al. Distal suprascapular nerve block—do it yourself: cadaveric feasibility study. J Shoulder Elbow Surg 2019;28(7):1291–7.
8. Eckmann M, Bickelhaupt B, Fehl J, et al. Cadaveric study of the articular branches of the shoulder joint. Reg Anesth Pain Med 2017;42(5):564–70.
9. Nasu H, Nimura A, Yamaguchi K, et al. Distribution of the axillary nerve to the subacromial bursa and the area around the long head of the biceps tendon. Knee Surg Sport Traumatol Arthrosc 2015;23(9):2651–7.
10. Gelber P, Reina F, Monllau J, et al. Innervation patterns of the inferior glenohumeral ligament: anatomical and biomechanical relevance. Clin Anat 2005;19(4):304–11.
11. Nam Y, Panchal K, Kim I, et al. Anatomical study of the articular branch of the lateral pectoral nerve to the shoulder joint. Knee Surg Sport Traumatol Arthrosc 2016;24(12):3820–7.
12. Akita K, Kawashima T, Shimokawa T, et al. Cutaneous nerve to the subacromial region originating from the lateral pectoral nerve. Ann Anat 2002;184(1):15–9.
13. Borbas P, Eid K, Ek ET, et al. Innervation of the acromioclavicular joint by the suprascapular nerve. Shoulder Elbow 2020;12(3):178–83.

# Shoulder Ablation Approaches

Angela Samaan, DO[1], David Spinner, DO, RMSK, CIPS, FAAPMR*

## KEYWORDS

- Radiofrequency ablation • Shoulder pain • Denervation

## KEY POINTS

- Radiofrequency ablation (RFA) of sensory-only articular branches to the shoulder complex could disrupt nociceptive pain pathways while preserving motor function.
- Currently, the identified peripheral nerves for ablation are the suprascapular nerve, axillary nerve, lateral pectoral nerve, and subscapular nerve.
- Needle accuracy is important in order to avoid postprocedural motor weakness, and proper placement has been widely studied in current literature.
- Ongoing research is needed in order to further distinguish the efficacy of ablative therapy, in comparison to conventional treatment, for management of chronic shoulder pain.

## BACKGROUND

Chronic shoulder pain is a common medical complaint that is associated with a reduction in patient function and significant health care cost.[1,2] Common causes include pain arising from the glenohumeral joint, acromioclavicular joint, or rotator cuff disease. Conservative treatment options, including physical therapy and pharmacotherapy, are first-line treatments; however, they may be ineffective in controlling pain symptoms. Invasive options, such as intra-articular steroid injections, are known to have temporary effects. For patients with refractory pain, surgical options may be considered; however, not all patients are appropriate surgical candidates. Radiofrequency ablation (RFA) may be indicated as an effective option in managing shoulder pain not responsive to conventional therapies.

Conflicts: A. Samaan reported no conflicts of interest. Role: A. Samaan participated in the conception of the review, acquisition, analysis, interpretation of data, and drafting the article. D. Spinner reported no conflicts of interest. Role: D. Spinner participated in the conception of the review, acquisition, analysis, interpretation of data, and drafting the article.
Department of Rehabilitation and Human Performance, Icahn School of Medicine at Mount Sinai, 10 Union Square East 5th Floor, Suite 5P, New York, NY 10003, USA
[1] Present address: One Gustave L. Levy Place Box 1240, New York, NY 10029, USA.
* Corresponding author.
E-mail address: dspinnerny@gmail.com

Phys Med Rehabil Clin N Am 32 (2021) 675–682
https://doi.org/10.1016/j.pmr.2021.07.002
1047-9651/21/© 2021 Elsevier Inc. All rights reserved.

RFA involves destruction of nerves using heat generated by a radiofrequency current. RFA of sensory-only articular branches to the shoulder complex could disrupt nociceptive pathways while sparing motor function. Many studies suggest a potential benefit of RFA in the treatment of patients with chronic shoulder pain.[3–5] One study retrospectively evaluated the effect of pulsed radiofrequency to the suprascapular nerve in 28 patients with shoulder pain lasting more than 1 month. Its findings suggest that pain relief appears to be long lasting with minimal side effects.[6] In this article, the authors discuss the option of RFA for the management of shoulder pain.

## INDICATIONS

RFA to the shoulder structures may be offered to patients with inadequate pain relief from conventional treatment options and patients with severe pain symptoms who are not considered for surgical intervention. Candidates should have evidence of symptomatic osteoarthritis and shoulder pain of peripheral origin. RFA of articular sensory nerves most likely has efficacy for pain that originates from the joint capsule, nearby ligaments, or directly from target nerves. Current evidence also shows that patients with rotator cuff injuries and pain after total shoulder arthroplasty may also benefit from ablative therapy.[7] Before ablation, a diagnostic block should be performed to determine prognostic value of RFA success. A goal of 50% or more pain relief after nerve block indicates a greater potential for benefit from RFA.[7] As with all pain interventions, it is important to inform patients of risks associated with this procedure, including nerve injury, joint infection, or bleeding. Special consideration should be given to patients with implanted cardiac devices, and strict cardiac device protection protocols should be executed in such patients who wish to proceed with this treatment option.[8]

## TARGETS FOR DENERVATION AND TECHNIQUE

At this time, identified peripheral nerves for ablative therapy include the suprascapular nerve, axillary nerve, lateral pectoral nerve, and subscapular nerve.[9–11] The safe zones for ablation have been defined as the area lateral to the spinoglenoid notch posteriorly (targeting suprascapular branches), at the inferior-posterior portion of the greater tubercle (targeting axillary branches), and over the coracoid process (targeting lateral pectoral branches).[11,12] Both ultrasound- and fluoroscopy-guided techniques have been described for RFA.

### Radiofrequency Ablation to the Suprascapular Nerve

After initial and successful diagnostic suprascapular nerve block, patients may proceed with RFA to the suprascapular nerve if pain persists in shoulder structures innervated by this peripheral nerve (anterior and inferior parts of the glenohumeral joint, acromioclavicular joint, subacromial bursa, and coracoclavicular ligament). This mixed motor-sensory nerve arises from the upper trunk of the brachial plexus and then courses inferiorly, laterally, and posteriorly to enter the supraspinatus fossa via the suprascapular notch (**Fig. 1**). It supplies the supraspinatus muscle and then courses around the spinoglenoid notch to innervate the infraspinatus muscle.[13]

To perform RFA, patients are placed prone with arms tucked to their side. Using C-arm fluoroscopy, the electrode is guided to the suprascapular notch, just proximal and medial to the coracoid process. As the coracoid process interferes with the view of the suprascapular notch, it is necessary for the C arm to be positioned in an oblique angle of 15° to 25° and further placed in a cephalocaudal angle of 15° to 25° in order to

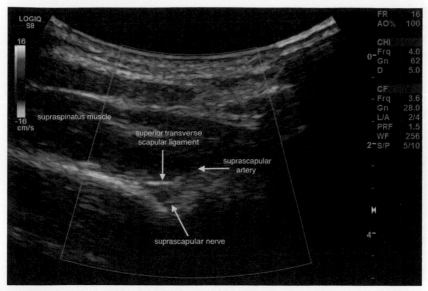

**Fig. 1.** Sonoanatomy of the suprascapular nerve entering the supraspinatus fossa via the suprascapular notch, under the superior transverse scapular ligament.

visualize the spine of the scapula.[9] Of note, there are 2 commonly described morphologies of the suprascapular notch: a symmetric U-shaped notch and a blunted V-shaped notch. When performing, the cannula will traverse the infraspinatus muscle; therefore, care should be taken by minimizing the number of needle passes. Sensory stimulation is performed at 50 Hz. Patients are asked to report if they feel paresthesia or sharp pains. Motor testing is performed at 1.5 to 2 V, and absence of muscle contractions should be confirmed.[14]

### Radiofrequency Ablation to the Axillary Nerve

RFA to the axillary nerve is performed in patients with pain in shoulder structures innervated by the axillary nerve (anterior and inferior parts of the glenohumeral joint). This mixed motor-sensory nerve arises from the posterior cord of the brachial plexus. The axillary nerve passes through the quadrangular space with the posterior circumflex humeral artery and then it is found inferior to the capsule of the shoulder joint where it courses medial to the surgical neck of the humerus (**Fig. 2**). The nerve will then divide into 2 branches under the deltoid muscle: the anterior branch of the axillary nerve innervates the deltoid muscle, and the posterior branch of the axillary nerve innervates the teres minor.[15]

To perform RFA, patients are placed prone with arms tucked at their side. Using C-arm fluoroscopy, the electrode is guided inferior to the greater tubercle, near the metaphyseal-diaphyseal junction of the humerus. Special caution should be taken, as many sensory fibers originate slightly medial to the posterior humeral head, and ablation to this area may increase the risk of postablation motor weakness. Therefore, it has been recommended to position the needle tip more laterally and superiorly to avoid motor denervation. Sensory stimulation is performed at 50 to 100 Hz. Patients are asked to report if they feel paresthesia or sharp pains. Motor testing is performed at 2 V, and absence of muscle contractions should be confirmed.[14]

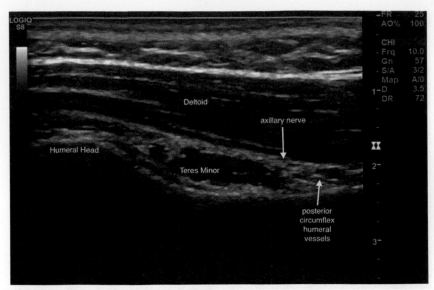

**Fig. 2.** Sonoanatomy of the axillary nerve at the surgical neck of the humerus, adjacent to the posterior circumflex humeral artery vessels.

## Radiofrequency Ablation to the Lateral Pectoral Nerve

RFA to the lateral pectoral nerve is performed in patients with pain in shoulder structures innervated by the lateral pectoral nerve (acromioclavicular joint, subacromial bursa, and anterior-superior glenohumeral joint).[16] The lateral pectoral nerve arises from the lateral cord of the brachial plexus and passes anterior to the axillary vein and artery. It then pierces though the claviopectoral fascia before terminating in the pectoralis muscle, which it innervates.[17]

To perform RFA, patients are placed supine with arms tucked to their side. Using C-arm fluoroscopy, the electrode is guided to the distal superior-lateral coracoid tip or superior-medial portion of coracoid process.[18] Notably, the target location is superficial; therefore, chemical neurolysis may be preferred. Furthermore, this procedure may be performed with ultrasound alone, in which the interfascial plane between the pectoralis major muscle and pectoralis minor muscle at the third rib (**Fig. 3**) serves as the target locations for the lateral pectoral nerve. Sensory stimulation is performed at 50 to 100 Hz. Patients are asked to report if they feel paresthesia or sharp pains. Motor testing is performed at 2 V, and absence of muscle contractions should be confirmed.[18]

## Radiofrequency Ablation to the Subscapular Nerve

The nerves to the subscapularis arise from the posterior cord of the brachial plexus. The upper subscapular nerve innervates the superior portion of the subscapularis muscle, and the inferior subscapular nerve innervates the inferior portion of the subscapularis muscle. There are limited data on RFA to the subscapular nerve.[19] One technique describes the patient positioned in the supine position. An electrode is guided to the upper lateral aspect of the anterior glenoid neck, superior to the coracoid process, as inferior to the coracoid process increases risk of injury to the brachial plexus. As with prior RFA techniques mentioned, sensory stimulation is performed at 50 to 100 Hz. Patients are asked to report if they feel paresthesia or sharp pains. Motor testing is performed at 2 V, and absence of muscle contractions should be confirmed.[8]

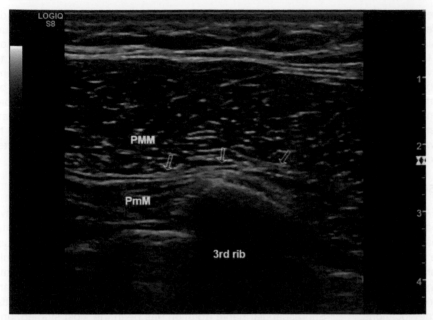

**Fig. 3.** Sonoanatomy of the interfascial plane (*arrows*) between the pectoralis major muscle (PMM) and the pectoralis minor muscle (PmM) at the third rib for lateral pectoral nerve target.

## CLINICAL EFFECTIVENESS AND SAFETY

RFA has been shown to be an effective option for managing chronic shoulder pain. In a randomized, single-blinded study, which compared RFA to intra-articular cortico-steroid injection, RFA was found to offer improved long-term relief. However, corti-costeroid injection was effective in providing short-term relief within the first few weeks of injection.[3] Another study retrospectively evaluated pain before RFA, imme-diately after procedure, and then at 1, 3, and 6 months. Compared with 1 group that received local anesthetic solution, patients who were treated with RFA reported significantly more pain relief at 6 months, concluding that ablative therapy appears to be long-lasting with minimal side effects.[6] Another randomized active placebo controlled, double-blind trial investigated 22 participants that were followed for a 6-month period and showed that pulsed radiofrequency may be beneficial in the management of chronic shoulder pain.[20] When compared with photobiomodulation therapy, suprascapular nerve ablation showed similar effectiveness when both treat-ment groups were treated with exercise treatment as well. In a randomized clinical trial by Korkmaz and colleagues,[21] there was no difference in effect between trans-cutaneous electrical nerve stimulation and pulsed radiofrequency treatment for man-agement of shoulder pain. Current literature certainly suggests that RFA is effective in managing chronic shoulder pain, and there is ongoing research to further evaluate this treatment option.

### Complications/Adverse Events

RFA is a relatively safe, nonsurgical treatment, with minimal risks of complications. Immediately following the procedure, patients may report hypersensitivity or burning over the injection site or in areas innervated by the target nerve. Other possible side effects patients may experience include superficial skin or joint infections, injury to surrounding vessels and nerves, heat damage to adjacent structures, or allergic reaction to the anesthetic used to numb the area. As previously mentioned, it is important to have needle accuracy in order to avoid postprocedural motor weakness. Motor testing should be performed immediately after the procedure, keeping in mind there may be some weakness depending on the amount of local anesthetic used. Furthermore, patients should be encouraged to begin passive range-of-motion exercises after treatment. Active range-of-motion exercises may be initiated as tolerated within 2 to 3 weeks after RFA treatment. Literature has shown improved range of motion after shoulder nerve ablation.[10]

## DISCUSSION

RFA to peripheral nerves of the shoulder joint serves as a promising and effective treatment option for patients with chronic shoulder pain, refractory to conventional treatment options. Denervation of motor nerves raises concern for postablation muscle weakness. RFA of sensory-only articular branches to the shoulder complex could disrupt nociceptive pain pathways while preserving motor function. Ablation-safe zones of the terminal sensory articular branches of the suprascapular nerve, axillary nerve, lateral pectoral nerve, and subscapularis nerve have been identified as potential target locations.[9,11,12] Suprascapular nerve ablation has been the most studied, and its technique has been the most described.[10,14,22–24] Studies of RFA for the management of chronic shoulder pain is limited. Nonetheless, current literature has demonstrated long-lasting positive outcomes, of up to 6 months.[22,25,26] Furthermore, an advantage of ablative therapy is the ability to repeat the procedure given preservation of tissue in the shoulder complex.

Although steroid injections for the management of shoulder pathologic condition and pain are commonly used, evidence for its effectiveness is unconvincing.[27] Furthermore, there are known deleterious effects of repetitive steroid use, including pain, rash, facial flushing, fat atrophy, skin irritation, and septic arthritis.[28] For this reason, alternative treatment options with long-last effects, such as RFA, may be more desirable. Despite a low number of side effects reported with ablative therapy, it is important that this procedure is performed using appropriate technique as guided by the current literature.

Shoulder pain has been shown to have a negative impact on physical, social, and emotional function as evidenced by lower SF-36 scores, a short-form measure of health status.[29,30] This common medical complaint is associated with significant morbidity and health care cost.[31] RFA may serve as an effective treatment option with long-term effects and positive outcomes in patients with chronic shoulder pain.

## DISCLOSURE

The authors declare that they have no conflicts of interest in the authorship or publication of this contribution.

## REFERENCES

1. Picavet HSJ, Schouten JSAG. Musculoskeletal pain in the Netherlands: prevalence, consequences and risk groups, the DMC (3)-study. Pain 2003;102:167–78.
2. Pope DP, Croft PR, Pritchard CM, et al. Prevalence of shoulder pain in the community: the influence of case definition. Ann Rheum Dis 1997;56:308–12.

3. Eyigor C, Eyigor S, Korkmaz OK, et al. Intra-articular corticosteroid injections versus pulsed radiofrequency in painful shoulder: a prospective, randomized, single-blinded study. Clin J Pain 2010;26:386–92.
4. Ökmen BM, Ökmen K. Comparison of photobiomodulation therapy and supra-scapular nerve-pulsed radiofrequency in chronic shoulder pain: a randomized controlled, single-blind, clinical trial. Lasers Med Sci 2017;32:1719–26.
5. Luleci N, Ozdemir U, Dere K, et al. Evaluation of patients' response to pulsed ra-diofrequency treatment applied to the suprascapular nerve in patients with chronic shoulder pain. J Back Musculoskelet Rehabil 2011;24:189–94.
6. Gabrhelik T, Michalek P, Adamus M, et al. Effect of pulsed radiofrequency therapy on the suprascapular nerve in shoulder pain of various aetiology. Ir J Med Sci 2010;179:369–73.
7. Eckmann MS, Johal J, Bickelhaupt B, et al. Terminal sensory articular nerve radio-frequency ablation for the treatment of chronic intractable shoulder pain: a novel technique and case series. Pain Med 2020;21(4):868–71.
8. Eckman M, Joshi M, Bickelhaupt B. How I do it: shoulder articular nerve blockade and radiofrequency ablation. ASRA 2020.
9. Tran J, Peng PWH, Agur AMR. Anatomical study of the innervation of glenohum-eral and acromioclavicular joint capsules: implications for image-guided interven-tion. Reg Anesth Pain Med 2019. https://doi.org/10.1136/rapm-2018-100152.
10. Simopoulos TT, Nagda J, Aner MM. Percutaneous radiofrequency lesioning of the suprascapular nerve for the management of chronic shoulder pain: a case series. J Pain Res 2012;5:91–7.
11. Bickelhaupt B, Eckmann MS, Brennick C, et al. Quantitative analysis of the distal, lateral, and posterior articular branches of the axillary nerve to the shoulder: im-plications for intervention. Reg Anesth Pain Med 2019. https://doi.org/10.1136/rapm-2019-100560.
12. Eckmann MS, Bickelhaupt B, Fehl J, et al. Cadaveric study of the articular branches of the shoulder joint. Reg Anesth Pain Med 2017;42(5):564–70.
13. Bird SJ. Suprascapular nerve. Encyclopedia Neurol Sci 2014;2:357–8.
14. Esparza-Miñana JM, Mazzinari G. Adaptation of an ultrasound-guided technique for pulsed radiofrequency on axillary and suprascapular nerves in the treatment of shoulder pain. Pain Med 2019;20(8):1547–50.
15. Rea P. Neck. Essential clinically applied anatomy of the peripheral nervous sys-tem in the head and neck. 2016;131-183.
16. Nam YS, Panchal K, Kim IB, et al. Anatomical study of the articular branch of the lateral pectoral nerve to the shoulder joint. Knee Surg Sports Traumatol Arthrosc 2016;24:3820–7.
17. Paul Rea MBChB, MSc, PhD, MIMI, RMIP, FHEA, FRSA, in Essential clinically applied anatomy of the peripheral nervous system in the limbs, 2015
18. Eckmann MS, Lai BK, Uribe MA 3rd, et al. Thermal radiofrequency ablation of the articular branch of the lateral pectoral nerve: a case report and novel technique. A A Pract 2019;13(11):415–9.
19. Sager B, Gates S, Collett G, et al. Innervation of the subscapularis: an anatomic study. JSES Open Access 2019;3(2):65–9.
20. Gofeld M, Restrepo-Garces CE, Theodore BR, et al. Pulsed radiofrequency of suprascapular nerve for chronic shoulder pain: a randomized double-blind active placebo-controlled study. Pain Pract 2013;13:96–103.
21. Korkmaz OK, Capaci K, Eyigor C, et al. Pulsed radiofrequency versus conven-tional transcutaneous electrical nerve stimulation in painful shoulder: a prospec-tive, randomized study. Clin Rehabil 2010;24:1000–8.

22. Sluijter ME, Teixeira A, Serra V, et al. Intra-articular application of pulsed radiofrequency for arthrogenic pain–report of six cases. Pain Pract 2008;8:57–61.
23. Kane TP, Rogers P, Hazelgrove J, et al. Pulsed radiofrequency applied to the suprascapular nerve in painful cuff tear arthropathy. J Shoulder Elbow Surg 2008;17:436–40.
24. Liliang PC, Lu K, Liang CL, et al. Pulsed radiofrequency lesioning of the suprascapular nerve for chronic shoulder pain: a preliminary report. Pain Med 2009; 10:70–5.
25. Shah RV, Racz GB. Pulsed mode radiofrequency lesioning of the suprascapular nerve for the treatment of chronic shoulder pain. Pain Physician 2003;6:503–6.
26. Gurbet A, Turker G, Bozkurt M, et al. Efficacy of pulsed mode radiofrequency lesioning of the suprascapular nerve in chronic shoulder pain secondary to rotator cuff rupture. Agri 2005;17:48–52.
27. Ekeberg OM, Bautz-Holter E, Tveita EK, et al. Subacromial ultrasound guided or systemic steroid injection for rotator cuff disease: randomised double blind study. BMJ 2009;338:a3112.
28. Shanahan EM, Ahern M, Smith M, et al. Suprascapular nerve block (using bupivacaine and methylprednisolone acetate) in chronic shoulder pain. Ann Rheum Dis 2003;62:400–6.
29. Beaton DE, Richards RR. Measuring function of the shoulder. A cross-sectional comparison of five questionnaires. J Bone Joint Surg Am 1996;78:882–90.
30. Gartsman GM, Brinker MR, Khan M, et al. Self-assessment of general health status in patients with five common shoulder conditions. J Shoulder Elbow Surg 1998;7:228–37.
31. Virta L, Joranger P, Brox JI, et al. Costs of shoulder pain and resource use in primary health care: a cost-of-illness study in Sweden. BMC Musculoskelet Disord 2012;13:17.

# The Use of Radiofrequency in the Treatment of Pelvic Pain

Caleb Seale, MD[a], B. Ryder Connolly, MD[a], Kendall Hulk, DO[a],
Gregory G. Yu, MD, PharmD, MBA, MPH[b],
Ameet S. Nagpal, MD, MS, MEd[b],*

## KEYWORDS

• Pelvic • Pain • Radiofrequency • Ablation

## KEY POINTS

• Radiofrequency ablation (RFA) and pulsed radiofrequency treatment of pelvic pain are relatively uncommon procedures to treat pelvic pain.
• The best evidence of efficacy of radiofrequency in the pelvis is for pudendal and inguinal neuralgia.
• Consider a transcoccygeal approach for RFA of the ganglion impar; RFA is preferred over pulsed radiofrequency treatment.

## INTRODUCTION

Radiofrequency (RF) has a long history as a method of pain relief. It was first described in the literature in the 1930s.[1] It was not until the 1950s, however, that the first commercial RF generator was available.[1] Currently, RF is used to treat numerous pain syndromes throughout the body, including facial, neck, back, abdominal, peripheral joint, sympathetic mediated, and pelvic pain.[2] This article focuses on the use of RF for the treatment of pelvic pain caused by a variety of etiologies.

Chronic pelvic pain has been defined as nonmalignant pain perceived in structures related to the pelvis of both men and women persisting for at least 6 months.[3] When evaluating a patient, a detailed history should be obtained with specific questions regarding aggravating and alleviating factors, such as dyspareunia, sexual interaction, urination, and defecation.[4] A numeric pain scale, Patient Health Questionnaire-9, and Quality of Life Scale all can be used to monitor and track a patient's response to treatments.[5,6] A physical examination, consisting of an abdominal, pelvic, and low back

[a] Department of Rehabilitation Medicine, University of Texas Health Science Center at San Antonio, 7703 Floyd Curl, Mail Code 7798, San Antonio, TX 78229, USA; [b] Department of Anesthesiology, University of Texas Health Science Center at San Antonio, 5282 Medical Drive, Suite 180, San Antonio, TX 78229, USA
* Corresponding author.
E-mail address: nagpala@uthscsa.edu

Phys Med Rehabil Clin N Am 32 (2021) 683–701
https://doi.org/10.1016/j.pmr.2021.05.006
1047-9651/21/© 2021 Elsevier Inc. All rights reserved.

examination, is vital. Patients will likely present to the pain clinic with a presumed diagnosis, laboratory test results, imaging, and a requested treatment by the referring provider. If not provided, however, a simple set of laboratory tests, such as a comprehensive metabolic panel, complete blood cell count with differential, erythrocyte sedimentation rate, urinalysis, sexually transmitted infection screen, and pregnancy test, should be obtained for further investigation. If there is question of the diagnosis, imaging, such as an ultrasound, radiograph, or magnetic resonance imaging, could be obtained. If a specific disorder is revealed, then the condition should be treated per specific guidelines.

## Technique

There are multiple RF techniques, including conventional/continuous RF ablation (RFA) and water-cooled RFA (cRFA). Continuous RFA typically involves heating an electrode to 80°C for 90 to 120 seconds, depending on the indication. For cRFA, sterile water is irrigated continuously around the active electrode at ambient temperature. The water actively cools the electrode, preventing the tip from acquiring the high surrounding tissue temperatures.[7] The current is applied for 150 seconds at 60°C; however, the surrounding tissues reach 80°C, which allows for a larger lesion compared with conventional RFA.[8] A larger lesion increases the likelihood of successfully ablating the target structure.

Differing from conventional RFA and cRFA, pulsed RF treatment (pRFT) is not ablative, although it is often referred to as pulsed radiofrequency ablation, which is a misnomer.[9] Podhajsky and colleagues examined the histologic effects of pRFT versus RFA on the sciatic nerve and dorsal root ganglion (DRG). They showed pRFT treatment heated the DRG to 42°C without causing destruction of the tissue compared with heating it to 80°C.[10] The exact mechanism of pain relief through pRFT has yet to be elucidated. Cahana and colleagues[11] proposed pRFT transiently inhibits synaptic activity which, in theory, impedes pain transmission. Alternatively, it has been proposed that pRFT alters neuropeptides in the dorsal root ganglion.[12] pRFT has been used to treat pudendal neuralgia; heating the probe to 42°C for 120 seconds in pulse mode has shown to effective.[13]

## Contraindications/Complications

Absolute contraindications for RF include patient refusal, sepsis, and local infection. There are many relative contraindications, however, including uncontrolled diabetes, coagulopathy/bleeding diatheses, oral anticoagulation, prior orthopedic surgery (such as fused L5-S1 or disc replacement for transdiscal approach), and pregnancy.[1] Each provider should weigh the risks versus the benefits prior to performing any procedure. As with any procedure, there are risks involved, such as increased nociceptive or neuropathic pain, infection, numbness, weakness, lack of pain relief, and superficial skin burns.

## Equipment/Staff

To perform the procedure safely, a variety of equipment are needed. A safe environment is required that is spacious enough to allow for safe movement of the patient, staff, and equipment. A procedure table that is able to adequately position the patient and fluoroscopic imaging equipment should be used. A vital sign device is required, with a monitor to ensure the patient is stable throughout the procedure. For the RFA lesioning needle electrodes, electric generator, and grounding pads are utilized. Should an emergency arise, the clinic also should have a crash cart in close proximity to the procedure room.[14]

These procedures do not require extensive personnel. The physician performing the procedure typically is a fellowship-trained pain medicine physician who completed residency in a variety of specialties, including physical medicine and rehabilitation, anesthesiology, emergency medicine, neurology, psychiatry, or radiology.[15] Other vital support staff include a circulating nurse to assist with drawing mediation, monitoring patient vitals, patient positioning, and operating the generator. Often a radiology technician is be employed to assist with manipulation of the fluoroscopic equipment. If sedation is used, then a medical professional with training in anesthesia should be present.

## DISCUSSION
### Radiofrequency for the Treatment of Chronic Pain due to Pudendal Neuralgia

The pudendal nerve, which provides sympathetic, sensory, and motor innervation to the pelvic region, is composed of the terminal branches of the ventral primary rami of the sacral plexus. When this nerve is injured, irritated, or compressed, pudendal neuralgia, a painful neuropathic condition, can arise. The International Pudendal Neuropathy Association estimates the incidence of this condition to be 1 out of every 100,000 people. However, a paucity of scientific evidence for the diagnosis of pudendal neuralgia, currently defined by the Nantes criteria, has led many physicians to believe the incidence may be higher.[16,17] Pudendal neuralgia is more likely to be diagnosed in patients who have given birth, underwent pelvic surgery or in those who engage in strenuous exercise.[18]

The pudendal nerve follows a complex course after its formation proximal to the sacrospinous ligament. It passes between the piriformis and coccygeus muscles

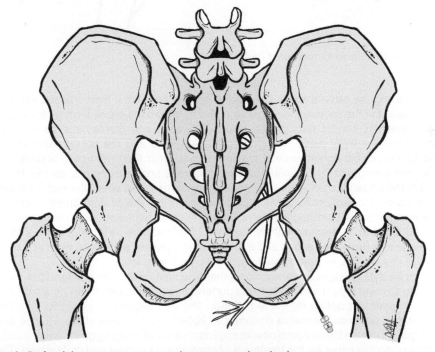

**Fig. 1.** Pudendal nerve RF treatment (posteroanterior view).

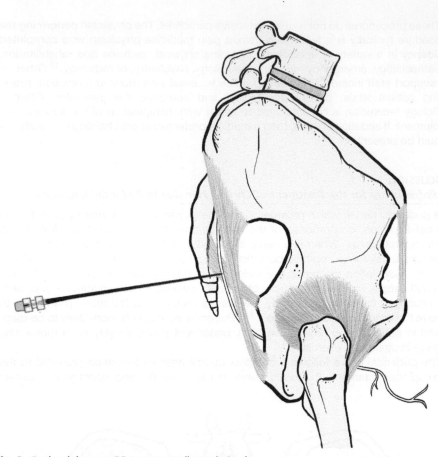

**Fig. 2.** Pudendal nerve RF treatment (lateral view).

before leaving the pelvis through the greater sciatic foramen. It then crosses over the lateral aspect of the sacrospinous ligament and re-enters the pelvis through the lesser sciatic foramen, travels through the pudendal canal, and divides into its terminal branches—the inferior rectal nerve, the perineal nerve, and the dorsal nerve of the penis in men, or the dorsal nerve of the clitoris in women. Common sites of pudendal nerve entrapment are (1) between the sacrotuberous and sacrospinus ligaments, (2) through the pudendal canal, and (3) at the base of the penis when the nerve passes through a tight osteofibrotic canal.[19] Depending on the site of entrapment, patients can experience pain involving the penis, scrotum, labia, perineum, or anorectal region in an S2, S3, and S4 dermatomal distribution.[15] Pudendal nerve impingement is often aggravated by prolonged sitting and thus can limit a patient's ability to work at a desk job, ride in a vehicle, or participate in activities such as biking.

When lifestyle changes, pharmacologic management, and other conservative measures fail to control pain associated with pudendal neuralgia, pRFT can be a safe and effective treatment option for many patients. The first reported use of pRFT for the treatment of pudendal neuralgia occurred in 2009.[20] In this case study, Rhame and colleagues[20] used a transvaginal needle approach without imaging guidance to modulate the pudendal nerve for the treatment of chronic left perineal and gluteal pain. The

**Table 1**
Details of studies reporting radiofrequency treatment for the management of pudendal neuralgia

| Study | Study Design | No. of Patients | Study Details | Adverse Events | Results |
|---|---|---|---|---|---|
| Collard et al,[25] 2019 | Retrospective analysis | 10 patients (18 total ablations) | Response to pRFT of pudendal nerve (42°C for 120 s) was compared with previously received perineural injection of anesthetic/corticosteroid. Four patients received bilateral treatments and 2 patients underwent the treatment twice. The procedures were performed using a fluoroscopically guided, transgluteal approach. | One patient reported interstitial cystitis flare, possibly related to the use of iodinated contrast. | 7 out of 10 patients experienced significant therapeutic benefit. pRFT was found to be at least as effective as perineural injection of anesthetic/corticosteroid but with longer duration of benefits. |
| Fang et al,[13] 2018 | Prospective, randomized controlled clinical trial | 80 | 80 patients diagnosed with pudendal neuralgia were divided randomly into a pRFT (42°C for 120 s) + nerve block (neurotropin, 2% lidocaine, 0.75% ropivvacaine, 0.9% NaCl) or nerve block alone group. The procedures were performed using an ultrasound-guided, transgluteal approach. Following the procedure, follow-up occurred at 2 wk, 1 mo, and 3 mo. | None | A total of 77 patients were followed up, 38 in the pRFT + nerve block group and 39 in the nerve block alone group. On postoperative d 1, the VAS scores were significantly decreased in both groups. The VAS score of pRFT group, however, was significantly lower than that of nerve block group at the 2-wk, 1-mo, and 3-mo follow-up appointments. The clinical effective rates for the pRFT and nerve block group 3 mo postprocedure were 92.1% and 35.9%, respectively. |
| Frank et al,[21] 2019 | Retrospective analysis | 7 | pRFT of pudendal nerve. 42°C for 90 s at a single site. The patient was positioned in the dorsal lithotomy position and the procedure was performed using a blind, intravaginal approach. | None | All 7 patients reported significant pain relief following pRFT. The average number of pRFT treatments was 4.43, and the duration of effect averaged 11.4 wk. |

(continued on next page)

**Table 1**
*(continued)*

| Study | Study Design | No. of Patients | Study Details | Adverse Events | Results |
|---|---|---|---|---|---|
| Hong et al,[23] 2016 | Case report | 2 | pRFT of pudendal nerve. 42°C for 120 s at 2 different sites. The procedures were performed using an ultrasound-guided, transgluteal approach. | None | Patient 1 reported NRS pain score reduction from 8/10–2/10 following procedure. Her pain relief remained stable at 10-mo follow-up appointment.<br><br>Patient 2 reported NRS pain score reduction from 8/10–3/10. Her pain relief remained stable at 6-mo follow-up appointment. |
| Petrov-Kondratov et al,[25] 2017 | Case report | 1 | pRFT of pudendal nerve. 42°C for 240 s at a single site. The procedure was performed using a fluoroscopically guided, transgluteal approach. | None | The patient reported >50% pain relief for at least 6 wk. |
| Rhame et al,[20] 2009 | Case report | 1 | pRFT of pudendal nerve. 42°C for 120 s at two different sites. The patient was positioned in the dorsal lithotomy position and the procedure was performed using a blind, intravaginal approach. | None | Prior to the procedure, the patient could only tolerate 1–2 h of sitting. Postprocedurally, the patient could tolerate 4–5 h of sitting. This benefit persisted at 18-mo follow-up appointment. |

*Abbreviations:* NRS, numeric rating scale; VAS, visual analog scale.

procedure was well tolerated without complications and allowed the patient to increase her sitting tolerance from 1 hours to 2 hours, to 4 hours to 5 hours, a benefit that was still seen 18 months following the procedure. In 2019, Frank and colleagues,[21] performed a retrospective analysis of patients who underwent pRFT for the treatment of pudendal neuralgia using a similar approach. All 7 patients in this study reported significant pain relief that lasted an average of 11.4 weeks.

pRFT of the pudendal nerve using a blind, intravaginal approach has the advantage of being relatively cost effective, easy to administer and can provide patients with pain relief. This approach cannot be performed for a male patient and may not be ideal for patients who are uncomfortable with an intravaginal procedure. Alternatively, a transgluteal approach can be used for the same purpose. This approach, originally described by Abdi and colleagues in 2004,[22] requires imaging guidance and, therefore, is more expensive and difficult to perform than an intravaginal approach but is more convenient for the patient and is thought to be safer. pRFT via a transgluteal approach with ultrasound guidance[13,23] or with fluoroscopic guidance[24,25] have been shown effective for the treatment of pudendal neuralgia. Although no studies have ever compared the efficacy and safety of pRFT of the pudendal nerve using ultrasound versus fluoroscopic guidance, Bellingham and colleagues[26] found no difference in the degree of neural blockade when using ultrasound or fluoroscopy for pudendal nerve blockade in a randomized, single blind, split plot study. Nevertheless, it has been hypothesized that because ultrasound imaging is limited by depth and field of view, CT-guided pudendal nerve ablations may be safer.[22] pRFT with both approaches have been shown to provide longer benefit than the use of anesthetics or corticosteroids for the treatment of pudendal neuralgia.[13,25] **Table 1** outlines the results and adverse events from the use of radiofrequency treatment for the management of pudendal neuralgia. **Figs. 1** and **2** depict the approach to the pudendal nerve from the posteroanterior and lateral views respectively.

*Clinics Care Points*

---

- pRFT of the treatment of chronic pain due to pudendal neuralgia has been shown to provide longer benefit than treatment with anesthetics and corticosteroids.

- pRFT can be performed using a blind transvaginal approach, ultrasound-guided transgluteal approach, or fluoroscopically guided transgluteal approach. The transvaginal approach is the most cost effective and requires the least amount of time but cannot be performed in a male patient and is the least convenient for the patient. Fluoroscopically guided injections cost more but provide the highest degree of safety and are faster than ultrasound-guided pudendal nerve ablations.

---

### Radiofrequency for the Treatment of Chronic Pain due to Inguinal Neuralgia

Cutaneous sensory innervation of the inguinal region arises from the T12-L2 spinal nerve roots and the upper lumbar plexus. The ilioinguinal nerve provides innervation to the skin over the proximal and medial aspects of the thigh, the scrotum and the root of the penis in men, and the mons pubis and labia majora in women. The iliohypogastric nerve provides sensation to the skin over the pubis and lateral gluteal region. Finally, the genitofemoral nerve provides cutaneous innervation to the scrotum in men and labia majora in women as well as the skin over the anteromedial thigh. These nerves can be damaged following trauma or abdominal surgeries that require a lower abdominal incision, such as testicular or gynecologic surgery, appendectomy, or hernia repair.[27] Approximately 12% of patients report neuropathic pain following inguinal herniorrhaphy in the United States.[28]

In 2006, Rozen and colleagues[29] reported using pRFT of the ilioinguinal nerve, which is the nerve injured most commonly in the inguinal region, to treat neuralgia following hernia repair. In this case series, 4 out of 5 patients reported significant pain relief that lasted from 4 months to 9 months. Since that time, several retrospective reviews have reported similar success with the use of RF neurotomy of the ilioinguinal nerve for the treatment of chronic inguinal pain following abdominal surgery.[30–32]

In 2012, Kastler and colleagues[30] found that CT-guided RFA of the ilioinguinal and iliohypogastric nerves to provide equivalent early inguinal pain relief to that of local injection with lidocaine, ropivacaine, and cortivazol. In this retrospective cohort study, patients receiving RFA reported an average of 12.5 months of pain relief compared with the local injection group, who reported only 1.6 months of pain relief. Microwave ablation of the ilioinguinal and iliohypogastric nerves using ultrasound also has been used to treat chronic inguinal pain successfully.[31] Ultrasound, which provides direct visualization of the target nerve, may provide more accurate placement of the ablation antenna but further research is needed to determine whether the imaging modality used for ablation of these nerves has an impact on patient outcomes.[32]

Although less common, the genitofemoral nerve also can be ablated for chronic inguinal pain.[31,33,34] Classically, this nerve is targeted at the pubic tubercle, where it is easily identified. This location may not be ideal, however, because the genitofemoral nerve is frequently injured at a more proximal point, such as within the inguinal canal or at the deep inguinal ring. Thus, an alternative transpsoas approach can be used to ablate the nerve prior to its entrance into the inguinal canal.[34]

Determining whether neuropathic pain arises from damage to the iliohypogastric, ilioinguinal, or genitofemoral nerve can be challenging, given their cutaneous sensory fields can overlap. On physical examination, reproduction of the patient's pain when tapping the affected area (ie, a positive Tinel sign) can be seen with ilioinguinal neuralgia but would not be expected with genitofemoral neuralgia.[29] Nerve blocks also may be performed on either nerve to determine which nerve is involved.[35]

**Table 2** outlines the results and adverse events from the use of radiofrequency treatment for the management of inguinal neuralgia.

## Clinics Care Points

- Ilioinguinal, iliohypogastric, and genitofemoral neuralgias can be seen following lower abdominal surgery. Of these nerves, the ilioinguinal nerve is damaged most frequently.

- Tinel sign and nerve blocks can be used to distinguish ilioinguinal neuralgia from genitofemoral neuralgia.

- RF neurotomy of each of these nerves has been successfully reported to treat chronic inguinal pain.

## Radiofrequency of the Ganglion Impar for the Treatment of the Pelvis and Perineum

The ganglion impar is the most distal ganglion in the sympathetic chain, and, as its name implies, is unpaired. It sits on the anterior surface of the sacrococcygeal junction and innervates the perineum, urethra, vulva, anus, vagina, coccyx, and the distal aspect of the rectum.[36]

**Table 2**
Details of studies reporting the use of radiofrequency for the treatment of inguinal neuralgia

| Study | Study Design | No. of Patients | Study Details | Adverse Events | Results |
|---|---|---|---|---|---|
| Kanwar et al,[33] 2017 | Retrospective review | 6 | RFA of ilioinguinal nerve. Only 3 of the 6 patients underwent RFA. | None | 2 of the 3 patients receiving RFA of ilioinguinal nerve reported good to excellent pain relief following procedure. |
| Kastler et al,[30] 2012 | Single-center, retrospective cohort study | 42 | 42 patients with chronic inguinal pain refractory to medication received treatment with either RFA (14 patients, 18 procedures) or local injection (28 patients) of the ilioinguinal and iliohypogastric nerves. RFA was performed using CT imaging. The visual analog scale was used to assess pain immediately before and after the procedures and at 1-mo, 3-mo, 6-mo, 9-mo, and 12-mo follow-up appointments. | None | Maximum early pain relief did not statistically differ between the RFA group (77%) and the injection group (81.5%). Mean duration of pain relief was significantly longer in the RF group (12.5 mo) vs the injection group (1.6 mo). |
| Lee et al,[31] 2019 | Retrospective review | 10 | 10 patients underwent a total of 12 microwave ablation procedures of either the ilioinguinal nerve, iliohypogastric nerve, or genitofemoral nerves for chronic inguinal pain. Ultrasound imaging was used to guide procedure. | One patient reported transient procedure-related pain at the skin entry site for 2–3 d. One patient had unmasking of meralgia paresthetica following procedure. | 12 mo postprocedure, 83.3% of the procedures resulted in had an average of 69% reduction in pain. |

*(continued on next page)*

**Table 2**
*(continued)*

| Study | Study Design | No. of Patients | Study Details | Adverse Events | Results |
|---|---|---|---|---|---|
| Parris et al,[34] 2010 | Case study | 1 | RFA of genitofemoral nerve. 80°C for 90 s each at 2 sites. The procedure was performed with CT imaging to guide a transpsoas approach. | None | The patient did not experience durable pain resolution following the procedure. |
| Rozen et al,[29] 2006 | Case series | 5 | pRFT of ilioinguinal nerve. 40°C for 120 s at 3 different sites (T12, L1, and L2). | None | 4 of 5 patients reported pain relief lasting from 4 mo to 9 mo. |

*Abbreviations:* CT, computed tomography; RFA, continuous RFA.

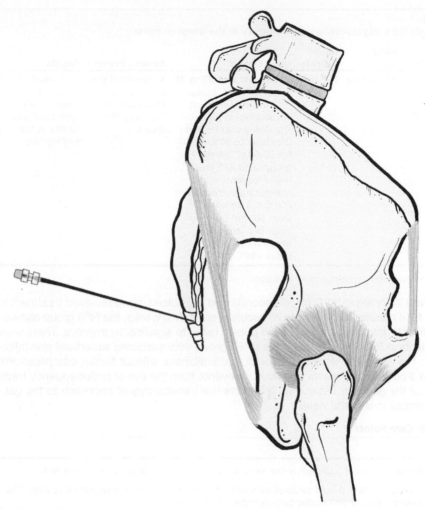

**Fig. 3.** Ganglion impar RF treatment.

There are several approaches to reach the ganglion, including anococcygeal, trans-sacrococcygeal, and transcoccygeal.[37–39] Oh and colleagues[40] evaluated 50 cadaver sacra and coccyges showing a varied location of the ganglion impar and implied the target for blockade/ablation should be cephalad to the junction of the first and second coccyx bones. This study infers that the transcoccygeal approach is more favorable. The transcoccygeal approach varies from the transsacrococcygeal approach as the instruments are passed through the coccygeal bones instead of the sacrococcygeal joint.

There have been several studies evaluating the use of RFA at the ganglion impar with positive results.[41,42] Usmani and colleagues[43] performed a prospective, random-ized, double-blind study to evaluate the use RFA versus pRFT to ablate the ganglion impar for the treatment of chronic perineal pain of nononcologic origin. There were 70 patients enrolled, 35 patients in each group. The 22-gauge RF needles were 10-cm long and had a 5-mm active tip. After confirming the needle placement, the RFA group

**Table 3**
Details the study reporting radiofrequency of the ganglion impar

| Study | Study Design | No. of Patients | Study Details | Adverse Events | Results |
|-------|--------------|-----------------|---------------|----------------|---------|
| Usmani et al,[43] 2018 | Prospective RCT | 70 | 35 patients in pRFT vs 35 patients in RFA group. Approach via the first intracoccygeal joint. The RFA group heated the tissue to 60°C–80°C for 60–90 s. The pRFT group used 420-kHz high-frequency alternating current at 200 mA is delivered in short (20-ms) bursts of twice per second, keeping the tissue <45°C. | 3 superficial skin infections in RFA group and 2 in the pRFT group | At 6 wk, 82.3% of RFA patients were satisfied with results vs 12.9% in the pRFT group |

*Abbreviation*: RFA, continuous RF ablation..

received lesioning at 80°C for 90 seconds and the pulsed group received treatment at 42°C for 4 minutes, 2 cycles of 120 seconds each. At 6 weeks, the RFA group showed significantly improved pain while the pulsed failed to significantly improve. There were 3 patients in RFA group and 2 in the pRFT group who sustained superficial skin infections. The infections were treated with oral antibiotics without further complications. **Table 3** outlines the results and adverse events from the use of radiofrequency treatment of the ganglion impar. **Fig. 3** depicts the transcoccygeal approach to the ganglion impair in a lateral view.

*Clinics Care Points*

- The transcoccygeal approach is the more favored approach for ganglion impar RFA.
- Conventional RFA should be used over pRFT for the treatment of nononcologic pain. The side-effect profile was similar between the 2 techniques.

*Radiofrequency of the Superior Hypogastric Plexus for the Treatment of the Pelvis and Perineum*

The superior hypogastric plexus (SHP) is a part of the sympathetic abdominopelvic nervous system. The location is well described as retroperitoneal at the level of the lower one-third of the fifth lumbar body and upper one-third of the first sacral vertebral body at the sacral promontory.[44] The SHP is the continuation of the aortic plexus and receives the lower two lumbar splanchnic nerves. It contains sympathetic fibers and visceral afferent fibers from most of the pelvic structures as well as the descending colon, rectum, and internal genitalia except the ovaries and fallopian tubes.[45] The inferior hypogastric plexus (IHP) is formed by the hypogastric, pelvic splanchnic, and sacral splanchnic nerves.[46] The IHP is located on either side of the rectum within presacral tissues ventral to the S2, S3, and S4 spinal segments. It contains sympathetic fibers, parasympathetic fibers, and visceral afferent fibers. It receives sensory innervation from the urinary bladder, uterus, uterine tubes, penis, vagina, anus, perineum, and rectum.[47,48] In clinical practice, blocking the IHP has been shown effective in treating lower pelvic visceral pain and pelvic cancer pain.[48,49] These investigators, however, were unable to identify literature which described RFA or pRFT of the IHP. This likely is due to its nebulous formation and proximity to the bowel, which make the IHP a challenging target. Because the SHP receives fibers from the IHP, the SHP instead is targeted, essentially treating both the SHP and IHP. The indications for SHP block are controversial; however, it has been shown to improve cancer-related pain.[2]

Although RFA has shown effective at the ganglion impar, there have been few studies showing the effectiveness of RF of the SHP. In 2016, Bharti and colleagues[49] published a case reporting using RFA to treat pelvic cancer pain. The patient described in this study had advanced stage cervical malignancy with severe pain not controlled by oral analgesics, including 150 oral morphine equivalents of morphine each day. After a diagnostic block, which resulted in short-term pain relief, RFA was performed. The traditional approach uses bilateral 6-inch or 7-inch, 22-gauge needles oriented 30° caudad and 45° medial to reach the anterolateral aspect of the L5 vertebral body.[50] The length of the active tip was not described. Antibiotic prophylaxis with ceftriaxone was given, to prevent discitis, and an L5-S1 transdiscal approach was executed. The ablation was performed at 90°C for 90 seconds, twice. Dexamethasone, 8 mg, and 2 mL of 2% lidocaine were injected following the ablation to reduce postprocedural edema and pain. At 6 weeks, the patient was no longer taking morphine and was only on diclofenac and pregabalin.

In 2016, Kim and colleagues[51] reported a case study of a patient with chronic pain due to interstitial cystitis, which was refractory to oral and intravesical medications. This patient's daily activities and sleep were greatly affected not only by pain but also by urinary urgency/frequency (every 15–60 min) and nocturia (10 voids a night). The diagnostic block was performed via L5-S1 transdiscal approach with 10% 1-mL mepivicaine and 5-mg dexamethasone. The therapeutic lesioning was done similarly to the traditional approach, described previously; however, the investigators did not state the needles were oriented 30° caudad, only 45° medial. The treatment was performed via pRFT at 42°C with a pulse frequency of 2-Hz width of 20 milliseconds (ms); it was repeated twice on both sides. After the first procedure, the patient had reduced pain, an increased urinary frequency interval

**Table 4**
Details the study reporting radiofrequency of the superior hypogastric plexus

| Study | Study Design | No. of Patients | Study Details | Adverse Events | Results |
|---|---|---|---|---|---|
| Bharti et al,[49] 2016 | Case report | 1 | RFA L5-S1 transdiscal approach. Ablation performed at 90°C for 90 s, twice. | None | At 6 wk, the patient had discontinued oral opioid medication |
| Kim et al,[51] 2016 | Case report | 1 | pRFT L5-S1 transdiscal approach. pRFT at 42°C with a pulse frequency of 2-Hz width of 20 ms, repeated twice on both sides | Did not discuss | Reduced pain, decreased nocturia, increased urinary frequency interval, decrease in oral medication use |

*Abbreviation*: RFA, continuous RFA.

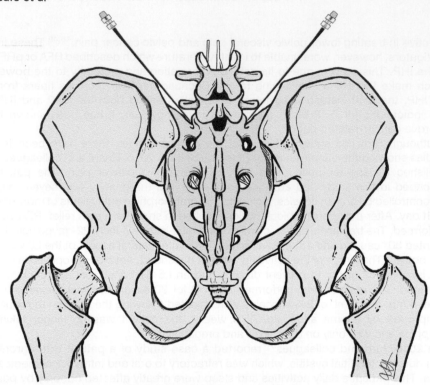

**Fig. 4.** SHP RF treatment (posteroanterior view).

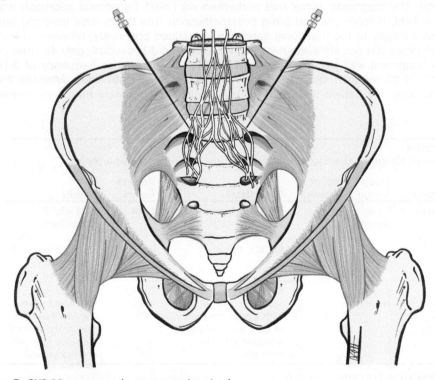

**Fig. 5.** SHP RF treatment (anteroposterior view).

(60–120 min), and decreased nocturia (1 void per night). In addition, her oral medication use decreased. These effects lasted for 3 months before returning. A repeat procedure then was performed. This time, the effects continued for 18 months, which was the last follow-up for the case. The investigators did not discuss any

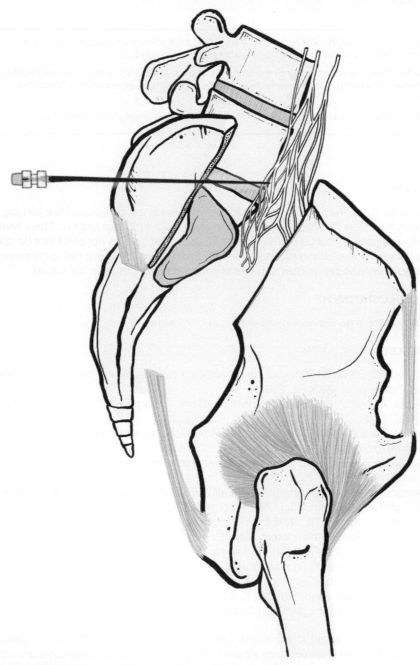

**Fig. 6.** SHP RF treatment (lateral view).

side effects. **Table 4** outlines the results and adverse events from the use of radio-frequency treatment of the superior hypogastric plexus. **Figs. 4–6** depict the approach to the superior hypogastric plexus from the posteroanterior, anteroposterior, and lateral views respectively.

*Clinics Care Points*

---

- Although blocks of the SHP commonly are used to treat pelvic pain, hypogastric RFA is not widely described in the literature, and more research is needed.

- The traditional approach to RF of the SHP uses bilateral 6-inch or 7-inch, 22-gauge needles oriented 30° caudad and 45° medial to reach the anterolateral aspect of the L5 vertebral body.

- If a transdiscal approach is used, the patient should receive prophylactic antibiotics.

---

## SUMMARY

Evidence for RF to treat pelvic pain is limited. The evidence consists of few randomized controlled trials (RCTs), case series, and even individual case studies. There were no meta-analyses, systematic reviews of RCTs or cohort studies nor can there be due to the paucity of available data. However, RF procedures are a promising treatment modality for chronic pelvic pain and warrant further investigation in the future.

## DISCLOSURE STATEMENT

The authors have no financial or nonfinancial disclosures.

## REFERENCES

1. Warfield C, Bajwa Z. Principles and practice of pain medicine. NY, USA: Mcgraw-Hill Professional; 2004. p. 226–7.
2. Gupta A, editor. Interventional pain medicine. Incorporated: Oxford University Press; 2012.
3. Fall M, Baranowski AP, Elneil S, et al. EAU guidelines on chronic pelvic pain. Eur Urol 2010;57(1):35–48.
4. Speer LM, Mushkbar S, Erbele T. Chronic Pelvic pain in women. Am Fam Physician 2016;93(5):380–7.
5. Burckhardt CS, Anderson KL. The Quality of Life Scale (QOLS): reliability, validity, and utilization. Health Qual Life Outcomes 2003;1:60.
6. Kroenke K, Spitzer RL, Williams JB. The PHQ-9: validity of a brief depression severity measure. J Gen Intern Med 2001;16(9):606–13.
7. Petersohn JD, Conquergood LR, Leung M. Acute histologic effects and thermal distribution profile of disc biacuplasty using a novel water-cooled bipolar electrode system in an in vivo porcine model. Pain Med 2008;9(1):26–32.
8. Ho KY, Hadi MA, Pasutharnchat K, et al. Cooled radiofrequency denervation for treatment of sacroiliac joint pain: two-year results from 20 cases. J Pain Res 2013; 6:505–11.
9. Gupta A, Huettner DP, Dukewich M. Comparative Effectiveness Review of Cooled Versus Pulsed Radiofrequency Ablation for the Treatment of Knee Osteoarthritis: A Systematic Review. Pain Physician 2017;20(3):155–71.

10. Podhajsky R, Sekiguchi Y, Kikuchi S, et al. The Histologic Effects of Pulsed and Continuous Radiofrequency Lesions at 42[degrees]C to Rat Dorsal Root Ganglion and Sciatic Nerve. Spine 2005;30(9):1008–13.
11. Cahana A, Vutskits L, Muller D. Acute differential modulation of synaptic transmission and cell survival during exposure to pulsed and continuous radiofrequency energy. J Pain 2003;4(4):197–202.
12. Higuchi Y, Nashold BS Jr, Sluijter M, et al. Exposure of the dorsal root ganglion in rats to pulsed radiofrequency currents activates dorsal horn lamina I and II neurons. Neurosurgery 2002;50(4):850–6.
13. Fang H, Zhang J, Yang Y, et al. Clinical effect and safety of pulsed radiofrequency treatment for pudendal neuralgia: a prospective, randomized controlled clinical trial. J Pain Res 2018;11:2367–74.
14. Bin Bilal Shafi B. Percutaneous Radiofrequency Ablation (RFA) of Liver Tumors Periprocedural Care: Equipment, Patient Preparation. 2020. Available at: https://emedicine.medscape.com/article/1390475-periprocedure.    Accessed November 2, 2020.
15. Arena A. Pain Management Fellowships. Pain Management EMRA. Available at: https://www.emra.org/books/fellowship-guide-book/18-pain-management/.    Accessed November 14, 2020.
16. Hibner M, Desai N, Robertson LJ, et al. Pudendal neuralgia. J Minim Invasive Gynecol 2010;17(2):148–53.
17. Labat JJ, Riant T, Robert R, et al. Diagnostic criteria for pudendal neuralgia by pudendal nerve entrapment (Nantes criteria). Neurourol Urodyn 2008;27(4):306–10.
18. Pérez-López FR, Hita-Contreras F. Management of pudendal neuralgia. Climacteric 2014;17(6):654–6.
19. Robert R, Prat-Pradal D, Labat JJ, et al. Anatomic basis of chronic perineal pain: role of the pudendal nerve. Surg Radiol Anat 1998;20(2):93–8.
20. Rhame EE, Levey KA, Gharibo CG. Successful treatment of refractory pudendal neuralgia with pulsed radiofrequency. Pain Physician 2009;12(3):633–8.
21. Frank CE, Flaxman T, Goddard Y, et al. The Use of Pulsed Radiofrequency for the Treatment of Pudendal Neuralgia: A Case Series. J Obstet Gynaecol Can 2019;41(11):1558–63.
22. Abdi S, Shenouda P, Patel N, et al. A novel technique for pudendal nerve block. Pain Physician 2004;7(3):319–22.
23. Hong MJ, Kim YD, Park JK, et al. Management of pudendal neuralgia using ultrasound-guided pulsed radiofrequency: a report of two cases and discussion of pudendal nerve block techniques. J Anesth 2016;30(2):356–9.
24. Petrov-Kondratov V, Chhabra A, Jones S. Pulsed Radiofrequency Ablation of Pudendal Nerve for Treatment of a Case of Refractory Pelvic Pain. Pain Physician 2017;20(3):E451–4.
25. Collard MD, Xi Y, Patel AA, et al. Initial experience of CT-guided pulsed radiofrequency ablation of the pudendal nerve for chronic recalcitrant pelvic pain. Clin Radiol 2019;74(11):897.e17–23.
26. Bellingham GA, Bhatia A, Chan CW, et al. Randomized controlled trial comparing pudendal nerve block under ultrasound and fluoroscopic guidance. Reg Anesth Pain Med 2012;37(3):262–6.
27. Bohrer JC, Walters MD, Park A, et al. Pelvic nerve injury following gynecologic surgery: a prospective cohort study. Am J Obstet Gynecol 2009;201(5):531.e1–5317.
28. Hall M. National Center for Health Statistics. Natl Health Statistic Rep 2017.

29. Rozen D, Ahn J. Pulsed radiofrequency for the treatment of ilioinguinal neuralgia after inguinal herniorrhaphy. Mt Sinai J Med 2006;73(4):716–8.
30. Kastler A, Aubry S, Piccand V, et al. Radiofrequency neurolysis versus local nerve infiltration in 42 patients with refractory chronic inguinal neuralgia. Pain Physician 2012;15(3):237–44.
31. Lee KS, Sin JM, Patil PP, et al. Ultrasound-Guided Microwave Ablation for the Management of Inguinal Neuralgia: A Preliminary Study with 1-Year Follow-up. J Vasc Interv Radiol 2019;30(2):242–8.
32. Eichenberger U, Greher M, Kirchmair L, et al. Ultrasound-guided blocks of the ilioinguinal and iliohypogastric nerve: accuracy of a selective new technique confirmed by anatomical dissection. Br J Anaesth 2006;97(2):238–43.
33. Kanwar S, Castellanos M. 528 - Radiofrequency Ablation of Ilioinguinal Nerve for the Management of Inguinodynia–Our Experience. The J Minimally Invasive Gynecol 2017;24(7):S185.
34. Parris D, Fischbein N, Mackey S, et al. A novel CT-guided transpsoas approach to diagnostic genitofemoral nerve block and ablation. Pain Med 2010;11(5):785–9.
35. Starling JR, Harms BA. Diagnosis and treatment of genitofemoral and ilioinguinal neuralgia. World J Surg 1989;13(5):586–91.
36. Benzon H. Chapter 56: peripheral and visceral sympathetic blocks. Practical management of pain. 5th ed. Saunders/Elsevier; 2014. p. 755–67.
37. Plancarte R, Amescua C, Patt RB, et al. Presacral blockade of the ganglion of Walther (ganglion Impar). Anesthesiology 1990;73:751.
38. Toshniwal GR, Dureja GP, Prashanth SM. Trans sacrococcygeal approach to ganglion Impar block for management of chronic perineal pain: A prospective observational study. Pain Physician 2007;10:661–6.
39. Foye PM. New approaches to ganglion Impar blocks via coccygeal joints. Reg Anesth Pain Med 2007;32:269.
40. Oh CS, Chung IH, Ji HJ, et al. Clinical implication of topographic anatomy on the ganglion Impar. Anesthesiology 2004;101:249–50.
41. Dolecek L, Michalek P, Stern M, et al. Long-term results of radiofrequency thermocoagulation of ganglion Impar in perineal pain. Reg Anesth Pain Med 2008;33:e197.
42. Abejon D, Pcheco MD, Cortina I, et al. Treatment of perineal pain with thermocoagulation of the ganglion Impar. Rev Soc Esp Dolor 2007;4:290–5.
43. Usmani H, Dureja GP, Andleeb R, et al. Conventional radiofrequency thermocoagulation vs pulsed radiofrequency neuromodulation of ganglion impar in chronic perineal pain of nononcological origin. Pain Med 2018 Dec 1;19(12):2348–56.
44. Kanazi GE, Perkins FM, Thakur R, et al. New technique for superior hypogastric plexus block. Reg Anesth Pain Med 1999;24(5):473–6.
45. Chung KW. Gross anatomy. 4th ed. Baltimore, Maryland: Lippincott Williams & Wilkins; 2000.
46. Eid S, Iwanaga J, Chapman JR, et al. Superior Hypogastric Plexus and Its Surgical Implications During Spine Surgery: A Review. World Neurosurg 2018;120:163–7.
47. Schultz DM. Inferior hypogastric plexus blockade: a transsacral approach. Pain Physician 2007;10(6):757–63.
48. Mohamed SA, Ahmed DG, Mohamad MF. Chemical neurolysis of the inferior hypogastric plexus for the treatment of cancer-related pelvic and perineal pain. Pain Res Manag 2013;18(5):249–52.

49. Bharti N, Singla N, Batra YK. Radiofrequency ablation of superior hypogastric plexus for the management of pelvic cancer pain. Indian J Pain 2016.
50. Plancarte R, Amescua C, Patt RB, et al. Superior hypogastric plexus block for pelvic cancer pain. Anesthesiology 1990;73:236–9.
51. Kim JH, Kim E, Kim BI. Pulsed radiofrequency treatment of the superior hypogastric plexus in an interstitial cystitis patient with chronic pain and symptoms refractory to oral and intravesical medications and bladder hydrodistension: A case report. Medicine (Baltimore) 2016;95(49):e5549.

# Sacroiliac Joint Anatomy

Shannon L. Roberts, PhD

## KEYWORDS

- Sacroiliac joint • Anatomy • Innervation • Landmarks • Blocks
- Radiofrequency ablation

## KEY POINTS

- Sacroiliac joint (SIJ) consists of 2 parts: a synovial joint (intraarticular part) and a syndesmosis (extraarticular part).
- Intraarticular part of the SIJ is innervated by both anterior and posterior sources but mainly by anterior source(s) (anterior sources: most frequently, branch(es) from the anterior rami of L4 and/or L5 or the lumbosacral trunk; posterior sources: the posterior sacral network [PSN]).
- Extraarticular part of the SIJ is innervated by posterior sources: the PSN, a fine nerve plexus formed by the lateral branches of the posterior rami of S1-S3 ± L5/S4.
- Interindividual and intraindividual variations exist in both anterior and posterior SIJ innervation.
- Posterior bony landmarks: (1) lateral branches: most common clock face positions as they emerge from the posterior sacral foramina identifiable with fluoroscopy; and (2) PSN: first to third transverse sacral tubercles of the lateral sacral crest identifiable with ultrasound and fluoroscopy.

 Video content accompanies this article at http://www.pmr.theclinics.com.

## INTRODUCTION

The sacroiliac joint (SIJ) consists of 2 parts: a synovial joint anteriorly (intraarticular part) and a syndesmosis posteriorly (extraarticular part).[1,2] There is histologic,[3–9] anatomic,[3,5,7,10–21] and physiologic[22,23] evidence that the SIJ is innervated and, therefore, could be a source of low back pain. Pain may arise from any one or combination of structures of the SIJ,[24] including the joint capsule[3,4] and surrounding ligaments.[3–5,8,9] Critical to identifying the source(s) of pain is a good anatomic understanding of SIJ innervation relative to bony landmarks. The innervation of the SIJ has been described as "complex and controversial,"[25] with wide variability both among and within individuals.[3,5,7,10–21] However, recent anatomic studies[11,17–21] have advanced our knowledge of SIJ innervation relative to bony landmarks identifiable with fluoroscopy and ultrasound. Diagnostic block/radiofrequency ablation (RFA) techniques based on anatomic evidence using precise, validated bony

PO Box 68508 Walmer, Toronto, Ontario M5S 3C9, Canada
*E-mail address:* shannon.roberts@mail.utoronto.ca

Phys Med Rehabil Clin N Am 32 (2021) 703–724
https://doi.org/10.1016/j.pmr.2021.05.007
pmr.theclinics.com

landmarks identifiable with fluoroscopy and/or ultrasound are essential for accurate diagnosis and effective treatment of sacroiliac pain.

The purpose of this review article is to summarize current anatomic evidence of the anterior and posterior innervation of the SIJ relative to bony landmarks identifiable with fluoroscopy and ultrasound. This article aims to provide clinicians with an anatomic basis for clinical application to diagnostic blocks and RFA for sacroiliac pain to optimize clinical outcomes.

## ANTERIOR INNERVATION OF THE SACROILIAC JOINT
### Histologic Evidence

Histologic studies have found nerve fibers[3] (myelinated and unmyelinated,[4] as well as substance P and calcitonin gene-related peptide [CGRP] positive[5]), mechanoreceptors,[3,5] and nociceptors[3,5] in the anterior sacroiliac ligament (ASL) and anterior SIJ capsule (**Table 1**), suggesting that the nerve fibers may transmit proprioceptive and pain signals from these structures. One study[6] found substance P and CGRP-positive "fiber-like structures" in the superficial layer of the articular cartilage of the sacrum and ilium and adjacent ligamentous tissue; however, these structures were not histologically confirmed to be nerve fibers.

### Anterior Sources of Innervation

Anatomic studies[3,5,7,10,11] have reported both interindividual and intraindividual variations in the innervation of the anterior aspect of the SIJ (**Table 2** and **Fig. 1**). Earlier anatomic studies[3,10] reported that the anterior aspect of the SIJ was innervated by the anterior rami of L4-S2 and the sacral plexus, with contributions from the anterior rami of L3 and S3 in some specimens and the superior gluteal nerve in one study. For example, Ikeda[3] found that the upper anterior part of the SIJ was mainly innervated by branch(es) from the anterior ramus of L5, whereas the lower anterior part

**Table 1**
**Histologic findings: anterior innervation of the sacroiliac joint**

| Study | n | Tissue Sample Type | Histologic Findings[a] |
|---|---|---|---|
| Ikeda,[3] 1991 | 6 | Cadaveric | • Nerve fibers (diameter: $0.2–2.5~\mu m^b$) and terminals (including free nerve endings) in anterior SIJ capsule and ASL |
| Fortin et al,[4] 1999 | 2 | Intraoperative biopsies[c] | • Myelinated and unmyelinated nerve fibers in capsular ligamentous tissue from anterior aspect of the SIJ |
| Szadek et al,[5] 2008 | 5 | Cadaveric | • Substance P and CGRP[d]-positive nerve fibers and receptors type II (mechanoreceptors) and type IV (nociceptors) in ASL |
| Szadek et al,[6] 2010 | 10 | Cadaveric | • Substance P and CGRP[d]-positive "fiber-like structures" in superficial layer of articular cartilage of sacrum and ilium and adjacent ligamentous tissue |

*Abbreviations:* ASL, anterior sacroiliac ligament; CGRP, calcitonin gene-related peptide.
[a] ASL is a thickening of the anterior SIJ capsule.[1,2,5,26]
[b] Diameter of nerve fibers reported for both the anterior and posterior aspects of the SIJ.
[c] Intraoperative biopsies from patients undergoing SIJ arthrodesis for chronic pain.
[d] Substance P and CGRP are pain neurotransmitters.

**Table 2**
Anterior sources of innervation to the sacroiliac joint

| | | Anterior Sources of Innervation, No. (%n) | | | | | | | | | |
|---|---|---|---|---|---|---|---|---|---|---|---|
| | | Anterior Ramus | | | | | | | | Sacral | | |
| Study | n | L3 | L4 | L5 | S1 | S2 | S3 | LST | Plexus | SGN | ON | FN |
| Solonen,[10] 1957 | 18 | 1 (5.6) | 17 (94.4) | 18 (100) | 11 (61.1) | 4 (22.2) | | | | 15 (83.3) | 0 (0) | 0 (0) |
| Ikeda,[3] 1991 | 26 | | | | | | | | | | | |
| UA | | 2 (7.7) | 4 (15.4) | 17 (65.4) | 5 (19.2) | 12 (46.2) | 3 (11.5) | | 11 (42.3) | | | |
| LA | | | | | | | | | 18 (69.2) | | | |
| Grob et al,[7] 1995 | 7 | | | | | | | | 0 (0) | | 0 (0) | |
| Szadek et al,[5] 2008 | 5 | | | | | | | 5 (100) | | | | |
| Cox et al,[11] 2017 | 24 | 4 (16.7) | 4 (16.7) | 18 (75) | 0 (0) | | | 0 (0) | 0 (0) | 0 (0) | 0 (0) | 0 (0) |

*Abbreviations:* FN, femoral nerve; LA, lower anterior part of the SIJ; LST, lumbosacral trunk (formed by anterior rami of L4 and L5); ON, obturator nerve; SGN, superior gluteal nerve; UA, upper anterior part of the SIJ.

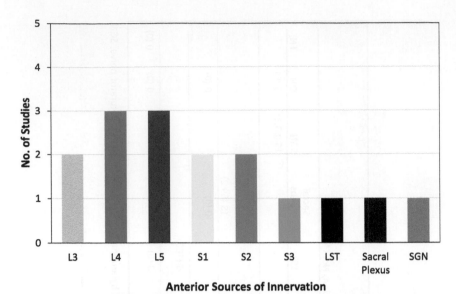

**Anterior Sources of Innervation**

**Fig. 1.** Anterior sources of innervation to the SIJ reported in anatomic studies. L3-S3, anterior rami; LST, lumbosacral trunk (formed by L4 and L5 anterior rami); SGN, superior gluteal nerve.

of the SIJ was mainly innervated by branches from the anterior ramus of S2 or the sacral plexus. In contrast, Grob and colleagues[7] did not find any branches from the sacral plexus innervating the anterior aspect of the SIJ and suggested that the SIJ is innervated exclusively by the lateral branches of the posterior rami of S1-S4.[4] However, this hypothesis has been refuted by more recent anatomic studies,[5,11] which have demonstrated that the anterior aspect of the SIJ is innervated by anterior sources. Szadek and colleagues[5] found small branches from the lumbosacral trunk (formed by the anterior rami of L4 and L5) innervating the ASL. In this study,[5] histologic examination demonstrated substance P and CGRP-positive nerve fibers, mechanoreceptors, and nociceptors in the ASL. Cox and colleagues[11] found small branch(es) from the anterior rami of L4 and/or L5 innervating the anterior aspect of the SIJ in 20 of 24 specimens (83.3%). These branches were examined histologically and found to be consistent with nerve tissue.[11] Cox and colleagues[11] did not find any branches from the anterior ramus of S1 innervating the anterior aspect of the SIJ in all 24 specimens. However, it should be noted that they did not investigate all possible anterior sources of innervation (see **Table 2**).[11] The anatomic and histologic findings that the anterior aspect of the SIJ is mainly innervated by anterior sources are supported by the physiologic findings of a randomized controlled trial (RCT) by Dreyfuss and colleagues[23] that multisite, multidepth sacral lateral branch blocks do not effectively anesthetize the intraarticular part of the SIJ, suggesting that it is innervated predominantly or additionally by anterior source(s).

In summary, the anterior aspect of the SIJ was most frequently found to be innervated by branch(es) from the anterior ramus of L5 (4/5 studies; 65.4%–100% of specimens), followed by the anterior ramus of L4 (4/5 studies; 15.4%–100% of specimens).[3,5,10,11] The branch(es) arose directly from the anterior rami of L4 and/or L5 in 3 studies[3,10,11] and from the lumbosacral trunk formed by the anterior rami of L4 and L5 in one study[5] (**Fig. 2**). These are the only branches that have been histologically identified as nerves.[11] Possible contributions from the anterior rami of S1-S3 and

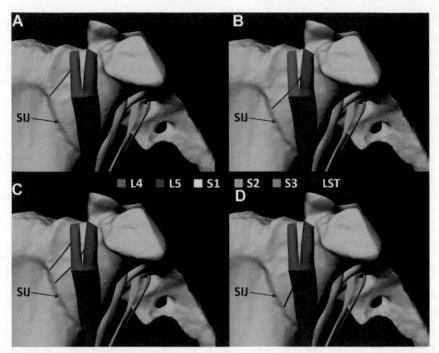

**Fig. 2.** Innervation of the anterior aspect of the SIJ, superoanterolateral views of 3-dimensional models. (A–D) Variations in innervation pattern: branch(es) from (A) L4 anterior ramus, (B) L5 anterior ramus, (C) both L4 and L5 anterior rami, and (D) lumbosacral trunk (LST, formed by L4 and L5 anterior rami). L4-S3, anterior rami.

the sacral plexus[3,10] have not been histologically confirmed. Further anatomic and histologic research is required to better understand the innervation of the anterior aspect of the SIJ.

### Number of Branches

Cox and colleagues[11] found 1 or 2 small branches from (see **Fig. 2A–C**)

- L4 anterior ramus (n = 2/24 [8.3%])
- L5 anterior ramus (n = 16/24 [66.7%])
- Both L4 and L5 anterior rami (1 branch each) (n = 2/24 [8.3%])

Szadek and colleagues[5] reported that small branches (not quantified) arose from the lumbosacral trunk (see **Fig. 2D**).

### Diameter and Length of Branches

Ikeda[3] found no difference in the diameter of branches innervating the 4 subdivisions of the SIJ (upper anterior, lower anterior, upper posterior, and lower posterior parts), which ranged from 0.292 to 0.997 mm (see **Table 2**). Cox and colleagues[11] found that the anterior rami of L4 and L5 had a diameter of less than 0.5 mm and a length of 5 to 31 mm (mean: 14 mm). Length increased from L4 to L5, but there was no statistically significant difference between sides or sexes.[11]

### Course

Cox and colleagues[11] found that 1 or 2 small branches arose from the posterior surface of the anterior rami of L4 and/or L5 and coursed laterally to the anterior aspect of the SIJ (see **Fig. 2**A–C). Szadek and colleagues[5] reported that small branches arose from the lumbosacral trunk at the level of the pelvic brim and coursed inferiorly to the ASL (see **Fig. 2**D).

### Distribution

Regardless of origin, the branches were found to innervate (see **Fig. 2**):[3,5,10,11]

- ASL
- Anterior SIJ capsule

Note that the ASL is a thickening of the anterior SIJ capsule (an intrinsic ligament).[1,2,5,26]

### Bony Landmarks

No precise, validated bony landmarks identifiable with fluoroscopy and ultrasound were found in the literature for the nerves innervating the anterior aspect of the SIJ.

## POSTERIOR INNERVATION OF THE SACROILIAC JOINT
### Histologic Evidence

Histologic studies have found nerve fibers[3] (myelinated and unmyelinated,[8] as well as CGRP positive[5]), mechanoreceptors,[3,5,8] nociceptors,[3,5] and substance P[9] in the posterior sacroiliac ligaments and/or interosseous sacroiliac ligament (ISL) (**Table 3**), suggesting that the nerve fibers may transmit proprioceptive and pain signals from these

**Table 3**
**Histologic findings: posterior innervation of the sacroiliac joint**

| Study | n | Tissue Sample Type | Histologic Findings |
|---|---|---|---|
| Ikeda,[3] 1991 | 6 | Cadaveric | • Nerve fibers (diameter: 0.2–2.5 μm[a]) and terminals (including free nerve endings) in posterior sacroiliac ligaments |
| Grob et al,[7] 1995 | 4 | Cadaveric | • Myelinated and unmyelinated nerve fibers in lateral branches of posterior rami of S1-S4 that innervated SPSL, LPSL, ISL, and STL |
| Vilensky et al,[8] 2002 | 6 | Intraoperative biopsies[b] | • Myelinated and unmyelinated nerve fibers and paciniform and nonpaciniform mechanoreceptors in posterior sacroiliac ligaments |
| Fortin et al,[9] 2003 | 2 | Intraoperative biopsies[b] | • Substance P[c] in posterior sacroiliac ligaments |
| Szadek et al,[5] 2008 | 5 | Cadaveric | • CGRP[c]-positive nerve fibers and receptors type II (mechanoreceptors) and type IV (nociceptors) in ISL |

*Abbreviations:* CGRP, calcitonin gene-related peptide; ISL, interosseous sacroiliac ligament; LPSL, long posterior sacroiliac ligament; SPSL, short posterior sacroiliac ligament; STL, sacrotuberous ligament.
[a] Diameter of nerve fibers reported for both the anterior and posterior aspects of the SIJ.
[b] Intraoperative biopsies from patients undergoing SIJ arthrodesis for chronic pain.
[c] Substance P and CGRP are pain neurotransmitters.

structures. One study[7] found myelinated and unmyelinated nerve fibers in the lateral branches of the posterior rami of S1-S4 that innervated the short posterior sacroiliac ligament (SPSL), long posterior sacroiliac ligament (LPSL), ISL, and sacrotuberous ligament (STL).

## Posterior Sources of Innervation

Anatomic studies[3,7,10,12–21] have found that the posterior aspect of the SIJ is innervated by the posterior sacral network (PSN), a fine nerve plexus receiving contributions from the lateral branches of the posterior rami of S1-S3 ± L5/S4 (**Fig. 3**). Variation was found in the contributions of the lateral branches of L5-S4 (**Table 4** and **Fig. 4**):[3,7,10,12–18]

- S1: consistent contribution (10/10 studies; 4%–100% of specimens, the differences in these findings may be explained by methodological differences; see **Table 4** footnotes)
- S2: consistent contribution (10/10 studies; 93.3%–100% of specimens)
- S3: consistent contribution (9/10 studies; 88%–100% of specimens)
- S4: highly variable contribution (8/10 studies; 4%–100% of specimens)
- L5: highly variable contribution (5/10 studies; 8%–100% of specimens)

Some studies reported that the lateral branch of L5 anastomosed with the lateral branch of S1 and contributed to the PSN that innervated the posterior aspect of the SIJ (see **Fig. 3**),[17,18] whereas other studies reported that the lateral branch of L5 innervated the posterior aspect of the SIJ directly[3] or both directly and via the PSN.[13] For example, Ikeda[3] found that the upper posterior part of the SIJ was mainly innervated directly by the lateral branch(es) of L5, whereas the lower posterior part of the SIJ was mainly innervated by branches that arose from a plexus formed by the lateral branches of S1-S4.

One study[17] reported that branches of the superior gluteal nerve "entered the lateral side of the long posterior sacroiliac ligament…[and] appeared to terminate in the SIJ" (n = 5/12 [41.7%]).

## Number of Lateral Branches

Interindividual and intraindividual variations in the number of lateral branches at each level (L5-S4) has been reported in anatomic studies (**Table 5** and **Fig. 3**).[13–15,17–21] Most studies found 1 or 2 lateral branches at each level from S1-S3, with variable contributions from L5 and S4 (1 branch each), innervating the posterior aspect of the SIJ. Cox and Fortin[17] reported the total number of lateral branches at each level and found that it ranged from 1 to 4. Most commonly, Cox and Fortin[17] found

- L5: 1 lateral branch anastomosed with the lateral branch of S1 and contributed to the PSN (n = 9/12 [75%])
- S1: 3 lateral branches (n = 8/12 [66.7%])
- S2: 1 lateral branch (n = 5/12 [41.7%])
- S3: 2 lateral branches (n = 6/12 [50%])
- S4: 2 lateral branches (n = 7/12 [58.3%])

Another study[18] reported the number of lateral branches at each level that contributed to the PSN and innervated the posterior aspect of the SIJ, which ranged from 1 to 3 (see **Fig. 3**). Most frequently, this study[18] found

- S1: 1 lateral branch (n = 15/25 [60%])
- S2: 2 lateral branches (n = 19/25 [76%])

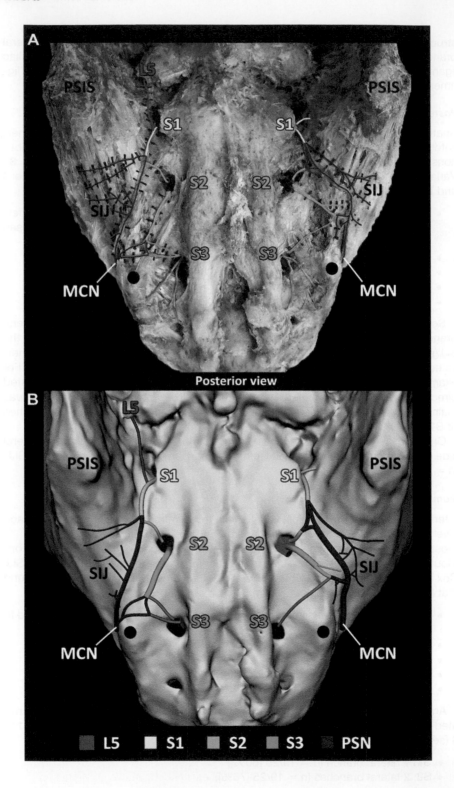

Posterior view

• S3: 1 lateral branch (n = 18/25 [72%])

The single lateral branch of L5 anastomosed with the lateral branch of S1 and contributed to the PSN in 2 of 25 specimens (8%).[18] In 23 of 25 specimens (92%), it did not contribute to the PSN; it remained superior to the SPSL.[18] The single lateral branch of S4 anastomosed with a lateral branch of S3 and contributed to the PSN in only 1 of 25 specimens (4%).[18]

### Diameter of Lateral Branches

The diameter of the lateral branches of L5-S4 was similar in anatomic studies, ranging from 0.292 to 0.997 mm in one study[3] and 0.21 to 1.51 mm in another study[18] (**Table 6**). A third study[13] reported that the diameter of the main trunks of the posterior rami of L5-S4 ranged from approximately 1/4 to 1 mm. The lateral branch of S2 was reported to have the largest mean diameter, followed by S1, L5, S3, and S4 in one study[18] (see **Table 6**).

### Course

After emerging from the posterior sacral foramina, the lateral branches of S1-S3 ± L5/S4 unite to form the PSN, coursing laterally on the posterior surface of the sacrum at the periosteal level and then on the posterior surface of the ISL (**Figs. 5 and 6** and Video 1).[7,12,13,15,18–21,27] At the S1 and S2 levels, the lateral branches and the PSN course deep to the SPSL (see **Fig. 5**).[7,12,13,18–21] Recent anatomic studies[18–21] have found a superior lateral branch of S1 that most commonly entered the ISL or occasionally the SPSL between the S1 and S2 levels in some specimens (n = 10/25 [40%] in one study[18]; **Figs. 3 and 5**). The PSN courses laterally toward and then deep to the LPSL (between the posterior superior iliac spine and the third transverse sacral tubercle [TST]) and the superficial lamina of the STL, on the ISL, where it gives off many branches that enter these ligaments (see **Figs. 5 and 6**).[7,12,13,15,18–21,27] The PSN also gives rise to the medial cluneal nerve(s) at this location, which course between the superficial and deep laminae of the STL, along the posterolateral surface of the sacrum, then penetrate the STL and gluteus maximus muscle and course superficially to become cutaneous (see **Fig. 3**).[7,12,16,18–21,27] Along their entire course, the lateral branches and the PSN are embedded within a layer of adipose and loose connective tissue, deep to arteries and veins, which each form their own plexuses (order of structures from superficial to deep: veins, arteries, nerves).[15,18–21,27,28]

### Distribution

The PSN was found to innervate (**Fig. 6**)[4,7,12–15,18–21]

• SPSL
• LPSL
• ISL
• Superficial lamina of STL

◀─────────────────────────────────────────────────

Fig. 3. Innervation of the posterior aspect of the SIJ by the posterior sacral network (PSN) formed by the lateral branches of the posterior rami of S1-S3 ± L5/S4. Photograph (*A*) and 3D model (*B*) of the same cadaveric specimen, posterior views. Black dots, third transverse sacral tubercle; MCN, medial cluneal nerve; PSIS, posterior superior iliac spine. (*Adapted from* Roberts SL, Burnham RS, Ravichandiran K, et al. Cadaveric study of sacroiliac joint innervation: Implications for diagnostic blocks and radiofrequency ablation. Reg Anesth Pain Med 2014;39(6):456-64; with permission from BMJ Publishing Group Limited.)

**Table 4**
**Posterior sources of innervation to the sacroiliac joint**

| | | Posterior Sources of Innervation, No. (%n) | | | | | | |
|---|---|---|---|---|---|---|---|---|
| | | Lateral Branch | | | | | | |
| Study | n | L5 | S1 | S2 | S3 | S4 | Plexus (S1-S4) | SGN |
| Horwitz,[12] 1939[a] | 60 | | 20 (33.3) | 56 (93.3) | 57 (95) | 8 (13.3) | | |
| Solonen,[10] 1957 | 18 | | 18 (100) | 18 (100) | | | | |
| Bradley,[13] 1974 | NR | NR (100) | NR (100) | NR (100) | NR (100) | | | |
| Ikeda,[3] 1991 | 14 | | | | | | | |
| UP | | 14 (100) | 3 (21.4) | | | | | |
| LP | | | | | 3 (21.4) | | 14 (100) | |
| Grob et al,[7] 1995 | 4 | | 4 (100) | 4 (100) | 4 (100) | 4 (100) | | |
| Yin et al,[14] 2003 | 3 | | 3 (100) | 3 (100) | 3 (100) | 1 (33.3) | | |
| McGrath and Zhang,[15] 2005[b] | 22 | | 1 (4) | 21 (96) | 22 (100) | 13 (59) | | |
| Willard et al,[16] 2009 | 19 | NR | NR | NR | NR | NR | | |
| Cox and Fortin,[17] 2014 | 12 | 9 (75) | 12 (100) | 12 (100) | 12 (100) | 9 (75) | | 5 (42) |
| Roberts et al,[18] 2014[c] | 25 | 2 (8) | 25 (100) | 25 (100) | 22 (88) | 1 (4) | | |

*Abbreviations:* LP, lower posterior part of the SIJ; NR, not reported; SGN, superior gluteal nerve; UP, upper posterior part of the SIJ.

[a] Horwitz[12] reported that the PSN consisted of a primary and secondary series of "loops" formed by the lateral branches. The primary series of loops was formed by the lateral branches of L5-S4, which anastomosed with each other after emerging from the posterior sacral foramina. The lateral branches of S1 and S2 were found to innervate the SPSL and LPSL. The secondary series of loops was formed variably by the lateral branches of S1-S4, deep to the LPSL and the superficial lamina of the STL, and gave rise to the medial cluneal nerve, which coursed within the STL and gave off branches to the surrounding ligaments. Horwitz[12] reported the frequency of contribution of the lateral branches to the secondary series of loops, which is included in this table.

[b] McGrath and Zhang[15] studied the relationship of the lateral branches to the LPSL only.

[c] Roberts and colleagues[18] reported the lateral branches of L5-S4 that contributed to the PSN and innervated the posterior aspect of the SIJ.

Willard and colleagues[16] reported that small branches of the PSN innervate the posteromedial SIJ capsule. Note that the posterior SIJ capsule is composed of irregular bands and has an opening to the intraarticular part of the SIJ (see **Fig. 6**).[29,30]

The medial cluneal nerves, which innervate the skin of the medial part of the buttock,[1,2,16] also arise from the PSN (see **Fig. 3**).[7,12,16,18–21,27]

***Bony Landmarks***

***Lateral branches: clock face positions as they emerge from the posterior sacral foramina***

Interindividual and intraindividual variations in the location of the lateral branches of S1-S4 as they emerge from the posterior sacral foramina has been reported in anatomic studies (**Table 7** and **Figs. 7 and 8**).[14,17–21] When the posterior sacral foramen is viewed as a clock face, lateral branch clock face positions ranged from 12:00 to 6:00 on the right and from 6:00 to 12:00 on the left.[14,17,18,21] One study[18] reported lateral branch quadrants of exit from the posterior sacral foramina and found that the lateral branch(es) most frequently emerged from

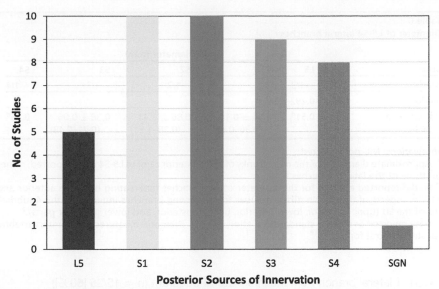

**Fig. 4.** Posterior sources of innervation to the SIJ reported in anatomic studies. L5-S4, lateral branches of posterior rami; SGN, superior gluteal nerve.

**Table 5**
**Number of L5-S4 lateral branches**

| Study | n | No. of Lateral Branches | | | | |
|-------|---|-----|-----|-----|-----|-----|
| | | L5[a] | S1 | S2 | S3 | S4 |
| Bradley,[13] 1974 | NR | 1 | 1 | 1 | 1 | 0 |
| Yin et al,[14] 2003[b] | 3 | | ≥1 | ≥1 | ≥1 | 0–1 |
| McGrath and Zhang,[15] 2005[c] | 22 | | 1–2 | 1–2 | 1–2 | 1–2 |
| Cox and Fortin,[17] 2014[d] | 12 | 0–1 | 2–4 | 1–4 | 1–4 | 0–3 |
| Roberts et al,[18] 2014[e] | 25 | 0–1 | 1–2 | 1–2 | 0–3 | 0–1 |

*Abbreviation:* NR, not reported.
 [a] Lateral branch of L5 anastomosed with the lateral branch of S1 and contributed to the PSN.
 [b] Yin and colleagues[14] reported the number of lateral branches at each level (L5-S4) that innervated the posterior aspect of the SIJ.
 [c] McGrath and Zhang[15] studied the relationship of the lateral branches to the LPSL only.
 [d] Cox and Fortin[17] reported the total number of lateral branches at each level (L5-S4).
 [e] Roberts and colleagues[18] reported the number of lateral branches at each level (L5-S4) that contributed to the PSN and innervated the posterior aspect of the SIJ. Note that most specimens in which the lateral branch of S3 did not contribute to the PSN and innervate the posterior aspect of the SIJ had an anatomic variation, such as L5 sacralization or a very prominent lateral sacral crest (eg, see **Fig. 3**E in Roberts and colleagues[19]).

**Table 6**
**Diameter of L5-S4 lateral branches**

| Study | n | L5 | S1 | S2 | S3 | S4 |
|---|---|---|---|---|---|---|
| | | Diameter (mm) | | | | |
| Bradley,[13] 1974[a] | NR | ~1/3 | ~1 | ~1/2 | ~1/3 | ~1/4 |
| Ikeda,[3] 1991 | 14 | 0.292–0.997[b] | | | | |
| Roberts et al,[18] 2014[c] | 20 | 0.51[d] | 0.64 ± 0.16 (0.36–0.85) | 0.86 ± 0.41 (0.28–1.51) | 0.38 ± 0.06 (0.21–0.48) | 0.36[d] |

*Abbreviations:* NR, not reported.
  [a] Approximate diameters of the main trunks of the posterior rami of L5-S4 were reported, rather than those of the lateral branches.[13]
  [b] Ikeda[3] reported a range for the diameter of all branches innervating both the anterior and posterior aspects of the SIJ. No difference was found among branches innervating the 4 subdivisions of the SIJ (upper anterior, lower anterior, upper posterior, and lower posterior parts).[3]
  [c] Data reported as mean ± standard deviation (range). Diameter measured at the intervertebral or posterior sacral foramina.[18]
  [d] n = 1.

- S1: 1 lateral branch from the inferolateral quadrant (n = 15/25 [60%])
- S2: 1 lateral branch from the superolateral quadrant and 1 lateral branch from the inferolateral quadrant (n = 11/25 [44%])
- S3: 1 lateral branch from the superolateral quadrant (n = 18/25 [72%])

The single lateral branch of S4 emerged from the superolateral quadrant and contributed to the PSN in only 1 of 25 specimens (4%).[18]

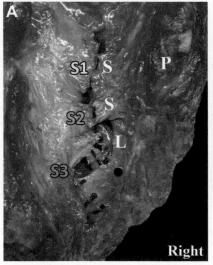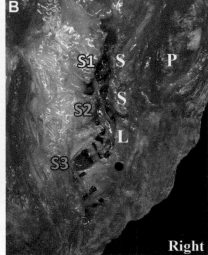

**Fig. 5.** Course of the lateral branches and posterior sacral network (PSN) relative to the posterior ligaments, posterior views. (*A*) At the S1 and S2 levels, the lateral branches and PSN course deep to the short posterior sacroiliac ligament (*S*). (*B*) S has been reflected to reveal the underlying lateral branches and PSN. The PSN courses laterally toward and then deep to the long posterior sacroiliac ligament (*L*) (between the posterior superior iliac spine [P] and the third transverse sacral tubercle [*black dot*]). S1-S3, lateral branches of posterior rami.

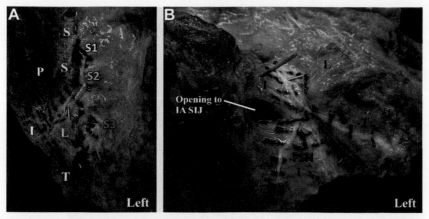

**Fig. 6.** Innervation of the posterior ligaments by the posterior sacral network (PSN), posterior (*A*) and lateral (*B*) views. I, interosseous sacroiliac ligament; IA SIJ, intraarticular part of the SIJ; L, long posterior sacroiliac ligament (reflected); P, posterior superior iliac spine; S, short posterior sacroiliac ligament (reflected); S1-S3, lateral branches of posterior rami; T, superficial lamina of the sacrotuberous ligament (reflected). (*From* Roberts SL, Stout A, Loh EY, et al. Anatomical comparison of radiofrequency ablation techniques for sacroiliac joint pain. Pain Med 2018;19(10):1924-43; with permission from Oxford University Press.)

**Table 7**
**Clock face positions of S1-S4 lateral branches as they emerge from posterior sacral foramina**

| Study | n | Lateral Branches | Clock Face Positions (%n) Left | Right |
|-------|---|------------------|--------------------------------|-------|
| Yin et al,[14] 2003 | 3 | S1-S3 | 6:00–10:00 | 2:00–6:00 |
| Cox and Fortin,[17] 2014 | 12 | S1-S4 | Average: 7:00–10:30 Range: 6:00–12:00 | Average: 1:30–5:00 Range: 12:00–6:00 |
| Roberts et al,[18] 2014[a] | 25 | S1 | IL (92%) SL & IL (8%) | |
| | | S2 | IL (52%) SL & IL (44%) SL (4%) | |
| | | S3 | SL (84%) SL & IL (4%) | |
| | | S4 | SL (4%) | |
| Stout et al,[21] 2018[b] | 40 | S1 | 6:00 & 7:30 | 4:30 & 6:00 |
| | | S2 | 6:30, 8:00, & 9:30 | 2:30, 4:00, & 5:30 |
| | | S3 | 9:30 & 11:00 | 1:00 & 2:30 |

*Abbreviations:* IL, inferolateral quadrant (left: 6:00–9:00; right: 3:00–6:00); SL, superolateral quadrant (left: 9:00–12:00; right: 12:00–3:00).

[a] Reported quadrants of exit from the posterior sacral foramina for both left and right sides. The lateral branch(es) of S3 contributed to the PSN and innervated the posterior aspect of the SIJ in n = 22/25 (88%) and the lateral branch of S4 in n = 1/25 (4%).[18]

[b] Clock face positions with the greatest number of lateral branches at each level (S1-S3), proposed by Stout and colleagues[21] as new fluoroscopic targets for cooled radiofrequency neurotomy of sacral lateral branches (targets located 10 mm lateral to center of posterior sacral foramen on posterior surface of sacrum).

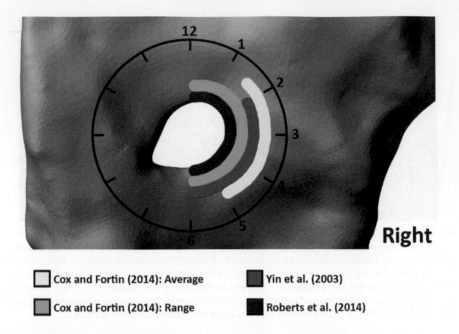

Right

■ Cox and Fortin (2014): Average     ■ Yin et al. (2003)

■ Cox and Fortin (2014): Range     ■ Roberts et al. (2014)

**Fig. 7.** Comparison of clock face positions of the S1-S4 lateral branches as they emerge from the posterior sacral foramina reported in anatomic studies, posterior view.

Stout and colleagues[21] determined the clock face positions with the greatest number of lateral branches at each level from S1-S3 and, based on the anatomic findings, proposed new fluoroscopic targets for cooled radiofrequency neurotomy of the sacral lateral branches (see **Table 7** and **Fig. 9**). These are precise, validated bony landmarks identifiable with fluoroscopy that can be used to localize the lateral branches.

**Posterior sacral network: first to third transverse sacral tubercles of the lateral sacral crest**
The first to third TSTs of the lateral sacral crest were found to be consistent bony landmarks for the PSN in a recent anatomic study (**Fig. 10**).[18] In this study,[18] most branches of the PSN coursed over the lateral sacral crest between TST1 and TST3, with the greatest number of branches between TST2 and TST3 (**Fig. 11**). Only 1 small branch coursed superior or inferior to these landmarks in 3 of 25 specimens (12%).[18] The lateral sacral crest and TST1-3 can be easily visualized with ultrasound.[19,31] TST1-3 are located on the lateral sacral crest at the level of the first to third posterior sacral foramina, respectively, and can be identified using the adjacent posterior sacral foramina.[19,31,32] These are precise, validated bony landmarks identifiable with ultrasound and fluoroscopy that can be used to localize the PSN.

**DISCUSSION**

A sound anatomic foundation is essential for accurate diagnosis and effective treatment of sacroiliac pain. Clinically, it is important to understand the difference between the intraarticular and extraarticular parts of the SIJ and their innervation. As Bogduk[33] stated, "for sacroiliac pain…there are at least two entities in question [pain from the SIJ itself and pain from the posterior ligaments]. The two are distinctly

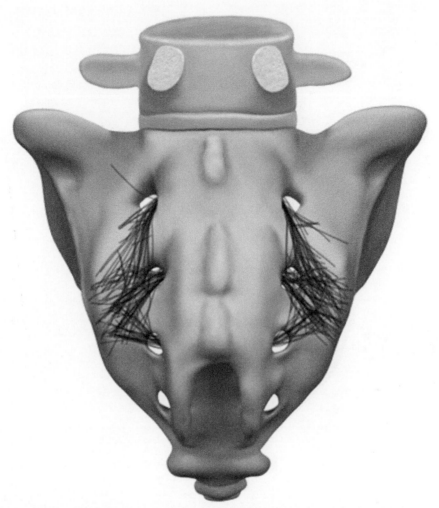

**Fig. 8.** Variations in clock face positions of the S1-S3 lateral branches as they emerge from the posterior sacral foramina reported by Stout and colleagues,[21] posterior view. Overlay of all S1-S3 lateral branches from 20 cadavers bilaterally. (*From* Stout A, Dreyfuss P, Swain N, et al. Proposed optimal fluoroscopic targets for cooled radiofrequency neurotomy of the sacral lateral branches to improve clinical outcomes: An anatomical study. Pain Med 2018;19(10):1916-23; with permission from Oxford University Press.)

different conceptually; each requires a different paradigm of diagnosis and treatment..." Specifically, Dreyfuss and colleagues[23] demonstrated that "Intra-articular blocks test for [sacroiliac] joint pain, and [lateral branch blocks] test for [posterior] ligament pain." This is critically important to understand because it impacts patient outcomes.

### Innervation of the Intraarticular Part of the Sacroiliac Joint

The intraarticular part of the SIJ (the SIJ itself/proper[14,22–24,33,34]) is a synovial joint: it consists of the articulation between the auricular surfaces of the sacrum and ilium,

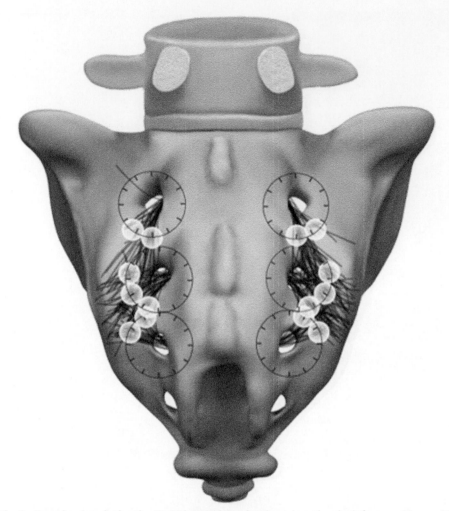

**Fig. 9.** Bony landmarks for the S1-S3 lateral branches based on the clock face positions with the greatest number of lateral branches, proposed by Stout and colleagues[21] as new fluoroscopic targets for cooled radiofrequency neurotomy of the sacral lateral branches, posterior view. Overlay of all S1-S3 lateral branches from 20 cadavers bilaterally with clock face and 8 mm lesions. (*From* Stout A, Dreyfuss P, Swain N, et al. Proposed optimal fluoroscopic targets for cooled radiofrequency neurotomy of the sacral lateral branches to improve clinical outcomes: An anatomical study. Pain Med 2018;19(10):1916-23; with permission from Oxford University Press.)

both covered with articular cartilage, and surrounded by a joint capsule.[1,2] The anterior SIJ capsule is a continuous sheet, whereas the posterior SIJ capsule is composed of irregular bands and has an opening to the intraarticular part of the SIJ.[29,30] Histologic evidence of nerve fibers, mechanoreceptors, and nociceptors in the anterior SIJ capsule[3,4] demonstrates that it is innervated and, therefore, could be a source of pain. No histologic studies were found in the literature that examined the posterior SIJ capsule. Substance P and CGRP-positive "fiber-like structures" were found in the superficial layer of the articular cartilage of the sacrum and ilium and adjacent

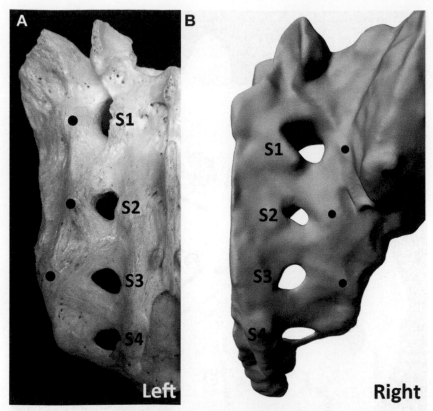

**Fig. 10.** Bony landmarks for the posterior sacral network (PSN): first to third transverse sacral tubercles (black dots) of the lateral sacral crest identifiable with ultrasound and fluoroscopy. Photograph of sacrum (*A*) and 3D model of the SIJ (*B*), posterior views.

ligamentous tissue in one histologic study[6] but not confirmed to be nerve fibers. Anatomic evidence demonstrates that the intraarticular part of the SIJ receives innervation from both anterior and posterior sources, but mainly from anterior source(s).[3,5,7,10,11] The anterior SIJ capsule was most frequently found to be innervated by branch(es) from the anterior rami of L4 and/or L5 directly[3,10,11] or from the lumbosacral trunk formed by the anterior rami of L4 and L5.[5] Possible contributions from the anterior rami of S1-S3 and the sacral plexus reported in some anatomic studies[3,10] have not been histologically confirmed. In contrast, the posteromedial SIJ capsule was reported to be innervated by the PSN formed by the lateral branches of the posterior rami of L5-S4 in one study.[16] Physiologic evidence is consistent with anatomic evidence that the intraarticular part of the SIJ is innervated by both anterior and posterior sources.[23] In an RCT, Dreyfuss and colleagues[23] found that multisite, multidepth sacral lateral branch blocks do not effectively anesthetize the intraarticular part of the SIJ, suggesting that it receives predominant or additional innervation from anterior source(s).

The ASL is a thickening of the anterior SIJ capsule.[1,2,5,26] Histologic evidence of nerve fibers (including substance P and CGRP positive[5]), mechanoreceptors, and nociceptors in the ASL[3-5] demonstrates that it is innervated and, therefore, could be a source of pain. Anatomic evidence demonstrates that the ASL receives

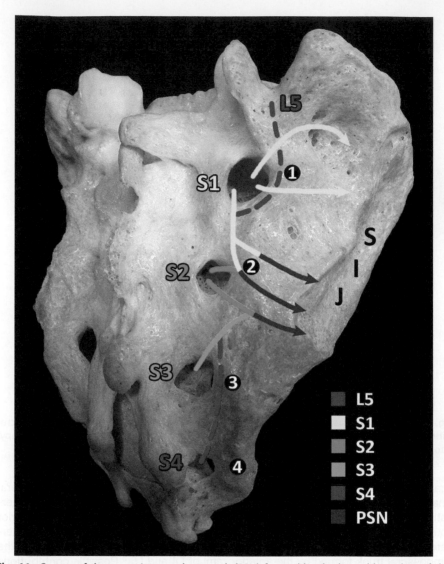

**Fig. 11.** Course of the posterior sacral network (PSN) formed by the lateral branches of the posterior rami of S1-S3 ± L5/S4 relative to the first to third transverse sacral tubercles (black dots) of the lateral sacral crest, posterolateral view. (*From* Roberts SL, Burnham RS, Ravichandiran K, et al. Cadaveric study of sacroiliac joint innervation: Implications for diagnostic blocks and radiofrequency ablation. Reg Anesth Pain Med 2014;39(6):456-64; with permission from BMJ Publishing Group Limited.)

innervation from anterior source(s), by the same nerve branches that innervate the anterior SIJ capsule,[3,5,10,11] because it is an intrinsic ligament.[1,2,5,26] Most frequently, the ASL was found to be innervated by branch(es) from the anterior rami of L4 and/or L5 or the lumbosacral trunk.[3,5,10,11] Possible contributions from the anterior rami of S1-S3 and the sacral plexus[3,10] have not been histologically confirmed, and further research is required.

## Innervation of the Extraarticular Part of the Sacroiliac Joint

The extraarticular part of the SIJ (the posterior ligaments[14,22–24,33,34]; described in anatomy textbooks[1,2] as a syndesmosis) includes the SPSL, LPSL, and ISL. Histologic evidence of nerve fibers, mechanoreceptors, nociceptors, and pain neurotransmitters (substance P and CGRP) in the posterior sacroiliac ligaments and ISL[3,5,7–9] demonstrates that these structures are innervated, and therefore, any one or combination of these structures could be a source of pain.[24] Anatomic evidence demonstrates that the extraarticular part of the SIJ receives innervation from posterior sources: the PSN formed by the lateral branches of the posterior rami of S1-S3 ± L5/S4.[3,7,10,12–21] Interindividual and intraindividual variations were reported in the number and location of the lateral branches as they emerge from the posterior sacral foramina.[13–15,17–21] Physiologic evidence is consistent with anatomic evidence that the extraarticular part of the SIJ is innervated by the PSN formed by the lateral branches. In an RCT, Dreyfuss and colleagues[23] found that multisite, multidepth sacral lateral branch blocks effectively anesthetize the posterior sacroiliac ligaments and ISL, demonstrating that these ligaments are innervated by the lateral branches. The PSN also innervates the superficial lamina of the STL[7,12,18–21] and gives rise to the medial cluneal nerves,[7,12,16,18–21,27] which innervate the skin of the medial part of the buttock.[1,2,16]

Precise, validated bony landmarks are important to identify and effectively treat the source(s) of pain. Stout and colleagues[21] proposed new fluoroscopic targets for cooled radiofrequency neurotomy of the sacral lateral branches based on the clock face positions with the greatest number of lateral branches as they emerge from the posterior sacral foramina at each level: on the right side, 4:30 and 6:00 at S1; 2:30, 4:00, and 5:30 at S2; and 1:00 and 2:30 at S3; and on the left side, 6:00 and 7:30 at S1; 6:30, 8:00, and 9:30 at S2; and 9:30 and 11:00 at S3 (targets located 10 mm lateral to the center of the posterior sacral foramen on the posterior surface of the sacrum; **Fig. 9**). A recent anatomic study[18] proposed new bony landmarks identifiable with ultrasound and fluoroscopy for the PSN: TST1-3 of the lateral sacral crest, based on the finding that most branches of the PSN coursed over the lateral sacral crest between TST1 and TST3, with the greatest number of branches between TST2 and TST3 (see **Fig. 11**). Diagnostic block/RFA techniques based on anatomic evidence using precise, validated bony landmarks identifiable with fluoroscopy and/or ultrasound to localize the target nerves are key to optimize clinical outcomes.

## SUMMARY

The SIJ consists of 2 parts: a synovial joint (intraarticular part) and a syndesmosis (extraarticular part). The intraarticular part of the SIJ receives innervation from both anterior and posterior sources, but mainly from anterior source(s) (anterior sources: most frequently, branch(es) from the anterior rami of L4 and/or L5 or the lumbosacral trunk; posterior sources: the PSN). The extraarticular part of the SIJ receives innervation from posterior sources: the PSN formed by the lateral branches of the posterior rami of S1-S3 ± L5/S4. Therefore, intraarticular and extraarticular SIJ pain require different techniques for diagnosis and treatment: intraarticular blocks/injections for the diagnosis and treatment of intraarticular SIJ pain (pain from the SIJ itself) versus lateral branch blocks for diagnosis and lateral branch RFA for treatment of extraarticular SIJ pain (pain from the posterior ligaments).[23,24,33,34] Rigorous diagnostic block and RFA techniques based on anatomic evidence using precise, validated bony landmarks identifiable with fluoroscopy and/or ultrasound are essential to identify and effectively treat the source(s) of pain to optimize clinically meaningful outcomes for each patient.

## CLINICS CARE POINTS

- SIJ consists of 2 parts: a synovial joint (intraarticular part) and a syndesmosis (extraarticular part).
- Interindividual and intraindividual variations exist in both anterior and posterior SIJ innervation (eg, source, number, location, and course of branches).

Intraarticular part of the SIJ:

- Innervated by both anterior and posterior sources but mainly by anterior source(s).
- Anterior sources: most frequently, branch(es) from the anterior rami of L4 and/or L5 or the lumbosacral trunk; possible contributions from the anterior rami of S1-S3 and the sacral plexus have not been histologically confirmed, and further research is required.
- Posterior sources: the PSN.

Extraarticular part of the SIJ:

- Innervated by posterior sources: the PSN, a fine nerve plexus formed by the lateral branches of the posterior rami of S1-S3 ± L5/S4.
- Bony landmarks: (1) lateral branches: most common clock face positions as they emerge from the posterior sacral foramina identifiable with fluoroscopy; and (2) PSN: first to third transverse sacral tubercles of the lateral sacral crest identifiable with ultrasound and fluoroscopy.

## DISCLOSURE

The author declares no conflicts of interest.

## FUNDING SOURCES

None.

## ACKNOWLEDGMENTS

The author would like to thank the individuals who donate their bodies and tissue for the advancement of education and research.

## SUPPLEMENTARY DATA

Supplementary data to this article can be found online at https://doi.org/10.1016/j.pmr.2021.05.007.

## REFERENCES

1. Standring S, Anand N, Birch R, et al. Gray's anatomy: the anatomical basis of clinical practice. 41st edition. New York: Elsevier; 2016.
2. Moore KL, Dalley AF, Agur AMR. Clinically oriented anatomy. 7th edition. Philadelphia: Wolters Kluwer Health/Lippincott Williams & Wilkins; 2014.
3. Ikeda R. Innervation of the sacroiliac joint. Macroscopical and histological studies. Nihon Ika Daigaku Zasshi 1991;58:587–96.
4. Fortin JD, Kissling RO, O'Connor BL, et al. Sacroiliac joint innervation and pain. Am J Orthop (Belle Mead NJ) 1999;28:687–90.
5. Szadek KM, Hoogland PV, Zuurmond WW, et al. Nociceptive nerve fibers in the sacroiliac joint in humans. Reg Anesth Pain Med 2008;33:36–43.

6. Szadek KM, Hoogland PV, Zuurmond WW, et al. Possible nociceptive structures in the sacroiliac joint cartilage: an immunohistochemical study. Clin Anat 2010;23: 192–8.
7. Grob KR, Neuhuber WL, Kissling RO. Die innervation des sacroiliacalgelenkes beim menschen. Z Rheumatol 1995;54:117–22.
8. Vilensky JA, O'Connor BL, Fortin JD, et al. Histologic analysis of neural elements in the human sacroiliac joint. Spine 2002;27:1202–7.
9. Fortin JD, Vilensky JA, Merkel GJ. Can the sacroiliac joint cause sciatica? Pain Physician 2003;6:269–71.
10. Solonen KA. The sacroiliac joint in the light of anatomical, roentgenological and clinical studies. Acta Orthop Scand Suppl 1957;27:1–127.
11. Cox M, Ng G, Mashriqi F, et al. Innervation of the anterior sacroiliac joint. World Neurosurg 2017;107:750–2.
12. Horwitz MT. The anatomy of (a) the lumbosacral nerve plexus—its relation to variations of vertebral segmentation, and (b), the posterior sacral nerve plexus. Anat Rec 1939;74:91–107.
13. Bradley KC. The anatomy of backache. Aust N Z J Surg 1974;44:227–32.
14. Yin W, Willard F, Carreiro J, et al. Sensory stimulation-guided sacroiliac joint radiofrequency neurotomy: technique based on neuroanatomy of the dorsal sacral plexus. Spine 2003;28:2419–25.
15. McGrath MC, Zhang M. Lateral branches of dorsal sacral nerve plexus and the long posterior sacroiliac ligament. Surg Radiol Anat 2005;27:327–30.
16. Willard FH, Carreiro JE, Yin W, et al. The dorsal sacral plexus and its relationship to ligaments of the sacroiliac joint. Pain Med 2009;10:953–4.
17. Cox RC, Fortin JD. The anatomy of the lateral branches of the sacral dorsal rami: implications for radiofrequency ablation. Pain Physician 2014;17:459–64.
18. Roberts SL, Burnham RS, Ravichandiran K, et al. Cadaveric study of sacroiliac joint innervation: implications for diagnostic blocks and radiofrequency ablation. Reg Anesth Pain Med 2014;39:456–64.
19. Roberts SL, Burnham RS, Agur AM, et al. A cadaveric study evaluating the feasibility of an ultrasound-guided diagnostic block and radiofrequency ablation technique for sacroiliac joint pain. Reg Anesth Pain Med 2017;42:69–74.
20. Roberts SL, Stout A, Loh EY, et al. Anatomical comparison of radiofrequency ablation techniques for sacroiliac joint pain. Pain Med 2018;19:1924–43.
21. Stout A, Dreyfuss P, Swain N, et al. Proposed optimal fluoroscopic targets for cooled radiofrequency neurotomy of the sacral lateral branches to improve clinical outcomes: an anatomical study. Pain Med 2018;19:1916–23.
22. Dreyfuss P, Snyder BD, Park K, et al. The ability of single site, single depth sacral lateral branch blocks to anesthetize the sacroiliac joint complex. Pain Med 2008; 9:844–50.
23. Dreyfuss P, Henning T, Malladi N, et al. The ability of multi-site, multi-depth sacral lateral branch blocks to anesthetize the sacroiliac joint complex. Pain Med 2009; 10:679–88.
24. King W, Ahmed SU, Baisden J, et al. Diagnosis and treatment of posterior sacroiliac complex pain: a systematic review with comprehensive analysis of the published data. Pain Med 2015;16:257–65.
25. Cohen SP, Chen Y, Neufeld NJ. Sacroiliac joint pain: a comprehensive review of epidemiology, diagnosis and treatment. Expert Rev Neurother 2013;13:99–116.
26. Poilliot AJ, Zwirner J, Doyle T, et al. A systematic review of the normal sacroiliac joint anatomy and adjacent tissues for pain physicians. Pain Physician 2019;22: E247–74.

27. McGrath C, Nicholson H, Hurst P. The long posterior sacroiliac ligament: a histological study of morphological relations in the posterior sacroiliac region. Joint Bone Spine 2009;76:57–62.
28. McGrath MC, Jeffery R, Stringer MD. The dorsal sacral rami and branches: sonographic visualisation of their vascular signature. Int J Osteopath Med 2012;15:3–12.
29. Forst SL, Wheeler MT, Fortin JD, et al. The sacroiliac joint: anatomy, physiology and clinical significance. Pain Physician 2006;9:61–7.
30. Vleeming A, Schuenke MD, Masi AT, et al. The sacroiliac joint: an overview of its anatomy, function and potential clinical implications. J Anat 2012;221:537–67.
31. Finlayson RJ, Etheridge JB, Elgueta MF, et al. A randomized comparison between ultrasound- and fluoroscopy-guided sacral lateral branch blocks. Reg Anesth Pain Med 2017;42:400–6.
32. Robinson TJG, Roberts SL, Burnham RS, et al. Sacro-iliac joint sensory block and radiofrequency ablation: assessment of bony landmarks relevant for image-guided procedures. Biomed Res Int 2016;2016:1432074.
33. Bogduk N. A commentary on appropriate use criteria for sacroiliac pain. Pain Med 2017;18:2055–7.
34. Bogduk N. Commentary on King W, Ahmed S, Baisden J, Patel N, MacVicar J, Kennedy DJ. Diagnosis of posterior sacroiliac complex pain: a systematic review with comprehensive analysis of the published data. Pain Med 2015;16:222–4.

# Sacroiliac Joint Diagnostic Block and Radiofrequency Ablation Techniques

Eldon Loh, MD, FRCPC[a,b,*], Taylor R. Burnham, MD, MSCI[c],
Robert S. Burnham, MSc, MD, FRCPC[d,e,f]

## KEYWORDS

- Sacroiliac joint • Radiofrequency ablation • Diagnostic blocks • Fluoroscopy
- Ultrasonography • Lateral branch • Innervation

## KEY POINTS

- The posterior sacral network is located between S2 and S3 in most cadaveric specimens, but could extend to just proximal to the S1 level; a lesion from the level of S2 to S3 is most important for strip lesions.
- The posterior innervation of the sacroiliac joint (SIJ) is at the level of the periosteum.
- Inclusion of L5 may not be necessary for alleviation of SIJ-specific pain.

## DIAGNOSTIC BLOCKS

- A single-depth block provides sufficient anesthetization of the SIJ and surrounding structures if appropriate locations along the lateral sacral crest are selected.

## RADIOFREQUENCY TECHNIQUES

- Multiple lesioning techniques (conventional thermal, cooled, multipolar, multilesion probes, multitined electrodes) have been described with various needle placements (linear strip lesion and periforaminal types).
- No current technique is clearly superior to other techniques based on clinical outcomes.
- Larger studies with appropriate selection criteria are necessary to allow meaningful clinical comparison between techniques.

[a] Department of Physical Medicine and Rehabilitation, Schulich School of Medicine and Dentistry, Western University, London, Ontario, Canada; [b] Parkwood Institute Research, Lawson Health Research Institute, London, Ontario, Canada; [c] Division of Physical Medicine and Rehabilitation, University of Utah, 590 Wakara Way, Salt Lake City, UT 84103, USA; [d] Division of Physical Medicine and Rehabilitation, Faculty of Medicine and Dentistry, University of Alberta, Canada; [e] Central Alberta Pain and Rehabilitation Institute, 1, 6220 - Highway 2A, Lacombe, Alberta T4L 2G5, Canada; [f] Vivo Cura Health, #100, 325 Manning Road NE Calgary, Alberta T2E 2P5, Canada
* Corresponding author. St. Joseph's Health Care London, Parkwood Institute (Main Building), PO Box 5777, STN B, London, Ontario N6A 4V2, Canada.
E-mail address: eldon.loh@sjhc.london.on.ca

Phys Med Rehabil Clin N Am 32 (2021) 725–744
https://doi.org/10.1016/j.pmr.2021.05.008
1047-9651/21/© 2021 Elsevier Inc. All rights reserved.

## BACKGROUND

Sacroiliac joint (SIJ) radiofrequency ablation (RFA) is a standard treatment of patients with recalcitrant SIJ pain. The SIJ accounts for 10% to 27% of lower back pain,[1] and prevalence increases with age and in the context of lower lumbar fusion.[2,3] SIJ RFA reduces pain through thermal coagulation of nerve fibers carrying afferent pain signals originating primarily from the SIJ.

SIJ RFA can effectively improve pain and function, and decrease health care use. A population-level study involving 4653 patients in Ontario, Canada, showed significant decreases in health care use following RFA for spinal pain, including SIJ RFA (which accounted for approximately 8% of the sample).[4] There was a 23.89% decrease in physician visits and an 85.7% decrease in spinal interventional procedures in the year following RFA. Of those with available prescription records and who received at least 1 opioid prescription in the year before RFA, 19.66% no longer required an opioid prescription in the year following RFA.

Recent meta-analyses have shown that SIJ RFA using different procedural techniques can decrease pain intensity and improve disability for up to 12 months postprocedure.[5–8] In general, success in individual studies has been variable; in 1 systematic review, 32% to 89% of patients achieved at least 50% pain relief for 6 months, whereas 11% to 44% of patients achieved 100% pain relief for the same period.[1] Outcome variability is likely the result of a paucity of high quality randomized controlled trials, small sample sizes, and heterogeneity in patient selection and technical protocols.[9,10] In general, the causal relationship between an intervention (eg, SIJ RFA) and outcome (eg, pain, function, health care use) is established when variables are tested in a specific population (eg, SIJ pain confirmed by block protocol) with a standardized intervention (eg, SIJ RFA technique) free of bias, confounders, or chance (eg, RCTs or extensive cohort studies).[11] At present, there are no uniform patient selection criteria or consensus on a single optimal technique for SIJ RFA, making it difficult to know the true efficacy of SIJ RFA.

Optimizing clinical outcomes of SIJ RFA requires an understanding of relevant SIJ posterior innervation, appropriate patient selection, and application of anatomically sound RFA procedural techniques. This article provides (1) a brief review of the innervation relevant to RFA of the SIJ, (2) a discussion on selection criteria and block techniques for SIJ RFA, and (3) a description of various procedural techniques for SIJ RFA.

## SACROILIAC JOINT INNERVATION AND RADIOFREQUENCY ABLATION

For a thorough description of the innervation of the SIJ, please see the Shannon L. Roberts' article, 'Sacroiliac Joint Anatomy," in this issue. Key points about SIJ innervation relevant to RFA and diagnostic blocks are summarized here.

The posterior innervation of the SIJ is mediated primarily by the posterior sacral network (PSN), a plexus of nerves that originates primarily from the S1 through S3 lateral branches, with occasional contribution from L5 and S4 (**Figs. 1** and **2**).[12] The location of these lateral branches as they exit the foramen is relevant for needle placement in periforaminal RFA techniques (discussed later). At the S1 level, the lateral branches primarily exit at the inferolateral quadrant of the posterior sacral foramen (PSF); at S2, there are up to 2 lateral branches exiting from the superolateral and/or inferolateral quadrants of the PSF; at S3, the lateral branches exit from the superolateral quadrant primarily (see **Fig. 2**).[12] After the lateral branches exit their respective foramen, they converge and form the PSN (see **Fig. 1**).

At the level of the lateral sacral crest (LSC), the PSN was found to extend from the second to just below the third transverse sacral tubercle (TST) most of the time (see

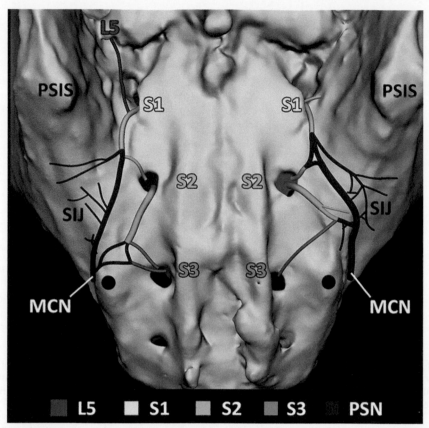

**Fig. 1.** A three-dimensional model of SIJ innervation via the PSN digitized from a cadaveric specimen. Black dots, third transverse sacral tubercle; MCN, medial clunial nerve; PSIS, posterior sacral iliac spine. (*Adapted from* BMJ Publishing Group Limited, Regional Anesthesia & Pain Medicine, Roberts SL et al, 39(6), 456-464, 2014, with permission.)

**Fig. 2**). Occasionally, a single branch separate from the PSN innervates the superior portion of the SIJ. This branch was usually located between the first and second transverse sacral tubercles, but it could travel just proximal to the first TST.[12] The PSN and the anatomic landmarks that define its borders are relevant to needle placement locations for linear strip lesion SIJ RFA techniques (discussed later). The medial clunial nerves arise from the PSN (see **Fig. 1**) [12]; therefore, numbness to the skin overlying the medial buttock is a potential consequence of SIJ RFA.

Note that the posterior innervation of the SIJ travels along the periosteum at the level of the LSC.[12] Therefore, a block or RFA lesion at the level of the periosteum is key to capturing the posterior innervation of the SIJ. Clinically, this concept is supported by a randomized trial that showed equivalent relief between an ultrasonography (US)-guided block at the lateral crest conducted at a single depth versus a fluoroscopy (FL)-guided multisite, multidepth protocol.[13]

A matter of controversy is the role of the L5 dorsal ramus in the innervation of the posterior SIJ. Practically, the main question is whether block or lesioning of the L5 dorsal ramus is necessary for diagnostic work-up or RFA of SIJ pain. A contribution from L5 to the posterior SIJ innervation is documented in some anatomic studies.[12,14–16]

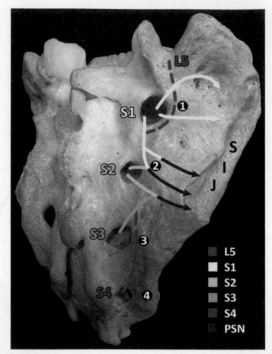

**Fig. 2.** Posterolateral overview of the posterior SIJ innervation. Black dots indicate transverse sacral tubercles (second tubercle is at level of PSIS). L5 and S4 are dashed given their inconsistent contribution to SIJ innervation. (*Adapted from* BMJ Publishing Group Limited, Regional Anesthesia & Pain Medicine, Roberts SL et al, 39(6), 456-464, 2014, with permission.)

However, anatomic studies that describe L5 involvement do not necessarily describe the course of this branch to the SIJ. One cadaveric study that describes the relevant course of the L5 lateral branch documents anastomosis of the L5 lateral branch to the PSN at the level of S1, just lateral to the S1 PSF.[12] Thus, a lesion at this level (lateral to the first PSF) would capture any L5 contribution to the SIJ, obviating a separate RFA lesion at the L5 dorsal ramus.

Clinical studies that explore the effect of lateral branch blocks on provoked pain from the SIJ and associated structures (eg, the dorsal sacroiliac ligaments, the interosseous sacroiliac ligament) provide further insight into the need for the inclusion of a targeted L5 block/RFA lesion.[13,17] A randomized trial that explored US-guided lateral branch blocks (without an L5 dorsal ramus block) versus a traditional FL-guided multisite, multidepth protocol (including L5 dorsal ramus block) found no difference in provoked pain postblock between the 2 techniques (discussed next).[13] This finding suggests that the L5 block is unnecessary to anesthetize the SIJ, the dorsal sacroiliac ligaments, and the interosseous sacroiliac ligament.

If a clinician finds that diagnostic block at L5 contributes to pain relief for RFA, it is not clear that block and subsequent RFA of the L5 dorsal ramus will denervate the SIJ or a separate structure innervated by the L5 dorsal ramus (eg, the L5/S1 facet).

## DIAGNOSTIC BLOCKS

Appropriate patient selection for SIJ RFA is critical for success. Diagnostic blocks targeting the SIJ posterior innervation are the recommended method for identifying appropriate SIJ RFA candidates. However, there is no consensus on which particular block protocol to use. Intra-articular block is not sufficient to select patients for SIJ RFA, given the possibility of extra-articular spread to surrounding structures from capsule defects and lack of anesthetization of relevant SIJ pain-generating structures (eg, dorsal sacroiliac and interosseous sacroiliac ligaments).[17] In addition, if the ventral innervation has a significant role in SIJ-mediated nociception for a particular patient, pain may improve following intra-articular block but would not be addressed with an existing SIJ RFA technique. Interestingly, most studies evaluating the effectiveness of SIJ RFA used intra-articular blocks as the diagnostic tool.[1,8] In addition, none of the studies using diagnostic blocks that targeted posterior innervation used the same block protocol.[18–21]

Two lateral branch block techniques have shown adequate anesthetization of the SIJ, and interosseous and dorsal sacroiliac ligaments. The multisite, multidepth lateral branch block technique used periforaminal injections of local anesthetic from S1 to S3 (right side, 2:30, 4, and 5 o'clock positions at S1 and S2 (**Fig. 3**);

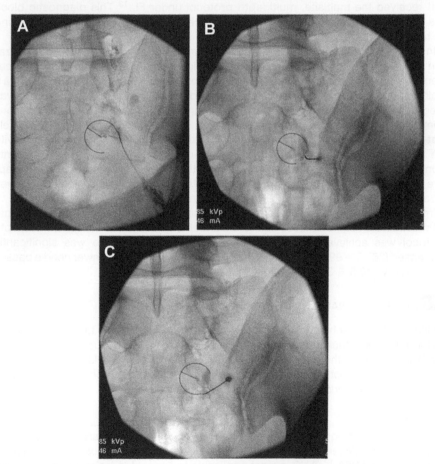

**Fig. 3.** Posteroanterior fluoroscopy views of injections of contrast medium from needles placed at various positions for S2 lateral branch blocks: (*A*) 2:30 position, (*B*) 4:00 position, (*C*) 5:30 position. (*From* Dreyfuss P et al. The Ability of Multi-Site, Multi-Depth Sacral Lateral Branch Blocks to Anesthetize the Sacroiliac Joint Complex. Pain Medicine 2009;10(4):679-688 with permission of Oxford University Press.)

2:30 and 4 o'clock positions at S3; equivalent positions on the left).[17] Fluoroscopy was used to guide needle placement. At each site, 0.2 mL of local anesthetic was injected at full depth; the needle was then withdrawn approximately 3 mm and the injection repeated. This technique was found to anesthetize interosseous and dorsal sacroiliac ligaments and the intra-articular portion of the SIJ in some patients compared with placebo.[17] Although this diagnostic protocol has been validated in asymptomatic individuals, it has not been used in any studies as a selection criterion for a patient receiving SIJ RFA.

The second technique used multiple local anesthetic injections along the LSC to anesthetize the PSN under US guidance: 1.5 mL of local anesthetic was injected at the midpoint between S2 and S3, whereas 0.5 mL of local anesthetic was injected immediately cephalad to S2 and at S1 (**Fig. 4**).[13] L5 was not blocked using this technique. Postinjection, anesthetization of the SIJ, interosseous sacroiliac ligament, and the dorsal sacroiliac ligament was achieved.[13] As mentioned earlier, there was no significant difference observed in provoked pain for a comparison group that received the multisite, multidepth protocol under FL.[13] This diagnostic block has also not been used within a study as a selection criterion for a patient going on to SIJ RFA.

In contrast, single-site, single-depth blocks under FL did not produce anesthetization of the dorsal sacral ligament, interosseous ligament, or SIJ postinjection.[22] Placement of the blocks was lateral to the 3 o'clock position of S1 to S3 on the right (with a 9 o'clock position on the left), and included L5 dorsal ramus block, and 0.2 mL was injected at each site. Given the posterior innervation of the SIJ, and the positions from which the lateral branches emerge from the S1 to S3 foramen, it is unlikely that the positions in this technique would capture the posterior SIJ innervation with the volume infused. In contrast, the US-guided block technique used placements along the lateral crest with a larger local anesthetic volume, which is more likely to capture the PSN. In particular, the largest local anesthetic volume was injected between S2 and S3, which is where the PSN is most often located.[12]

Importantly, although US-guided lateral branch block was done at a single depth without inclusion of the L5 level, equivalent anesthetization to the multisite, multidepth protocol was achieved.[13] As a consequence, procedural time was significantly decreased (267.5 ± 99.3 seconds vs 628.7 ± 120.3 seconds) and fewer needle passes (4.3 ± 1.1. vs 16.3 ± 3.9) were required with this technique.[13]

## SACROILIAC JOINT RADIOFREQUENCY ABLATION TECHNIQUES

Multiple SIJ RFA techniques have been described. They vary in target visualization method, lesioning technique used, and target sites. The key to success of any technique is ultimately the maximal denervation of the posterior SIJ innervation. The different variables that affect SIJ RFA and their potential impacts on the effective capture of the SIJ posterior innervation are described next.

### Guidance Techniques

Most SIJ RFA techniques use FL imaging. The PSFs are the primary landmarks used to guide needle placement under FL. US guidance has been proposed as an imaging modality for SIJ RFA.[12,23] US is most applicable to linear strip lesion techniques, and allows visualization of the TSTs, PSF, and LSC, which are important anatomic landmarks for localizing the PSN (**Fig. 5**). Advantages of US include the lack of ionizing radiation, increased accessibility, and reduced equipment costs. The LSC, which is a helpful landmark to guide linear strip lesion techniques, cannot be visualized under FL.

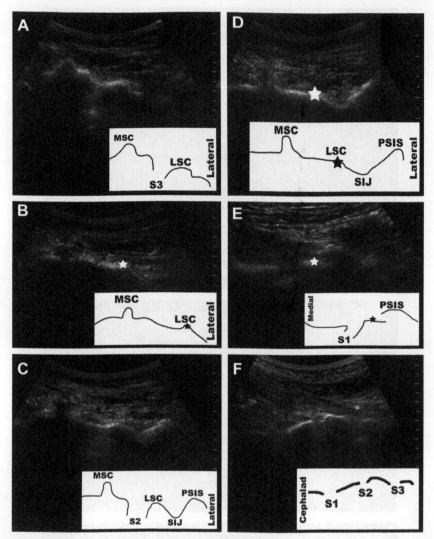

Fig. 4. US images of the posterior sacrum depicting the views required for US-guided lateral branch block. Injection points are marked by a star (★). (A) Transverse sonographic view of the lower sacrum showing the median sacral crest (MSC), posterior foramen of S3 (S3), and LSC. (B) Transverse scan of the lower sacrum depicting the injection point on the LSC, midpoint between the posterior foramina of S3 and S2. (C) Transverse scan at the level of the S2 posterior foramen (S2) showing the caudad aspects of the SIJ and PSIS. (D) Transverse scan of the posterior sacrum showing the injection point on the LSC cephalad to the S2 posterior foramen. (E) Transverse scan of the sacrum showing the injection point lateral to the S1 posterior foramen (S1). (F) Sagittal sonographic view of the sacrum with visualization of the posterior foramina of S1, S2, and S3. (Adapted from BMJ Publishing Group Limited, Regional Anesthesia & Pain Medicine, Finlayson RJ et al, 39(6), 456-464, 2014, with permission.)

The addition of endoscopy to aid in direct visualization of target structures for SIJ RFA has been described in case reports and series, but use of this modality is in its infancy.[24,25]

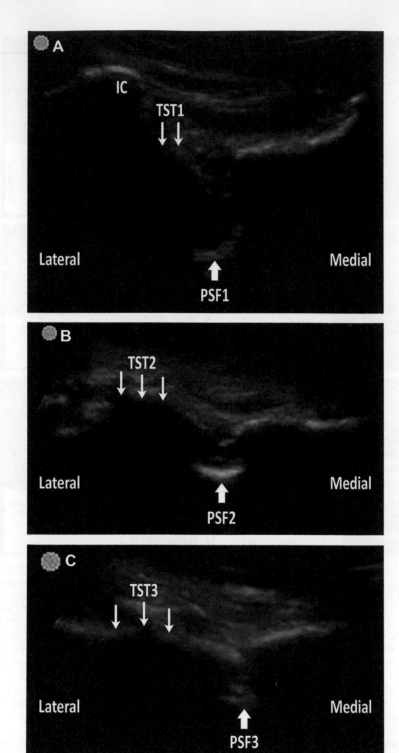

## Lesioning Techniques

A variety of lesioning techniques have been explored for SIJ RFA, including conventional thermal, pulsed, and cooled RFA. Conventional thermal RFA with a single conventional radiofrequency (RF) cannula (ie, monopolar lesioning) generates an ellipsoid lesion around the uninsulated cannula tip with minimal lesioning beyond the tip of the cannula (**Fig. 6**).[26] However, lesion size (including extension beyond the cannula's distal end) could be maximized by varying tip diameter, tip length, RFA temperature, and RFA time.[27] Most placements of RF cannulae are perpendicular to the sacrum; the distal RFA lesion generated by conventional monopolar RFA at the sacral surface is therefore expected to be smaller than the lateral extent of the lesion around the cannula tip. Because the posterior innervation traverses along the periosteum, less of the innervation may be captured with conventional monopolar RFA. Alternatively, if the cannula is placed along (ie, parallel to) the periosteum, a larger lesion at the sacral surface could be generated.

Pulsed RFA is a nonneurolytic technique that uses short bursts of RFA current[28] to create a large electromagnetic field with a target area that may be larger than conventional RFA.[29] The analgesic mechanism of pulsed RFA is not known.[28,30] At present, there are only smaller studies that evaluate the effectiveness of pulsed RFA. Although outcomes are positive, the evidence is limited.[28,29,31]

Cooled RFA generates a slightly oblate ellipsoid lesion, with an average length and width of 9.9 mm and 8.9 mm respectively (given an 18-gauge, 4-mm tip heated to 60°C over 2.5 minutes and 45 seconds of precooling).[27] Importantly, the lesion extends significantly beyond the tip of the needle compared with conventional monopolar RFA (see **Fig. 6**). This treatment results in a larger lesion at the sacral surface compared with conventional thermal RFA; therefore, there is a greater chance of capturing more of the posterior innervation with cooled RFA. Cooled RFA lesion sizes are also affected by tip and RFA parameters; careful attention should be paid to these factors to maximize clinical outcomes. Two exploratory (sham-controlled) trials show that cooled RFA is more efficacious than sham at 1 and 3 months. Pooled, the between-group comparison revealed that patients treated with cooled RFA were 4 times more likely to have 50% or greater pain reduction at 3 months compared with sham (proportion rate ratio/relative risk, 4.84; 95% confidence interval, 1.19–19.73).[19,20]

Different cannula designs have been used to improve lesion morphology for different RFA techniques, including SIJ RFA. Multitined electrodes result in pyramidal[32]/elongate spheroid[33] lesions with a wide-based lesion beyond the end of the cannula compared with conventional RFA cannulae (**Fig. 7**). Given their lesion morphology, multitined electrodes may increase nerve capture along the periosteum with perpendicular placement. Practical use of cooled RFA and multitined electrodes can be limited by cost. Both options are more expensive than conventional RF cannulae, with cooled RFA being the most expensive.

A multilesion probe that generates a series of monopolar and bipolar lesions in a preprogrammed sequence has also been evaluated (eg, Simplicity III probe).[18,21,34–38]

**Fig. 5.** Transverse US scans of TSTs used to localize placement along the left LSC. (*A*) At the level of TST1. (*B*) At the level of TST2. (*C*) At the level of TST3. IC, iliac crest; PSF, posterior sacral foramen; TST, transverse sacral tubercle. (Adapted by permission from BMJ Publishing Group Limited, Regional Anesthesia & Pain Medicine, Roberts SL et al, 42(1):69-74, 2017.)

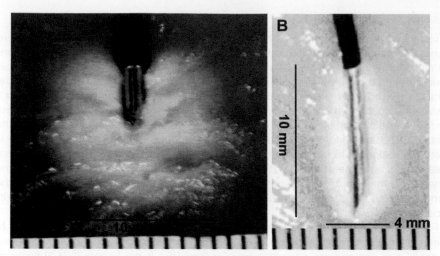

**Fig. 6.** Radiofrequency lesions generated by (A) cooled and (B) conventional thermal RF in chicken meat. Small lines indicate 1-mm divisions. (From Cohen SP, Hurley RW, Buckenmaier CC, Kurihara C, Morlando B, Dragovich A. Randomized Placebo-controlled Study Evaluating Lateral Branch Radiofrequency Denervation for Sacroiliac Joint Pain. Anesthesiology. 2008;109(2):279-288. https://pubs.asahq.org/anesthesiology, with permission)

The probe is placed along the sacral surface and is thought to form a linear strip lesion along the periosteum that is larger than that obtained with conventional RFA[35] (**Fig. 8**).

The use of multiple electrodes simultaneously (in a bipolar or multipolar configuration) also affects the lesion generated. Using conventional RFA cannulae in a multipolar configuration, a rounded rectangular RFA lesion would be generated between electrodes (**Fig. 9**). Conventional RFA cannulae (assuming an 18 or 20 gauge and a 10–15-mm uninsulated tip, a temperature of 80–90°C, and lesion time of 2–3 minutes) should be placed 8 to 12 mm apart.[39] Care must be taken to ensure the cannulae are not too far apart at the surface of the sacrum so that a confluent lesion is generated; this can be accomplished by assuring that RF cannulae are inserted as parallel to each other as possible, in the same plane. A series of consecutive bipolar and multipolar lesions created in a leapfrogging manner (by moving proximal needles distal to the most distal needle in sequence) can be used to create a linear strip lesion over the intended target area. Multitined electrodes can also be used in a multipolar configuration. Given the larger lesion area created by these electrodes, they can be placed further apart than conventional RFA cannulae (estimated 15 mm to 20 mm).[33]

The sacrum's undulating surface might result in a discontinuous lesion at the sacral surface, despite appropriate tip spacing. Tip offset (ie, tips that are not at the same depth) increases the chances of creating 2 monopolar lesions surrounding each tip rather than a continuous bipolar lesion.[39] Because the surface of the sacrum is not a flat, uniform plane, tip offset may be a significant issue that results in incomplete nerve capture as a result of the generation of discrete, monopolar lesions. One possible way to minimize tip offset caused by the dorsal sacral contour is to move the strip lesions slightly medial to the LSC (but remaining lateral to the PSF). The dorsal sacrum is most undulated along the LSC as a result of the sacral tubercles; moving the strip lesions slightly medial to the lateral sacral crest usually places the needles on a smooth sacral surface. The consistency of bipolar lesion morphology in vivo for SIJ RFA has not been explored.

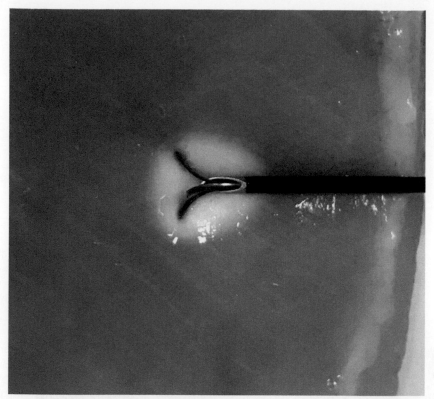

**Fig. 7.** RF lesion generated by a multitined electrode (Diros Trident RF Cannula) in chicken breast. (With permission from Diros Technology, Inc.)

Regardless of the lesioning technique chosen for SIJ RFA, the goal is to ensure that an adequate lesion is generated that encompasses the targeted areas at the periosteal level. Lesioning techniques in a multipolar linear strip lesion configuration may better capture the posterior innervation of the SIJ based on estimated RFA lesion sizes that are applied to an anatomic model,[40] but technical factors (tip spacing, tip offset, tip skew, and so forth) may affect the morphology of lesions generated in a clinical setting and affect clinical outcomes.

### Radiofrequency Ablation Needle Placement

Different target locations have been used for SIJ RFA. In general, these needle placements are either in a strip along the sacrum or periforaminal. An intraforaminal technique has been described but is not commonly used in clinical practice given probe placement within the foramen.[41] Specific approaches for linear strip lesion and periforaminal techniques are described next.

#### Linear strip lesion techniques

Linear strip lesion techniques use an extensive continuous lesion along the sacrum to capture the posterior innervation of the SIJ as it traverses from the PSF to the SIJ. Needle placements for strip lesion techniques have been described along the lateral crest (only visualized under US),[12] lateral to the PSF,[42,43] and over the posterior SIJ.[44]

The extent of the strip lesions varies, with placements extending as far proximal as the S1 superior articular process and as far distal as the fourth PSF.[40] Using the US-

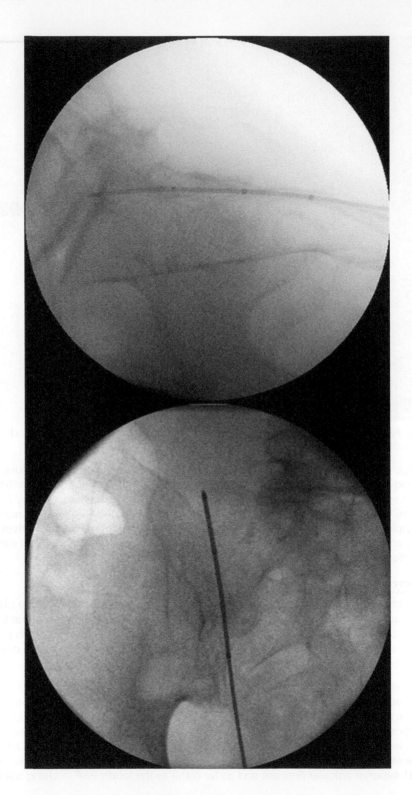

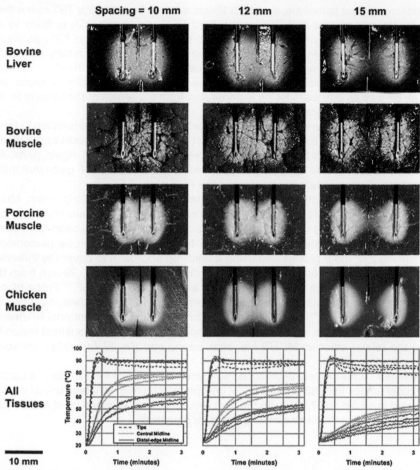

**Fig. 9.** Cross-sectional photographs of bipolar lesions in ex vivo bovine liver, bovine muscle, porcine muscle, and chicken muscle. Intratip and intertip temperatures are plotted over the same time axis for each spacing. The midline temperatures decline with increased spacing. Configuration: variable spacing, 20-gauge diameter, 10-mm tip length, 90°C tip temperature, 3-minute lesion time. (*Adapted from* Cosman ER et al, Bipolar radiofrequency lesion geometry: Implications for palisade treatment of sacroiliac joint pain. Pain Practice. 2011;11(1):3–22. with permission of Wiley.)

**Fig. 8.** Radiographic imaging of Simplicity III probe placement, lateral (*top*) and anteroposterior (*bottom*) views. (Adapted by permission from Springer Nature Customer Service Centre GmbH: Springer, Neurosurgical Review, Bayerl SH et al, Radiofrequency denervation for treatment of sacroiliac joint pain—comparison of two different ablation techniques, 2018, with permission.)

guided lateral crest technique, if an RFA lesion extends from the first TST to the third TST (ie, lateral from the first PSF to the third PSF), the entire PSN is likely to be captured.[40] As the PSN extends primarily from the second to third TST, particular attention should be given to this region during RFA. If RFA is technically difficult to manage at the level of the first TST (which could be the case given the close location of the iliac crest, particularly in men), it may still be possible to complete a successful RFA as long as an adequate lesion is generated from the region of the second to the third TST, along the lateral crest.

Under FL, although the lateral crest cannot be visualized, a linear strip lesion extending from the first PSF to the third PSF that is just lateral to the PSF should approximate the intended target levels for the PSN lateral crest technique (**Fig. 10**). Again, particular attention should focus on the area lateral to the second and third PSF given that these levels more often delineate the borders of the PSN at the LSC.[12]

Different lesioning techniques have been used to create a linear strip lesion. Multipolar needle placements perpendicular to the posterior sacrum are common, but needle placement along (ie, parallel to) the sacral surface has also been described. In the multipolar scenario, approximately 5 to 7 conventional probe placements (often using 2 or more probes and using a leapfrog approach to cover the intended length) would be required based on a mean distance of $52.68 \pm 5.99$ mm from the most proximal part of the S1 PSF to the distal aspect of the third PSF.[45] Probe placement along the sacral surface has been accomplished with a multilesion probe (eg, Simplicity probe).[18,21,34–38] An alternative technique using a conventional RF needle with a 20-mm active tip, placed along the sacral surface, with sequential lesioning along the lateral crest under US has also been used (Dr JP Etheridge, personal communication, 2018).

Estimated capture of lateral branches with linear strip lesion techniques in a cadaveric model ranges from 93.4% to 99.7%; complete capture of all lateral branches was estimated in 62.5% to 97.5%, with the best results for the US lateral crest and FL palisade techniques, which use similar probe placements.[40]

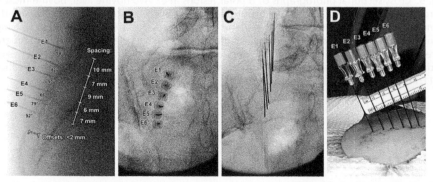

**Fig. 10.** Example of needle placement for an FL-guided SIJ strip lesion technique (palisade). Six straight RF cannulae (20 gauge, 10-mm tip length) are placed between the S1, S2, and S3 dorsal sacral foramina and the ipsilateral SIJ 10 mm apart. (*A*) Lateral view. Electrode-to-surface angles are estimated relative to lines connecting the distal ends of the cannulae. (*B*) Needle view. (*C*) Anteroposterior view. (*D*) External view. (*Adapted from* Cosman ER et al, Bipolar radiofrequency lesion geometry: Implications for palisade treatment of sacroiliac joint pain. Pain Practice. 2011;11(1):3–22. with permission of Wiley.)

Despite fairly comprehensive capture of the lateral branches predicted in the cadaveric model, clinical outcomes are not as robust: 38% to 69% obtain 50% relief of pain at 6 months.[40]

### Periforaminal techniques

These techniques focus on needle placement around the lateral margin of the PSF, and have only been described under FL. Needle placements are semicircumferential and often defined relative to a clock face with needle placements ranging from the 12 to 6 o'clock position[19,20,46–48] (**Fig. 11**). Estimated needle placement from the lateral margin of the foramen has been described from 1 to 10 mm, depending on the study.[40]

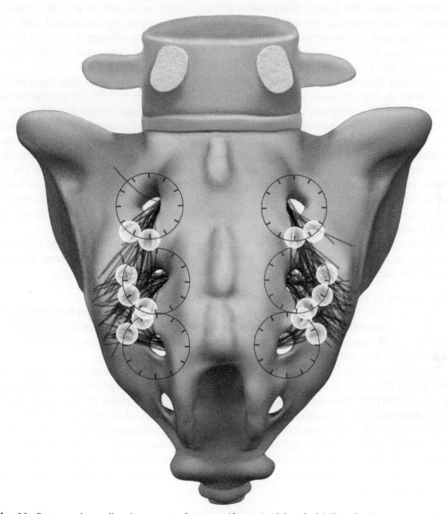

**Fig. 11.** Proposed needle placements for a periforaminal (cooled RF) technique on a cadaveric model. Clockface and lateral branches of all specimens included in the study are overlaid with 8-mm lesion sites. (*From* Stout A et al. Proposed optimal fluoroscopic targets for cooled radiofrequency neurotomy of the sacral lateral branches to improve clinical outcomes: An anatomical study. Pain Medicine 2018;19(10):1916-1923 with permission of Oxford University Press.)

A steel circular ruler (epsilon) is sometimes used to assist with positioning and to measure a fixed distance from the foramen.

Cooled RF needle placements have been previously described at the 2:30, 4:00, and 5:30 positions on the right at S1 and S2 and 2:30 and 4:00 at S3, with equivalent mirrored positions on the left.[46,49,50] A cadaveric study that modeled estimated lesions over the dissected nerves supplying the SIJ found that only 60% of 40 specimens would be completely denervated using these needle placements.[49]

Based on cadaveric innervation patterns visualized under FL (using radiopaque wires), new cooled RF probe placements were proposed at 4:30 and 6:00 (S1); 2:30, 4:00, and 5:30 (S2); and 1:00 and 2:30 (S3) on the right, and mirrored positions on the left (see **Fig. 11**). These positions would target quadrants around the S1 to S3 foramen, where the lateral branches are most often expected to exit (discussed earlier).[12] Complete capture in 95% of cadaveric specimens was estimated with the new proposed RF placement locations.[49] Segment-specific imaging through each vestigial disc space from S1-2 to S3-4 was found to worsen miss rates and is unnecessary for this technique.

Lesioning techniques used with periforaminal needle placements that have been evaluated in the literature include cooled monopolar,[19,20,38,46,48,51,52] conventional monopolar,[20,50] and bipolar conventional[47] techniques. Bipolar conventional lesioning was estimated to capture the highest percentage of lateral branches in a cadaveric model (mean capture rate of 98.6%–98.9% of lateral branches, with complete capture in 90.0%–92.5% of specimens).[40] Cooled RF monopolar techniques (excluding the new proposed technique described earlier) captured between 79.0% and 99.1% of lateral branches, with complete capture in 20.0% to 92.5% of specimens.[40] Conventional monopolar techniques were estimated to capture a mean of 49.6% to 64.6% of lateral branches, and completely capture the lateral branches in 2.5% to 12.5% of specimens.[40]

Despite the variability in estimated lateral branch capture rates between different periforaminal techniques, significant differences between clinical outcomes are not evident in clinical studies.[8,40]

### Comparison of periforaminal and linear strip lesion techniques

In general, linear strip lesion RFA techniques are estimated to have better capture of the lateral branches compared with periforaminal techniques.[40] However, clinical outcomes across various techniques are variable, with 32% to 89% obtaining 50% relief at 6 months, and only 11% to 44% at 12 months.[1]

The distance from the first PSF to the first TST is on average only 6.34 ± 1.36 mm, and at the S3 level is 9.45 ± 2.16 mm.[45] Most FL-guided periforaminal and linear strip lesion techniques situate probes less than 10 mm from the lateral margin of the PSF. Thus, even without US imaging, these placements are likely at or near the lateral crest. The semicircumferential orientation of periforaminal techniques may be less important than the fact that a lesion is generated at the level of the lateral crest adjacent to the foramen. Periforaminal techniques may result in short, discrete lesions on the lateral crest, rather than a continuous linear strip lesion, which is more likely to capture all the lateral branches.

### SUMMARY

Recent anatomic studies have helped to delineate the SIJ posterior innervation and have revealed targetable diagnostic and therapeutic structures. More extensive studies with more robust selection criteria and the application of anatomically sound diagnostic block and SIJ RFA techniques may allow a better understanding of the real efficacy of SIJ RFA and differentiation between SIJ RFA techniques in the future.

## CLINICS CARE POINTS

- For multipolar approaches using a perpendicular placement, probes should be placed as parallel to each other as possible to ensure consistent lesioning.
- If cannula placement lateral to the S1 foramen is challenging given proximity of the posterior superior iliac spine, ensuring an adequate lesion from S2 to S3 may be sufficient for relief.
- L5 dorsal ramus RFA may be performed if this is thought to contribute to a patient's pain presentation, but may not be necessary.
- Under FL, only the superior endplate of S1 needs to be squared off; squaring of the vestigial S1/S2, S2/S3, and S3/S4 disc spaces may decrease the capture rate of SIJ RFA.
- Numbness to the skin over the medial buttock is expected post-RFA and post-block given capture of the medial clunial nerve.

## DISCLOSURE

Dr E. Loh has received in-kind contributions of RF cannulae for research studies from Diros Technology Inc and Nimbus Concepts LLC. Dr R. Burnham has received in-kind contributions of RF cannulae from Nimbus Concepts LLC for research studies. Dr T.R. Burnham has no conflicts to declare.

## REFERENCES

1. King W, Ahmed SU, Baisden J, et al. Diagnosis and treatment of posterior sacro-iliac complex pain: a systematic review with comprehensive analysis of the published data. Pain Med 2015;16(2):257–65.
2. Weiner DK, Sakamoto S, Perera S, et al. Chronic low back pain in older adults: prevalence, reliability, and validity of physical examination findings. J Am Geriatr Soc 2006;54(1):11–20.
3. DePalma MJ, Ketchum JM, Saullo T. What is the source of chronic low back pain and does age play a role? Pain Med 2011;12(2):224–33.
4. Loh E, Reid JN, Alibrahim F, et al. Retrospective cohort study of healthcare utilization and opioid use following radiofrequency ablation for chronic axial spine pain in Ontario, Canada. Reg Anesth Pain Med 2019;44(3):398–405.
5. Chen CH, Weng PW, Wu LC, et al. Radiofrequency neurotomy in chronic lumbar and sacroiliac joint pain: a meta-analysis. Medicine (Baltimore) 2019;98(26): e16230.
6. Sun HH, Zhuang SY, Hong X, et al. The efficacy and safety of using cooled radiofrequency in treating chronic sacroiliac joint pain: a PRISMA-compliant meta-analysis. Medicine (Baltimore) 2018;97(6):e9809.
7. Shih CL, Shen PC, Lu CC, et al. A comparison of efficacy among different radiofrequency ablation techniques for the treatment of lumbar facet joint and sacroiliac joint pain: a systematic review and meta-analysis. Clin Neurol Neurosurg 2020;195:105854.
8. Aydin SM, Gharibo CG, Mehnert M, et al. The role of radiofrequency ablation for sacroiliac joint pain: a meta-analysis. PM R 2010;2(9):842–51.

9. Yang AJ, McCormick ZL, Zheng PZ, et al. Radiofrequency ablation for posterior sacroiliac joint complex pain: a narrative review. PM R 2019;11(Suppl 1): S105–13.

10. Schneider BJ, Rosati R, Zheng P, et al. Challenges in diagnosing sacroiliac joint pain: a narrative review. PM R 2019;11(Suppl 1):S40–5.

11. Speckman RA, Burnham TR. Summary measures and measures of effect: summarizing and comparing outcomes in rehabilitation research. part 2: binary outcomes. PM R 2020;12(9):933–9.

12. Roberts SL, Burnham RS, Ravichandiran K, et al. Cadaveric study of sacroiliac joint innervation: implications for diagnostic blocks and radiofrequency ablation. Reg Anesth Pain Med 2014;39(6):456–64.

13. Finlayson RJ, Etheridge J, Elgueta MF, et al. A randomized comparison between ultrasound- and fluoroscopy-guided sacral lateral branch blocks. Reg Anesth Pain Med 2017;42(3):400–6.

14. Ikeda R. [Innervation of the sacroiliac joint. Macroscopical and histological studies]. Nihon Ika Daigaku Zasshi 1991;58(5):587–96.

15. Bradley KC. The anatomy of backache. Aust N Z J Surg 1974;44(3):227–32.

16. Cox RC, Fortin JD. The anatomy of the lateral branches of the sacral dorsal rami: implications for radiofrequency ablation. Pain Physician 2014;17(5):459–64.

17. Dreyfuss P, Henning T, Malladi N, et al. The ability of multi-site, multi-depth sacral lateral branch blocks to anesthetize the sacroiliac joint complex. Pain Med 2009; 10(4):679–88.

18. Mehta V, Poply K, Husband M, et al. The effects of radiofrequency neurotomy using a strip-lesioning device on patients with sacroiliac joint pain: results from a single-center, randomized, sham-controlled trial. Pain Physician 2018;21(6): 607–18.

19. Patel N, Gross A, Brown L, et al. A randomized, placebo-controlled study to assess the efficacy of lateral branch neurotomy for chronic sacroiliac joint pain. Pain Med 2012;13(3):383–98.

20. Cohen SP, Hurley RW, Buckenmaier CC, et al. Randomized placebo-controlled study evaluating lateral branch radiofrequency denervation for sacroiliac joint pain. Anesthesiology 2008;109(2):279–88.

21. van Tilburg CWJ, Schuurmans FA, Stronks DL, et al. Randomized sham-controlled double-blind multicenter clinical trial to ascertain the effect of percutaneous radiofrequency treatment for sacroiliac joint pain: Three-month results. Clin J Pain 2016;32(11):921–6.

22. Dreyfuss P, Snyder BD, Park K, et al. The ability of single site, single depth sacral lateral branch blocks to anesthetize the sacroiliac joint complex. Pain Med 2008; 9(7):844–50.

23. Roberts SL, Burnham RS, Agur AM, et al. A cadaveric study evaluating the feasibility of an ultrasound-guided diagnostic block and radiofrequency ablation technique for sacroiliac joint pain. Reg Anesth Pain Med 2017;42(1):69–74.

24. Ibrahim R, Telfeian AE, Gohlke K, et al. Endoscopic radiofrequency treatment of the sacroiliac joint complex for low back pain: a prospective study with a 2-year follow-up. Pain Physician 2019;22(2):E111–8.

25. Choi W-S, Kim J-S, Ryu K-S, et al. Endoscopic radiofrequency ablation of the sacroiliac joint complex in the treatment of chronic low back pain: a preliminary study of feasibility and efficacy of a novel technique. Biomed Res Int 2016; 2016:2834259.

26. Bogduk N, Macintosh J, Marsland A. Technical limitations to the efficacy of radiofrequency neurotomy for spinal pain. Neurosurgery 1987;20(4):529–35.

27. Cosman ER Jr, Dolensky HRA, Cosman ER, et al. Factors that affect radiofrequency heat lesion size. Pain Med 2014;15(12):2020–36.
28. Vallejo R, Benyamin RM, Kramer J, et al. Pulsed radiofrequency denervation for the treatment of sacroiliac joint syndrome. Pain Med 2006;7(5):429–34.
29. Dutta K, Dey S, Bhattacharyya P, et al. Comparison of efficacy of lateral branch pulsed radiofrequency denervation and intraarticular depot methylprednisolone injection for sacroiliac joint pain. Pain Physician 2018;21(5):489–96.
30. Shanthanna H, Chan P, McChesney J, et al. Pulsed radiofrequency treatment of the lumbar dorsal root ganglion in patients with chronic lumbar radicular pain: a randomized, placebo-controlled pilot study. J Pain Res 2014;7:47–55.
31. Chang MC, Cho YW, Ahn SH. Comparison between bipolar pulsed radiofrequency and monopolar pulsed radiofrequency in chronic lumbosacral radicular pain: a randomized controlled trial. Medicine (Baltimore) 2017;96(9):e6236.
32. Diros Technology Inc. Diros Trident RF Cannula. Available at: https://dirostech.com/product-details/rf-tridenttrident-hybrid-cannulae/. Accessed November 26, 2020.
33. Wright RE, Allan KJ, Kraft M, et al. Radiofrequency Ablation Using a Novel Multitined Explandable Electrode: Device Description and Research Study. MISP 2012;1(1):41–53.
34. Schmidt PC, Pino CA, Vorenkamp KE. Sacroiliac joint radiofrequency ablation with a multilesion probe: a case series of 60 patients. Anesth Analg 2014; 119(2):460–2.
35. Anjana Reddy VS, Sharma C, Chang K-Y, et al. Simplicity' radiofrequency neurotomy of sacroiliac joint: a real life 1-year follow-up UK data. Br J Pain 2016; 10(2):90–9.
36. Bellini M, Barbieri M. Single strip lesions radiofrequency denervation for treatment of sacroiliac joint pain: two years' results. Anaesthesiol Intensive Ther 2016;48(1):19–22.
37. Hegarty D. Clinical outcome following radiofrequency denervation for refractory sacroiliac joint dysfunction using the Simplicity III Probe: a 12- month retrospective evaluation. Pain Physician 2016;19:E129–35.
38. Tinnirello A, Barbieri S, Todeschini M, et al. Conventional (Simplicity III) and cooled (SInergy) radiofrequency for sacroiliac joint denervation: one- year retrospective study comparing two devices. Pain Med 2017;18(9):1731–44.
39. Cosman ER Jr, Dolensky JR, Cosman ER Jr, et al. Bipolar radiofrequency lesion geometry: implications for palisade treatment of sacroiliac joint pain. Pain Pr 2011;11(1):3–22.
40. Roberts SL, Stout A, Loh EY, et al. Anatomical comparison of radiofrequency ablation techniques for sacroiliac joint pain. Pain Med 2018;19(10):1924–43.
41. Buijs EJ, Kamphuis ET, Groen GJ. Radiofrequency treatment of sacroiliac joint-related pain aimed at the first three sacral dorsal rami: a minimal approach. Pain Clin 2004;16(2):139–46.
42. Cánovas Martínez L, Orduña Valls J, Paramés Mosquera E, et al. Sacroiliac joint pain: prospective, randomised, experimental and comparative study of thermal radiofrequency with sacroiliac joint block. Rev Esp Anestesiol Reanim 2016; 63(5):267–72.
43. Cheng J, Chen SL, Zimmerman N. A new radiofrequency ablation procedure to treat sacroiliac joint pain. Pain Physician 2016;19:603–15.
44. Ferrante FM, King LF, Roche EA. Radiofrequency sacroiliac joint denervation for sacroiliac syndrome. Reg Anesth Pain Med 2001;26(2):137–42.

45. Robinson TJ, Roberts SL, Burnham RS, et al. Sacro-Iliac Joint Sensory Block and Radiofrequency Ablation: Assessment of Bony Landmarks Relevant for Image-Guided Procedures. Biomed Res Int 2016;2016:1432074.

46. Karaman H, Kavak GO, Tüfek A, et al. Cooled radiofrequency application for treatment of sacroiliac joint pain. Acta Neurochir (Wien) 2011;153(7):1461–8.

47. Burnham RS, Yasui Y. An alternate method of radio- frequency neurotomy of the sacroiliac joint: a pilot study of the effect on pain, function, and satisfaction. Reg Anesth Pain Med 2007;32(1):12–9.

48. Cheng J, Pope JE, Dalton JE, et al. Comparative outcomes of cooled versus traditional radiofrequency ablation of the lateral branches for sacroiliac joint pain. Clin J Pain 2013;29(2):132–7.

49. Stout A, Dreyfuss P, Swain N, et al. Proposed optimal fluoroscopic targets for cooled radiofrequency neurotomy of the sacral lateral branches to improve clinical outcomes: an anatomical study. Pain Med 2018;19(10):1916–23.

50. Yin W, Willard F, Carreiro J, et al. Sensory stimulation-guided sacroiliac joint radio-frequency neurotomy: technique based on neuroanatomy of the dorsal sacral plexus. Spine (Phila Pa 1976) 2003;28(20):2419–25.

51. Kapural L, Nageeb F, Kapural M, et al. Cooled radiofrequency system for the treatment of chronic pain from sacroiliitis: the first case-series. Pain Pract 2008; 8(5):348–54.

52. Cheng J, Chen SL, Zimmerman N, et al. Prospective evaluation a new radiofrequency ablation procedure to treat sacroiliac joint pain. Pain Physician 2016; 19:603–15.

# Overview of the Innervation of the Hip Joint

Jessi Jo G. Barnett[a,b,*,1], Shayan Shakeri[a,b,1], Anne M.R. Agur, BSc(OT), MSc, PhD[b]

## KEYWORDS

- Hip joint • Innervation • Anatomy • Denervation

## KEY POINTS

- The innervation of the hip joint is multifaceted, with articular nerves originating from many sources in close proximity to and distant from the hip joint.
- Articular branches of the femoral, obturator, and accessory obturator nerves supply the anterior hip joint capsule.
- The posterior hip joint capsule receives innervation from the nerve to quadratus femoris/inferior gemellus, superior gluteal nerve, and/or directly from the sciatic nerve.
- Further investigation is necessary to optimize anatomic landmarks for image-guided procedures.

## INTRODUCTION

The sensory nerve supply of the hip joint has been a topic of study for several centuries. Over this period of time, 32 cadaveric studies were identified in the literature that explored the innervation of the hip joint capsule. The innervation patterns were found to be complex and the articular branches small, requiring meticulous dissection. Kaplan[1] stated that "Dissection of the articular branches … is technically very difficult and requires fine and patient search with the aid of magnification." The frequency and course of the articular nerves innervating the anterior aspect of the hip joint will be discussed first followed by the posterior aspect.

### Innervation of the Anterior Hip Joint

The anterior hip joint has been found to be innervated by articular branches of the femoral (FN),[1–18] obturator (ON),[1–3,5–17,19–23] and accessory obturator nerve (AON).[5–9,11,12,15,16,19,21,24–31] Of the 32 studies found, 31 investigated the innervation of anterior hip joint.

[a] School of Medicine, St. George's University, Grenada, West Indies; [b] Division of Anatomy, Department of Surgery, Temerty Faculty of Medicine, University of Toronto, 1 King's College Circle, Room 1158, Toronto, Ontario M5S 1A8, Canada
[1] Co-first authors.
* Corresponding author. Division of Anatomy, Department of Surgery, Temerty Faculty of Medicine, University of Toronto, 1 King's College Circle, Room 1158, Toronto, Ontario M5S 1A8, Canada
E-mail address: jessi.barnett@live.ca

Phys Med Rehabil Clin N Am 32 (2021) 745–755
https://doi.org/10.1016/j.pmr.2021.05.009
1047-9651/21/© 2021 Elsevier Inc. All rights reserved.

### Femoral nerve

Articular branches originating from the FN were identified in 17 of 31 cadaveric studies (**Table 1**). Of the 6 studies that reported innervation frequency, 2 studies found FN supply in all specimens.[16,17] In the other 4 studies, the frequency ranged from 8.7% to 90% (see **Table 1**).

Articular branches have been found to originate from the main trunk of the FN superior or inferior to its branching at the level of the inguinal ligament (**Fig. 1**). The articular nerves originating from the main trunk coursed intramuscularly or deep to the iliacus (iliopsoas) muscle to the anterior hip joint capsule (see **Fig. 1**B).[5,10,14,16–18] More distally, these branches lay on the periosteal surface of the pubis between the anterior superior iliac spine and the medial aspect of the iliopubic eminence, before innervating the anterior hip joint.[16]

Articular nerves originating distal to the branching of the FN have been reported to emerge from the muscular branches to pectineus, rectus femoris, vastus lateralis, and vastus medialis.[2,7–11,13,18] Some of these branches were found to pierce iliopsoas and travel laterally to innervate the anterior hip joint (see **Fig. 1**C).[5,8,14] Other branches were found to course inferiorly before recurring superiorly to supply the capsule (see **Fig. 1**A).[2,4,7,8,10,13,16]

### Obturator nerve

Twenty-one studies were found that reported ON innervation of the anterior hip joint (see **Table 1**). The frequency of innervation of the ON was documented in 7 studies. In 6 studies, the ON had a high prevalence of capsular innervation, ranging from 83.3% to 100% of specimens, and in one study, a lower prevalence of 64.3% (see **Table 1**).

Articular branches have been reported to emerge from the ON within or just superior to the obturator canal in 13 studies and/or more inferiorly from the anterior and posterior divisions in 16 studies. Origin from the anterior division (12 studies) was found more frequently than from the posterior division (9 studies).

The articular branches emerging from the ON at the obturator canal have been described by Kaiser[21] as "hugging the lateral bony aspect ... adjacent to the outlet of the obturator canal." These branches continued to course laterally to supply the anteromedial/inferomedial aspect of the capsule (**Fig 2**A). Articular branches originating from the anterior and/or posterior divisions of the ON also coursed laterally to terminate in the same capsular region (see **Fig. 1**A; **Fig. 2**B).

Anatomic landmarks to localize the articular branches of ON were identified in 4 studies.[16,20,21,23] Locher and colleagues[23] described the location of the articular branches of the ON as "... located immediately below the teardrop silhouette formed by the anterior inferior [aspect] of the acetabulum." This landmark was also described by Short and colleagues[16] In addition, Minne and Depreux[20] and Kaiser[21] suggested that the opening of the obturator canal could also be used to target articular branches of the ON.

### Accessory obturator nerve

The AON was initially described by J.A. Schmidt[24] in 1794 and subsequently investigated throughout the twentieth and twenty-first centuries (see **Table 1**). Nineteen of the 23 studies investigating the AON found articular branches to the hip joint, 4 did not. The frequency of capsular innervation by AON was the lowest of all the nerves, ranging from 2% to 53.8%. Birnbaum and colleagues,[14] who did not find any AON innervation, stated "It is possible that these articular branches passing through the iliac m. were misunderstood as motor n. fibers of the iliac m."

**Table 1**
Previous dissection studies of the innervation of the anterior hip joint

| Author | N | FN | ON | AON | Author | N | FN | ON | AON |
|---|---|---|---|---|---|---|---|---|---|
| Schmidt,[24] 1794 | NS | N/A | N/A | ✓ | Tavernier and Pellenda,[9] 1949 | 77 | ✓ | ✓ | 6.5% |
| Rüdinger,[2] 1857 | NS | ✓ | ✓ | N/A | Poulhés et al,[10] 1949 | NS | ✓ | ✓ | X |
| Beaunis and Bouchard,[3] 1879 | NS | ✓ | ✓ | N/A | Wertheimer,[11] 1952 | 50 | 8.7% | 98% | 2% |
| Cruveilhier,[19] 1844 | NS | X | ✓ | ✓ | Poláček,[28] 1958 | 30 | N/A | N/A | 16.6% |
| Chandelux,[4] 1886 | NS | ✓ | X | N/A | Woodburne,[29] 1960 | 550 | N/A | N/A | 8.7% |
| Duzêa,[5] 1886 | NS | ✓ | X | ✓ | Poláček,[12] 1963 | 30 | 90% | 90% | 16.7% |
| Eisler,[25] 1892 | 120 | X | X | 29% | Katritis et al, 1963 | 1000 | N/A | N/A | 13.2% |
| Patterson,[26] 1894 | 24 | X | X | ✓ | Dee,[13] 1969 | 41 | ✓ | ✓ | X |
| Ancel and Sencert,[27] 1901 | 64 | N/A | N/A | 6.2% | Birnbaum et al,[14] 1997 | 11 | ✓ | ✓ | X |
| Bardeen and Elting,[6] 1901 | 246 | ✓ | ✓ | 8.5% | Kampa et al,[15] 2007 | 20 | ✓ | ✓ | 5% |
| Billet et al,[7] 1947 | 12 | 50% | 83.3% | 16.5% | Locher et al,[23] 2008 | 14 | N/A | 85.7% | N/A |
| Minne and Depreux,[20] 1947 | 12 | X | ✓ | X | Akkaya et al,[31] 2008 | 24 | N/A | N/A | 12.5% |
| Gardner,[8] 1948 | 15 | ✓ | ✓ | 26.6% | Short et al,[16] 2018 | 13 | 100% | 100% | 53.8% |
| Kaplan,[1] 1948 | 28 | N/A | ✓ | N/A | Nielsen et al,[17] 2018 | 15 | 100% | N/A | N/A |
| Kaiser,[21] 1949 | 24 | N/A | ✓ | 8.3% | Sakamoto et al,[18] 2018 | 14 | 71.4% | 64.3% | N/A |
| Larochelle and Jobin,[22] 1949 | 106 | N/A | 91.5% | N/A | | | | | |

*Abbreviations:* N, number of specimens; N/A, did not study; NS, not stated; X, did not find.

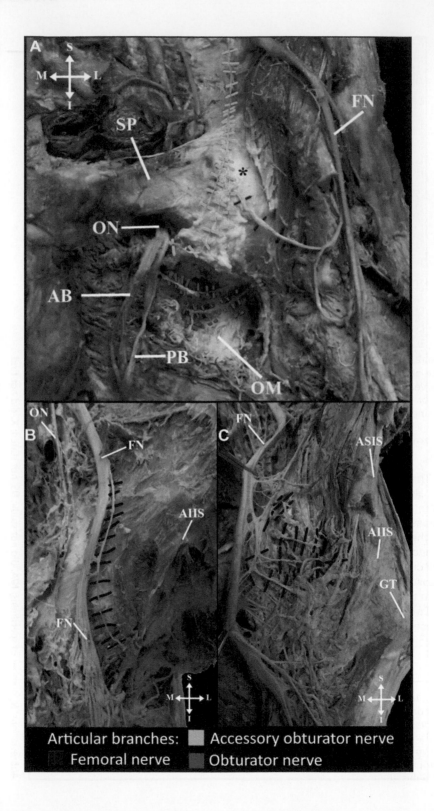

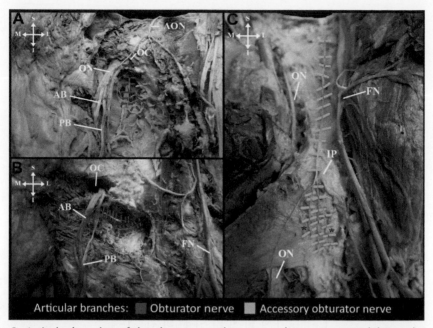

Fig. 2. Articular branches of the obturator and accessory obturator nerves. (A) Branches of the obturator nerve in the obturator canal. (B) Branches from divisions of the obturator nerve. (C) Branches of the accessory obturator nerve. AB, anterior division (branch) of obturator nerve; AON, accessory obturator nerve; FN, femoral nerve; I, inferior; IP, iliopubic eminence; L, lateral; M, medial; OC, obturator canal; ON, obturator nerve; PB, posterior branch of obturator nerve; S, superior. (Reproduced with permission from Philip Peng Educational Series.)

The origin of AON, when documented, was primarily from the anterior rami of L3 and L4. However, Katritsis[30] reported additional origin from L2, and Eisler[25] and Schmidt[24] from L5. In all studies, AON was described as a single nerve that coursed deep to psoas along its medial aspect, parallel to the ON. Distally, the AON passed superficial to the superior ramus of pubis and continued to course deep to pectineus before branching into 3 to 5 articular branches (Fig. 2C).[5,9,19,29,30] These branches were described as "small twigs" by Gardner[8] that directly supplied the anterior hip joint capsule. One of the articular branches was found to course medially to anastomose with the ON or its anterior/posterior divisions (see Fig. 1A).[5,8,16,19,21,26,27,31]

Two bony landmarks related to the AON were identified in the literature. One of these landmarks was the superior ramus of the pubis, in the region of the pecten pubis.[27,29–31] The other key landmark was the iliopectineal (iliopubic) eminence.[8,16,19,21]

Fig. 1. Innervation of the anterior hip joint, anterior views. (A) Articular branches of the femoral, obturator, and accessory obturator nerves. (B) Superior articular branch of femoral nerve. (C) Inferior articular branches of femoral nerve. *, Iliopubic eminence; AB, anterior division (branch) of obturator nerve; ASIS, anterior superior iliac spine; FN, femoral nerve; GT, greater trochanter; I, inferior; L, lateral; M, medial; OM, obturator membrane; ON, obturator nerve; PB, posterior division (branch) of obturator nerve; S, superior; SP, superior ramus of pubis. (Reproduced with permission from Philip Peng Educational Series.)

**Table 2**
**Previous dissection studies of the innervation of the posterior hip joint**

| Author | N | NQF | SGN | SN | Author | N | NQF | SGN | SN |
|---|---|---|---|---|---|---|---|---|---|
| Cruveilhier,[19] 1844 | NS | ✓ | X | X | Larochelle and Jobin,[22] 1949 | 106 | 84.9% | N/A | N/A |
| Rüdinger,[2] 1857 | NS | X | ✓ | ✓ | Tavernier and Pellanda,[9] 1949 | 22 | 86.4% | N/A | 13.6% |
| Beaunis and Bouchard,[3] 1879 | NS | ✓ | X | ✓ | Poulhés et al,[10] 1949 | NS | ✓ | X | X |
| Chandelux,[4] 1886 | NS | ✓ | X | ✓ | Wertheimer,[11] 1952 | 53 | 100% | NS | 3.8% |
| Duzêa,[5] 1886 | 1 | 100% | X | 100% | Poláček,[12] 1963 | 30 | X | 43.3% | ✓ |
| Sadovsky,[32] 1933 | X | ✓ | ✓ | ✓ | Dee,[13] 1969 | 41 | ✓ | 4.9% | X |
| Billet et al,[7] 1947 | 12 | 100% | ✓ | ✓ | Birnbaum et al,[14] 1997 | 11 | ✓ | 36.4% | 9.1% |
| Gardner,[8] 1948 | 15 | ✓ | X | X | Kampa et al,[15] 2007 | 20 | ✓ | ✓ | ✓ |
| Kaplan,[1] 1948 | 28 | ✓ | X | ✓ | | | | | |

*Abbreviations:* N, number of specimens; N/A, did not study; NS, not stated; X, did not find.

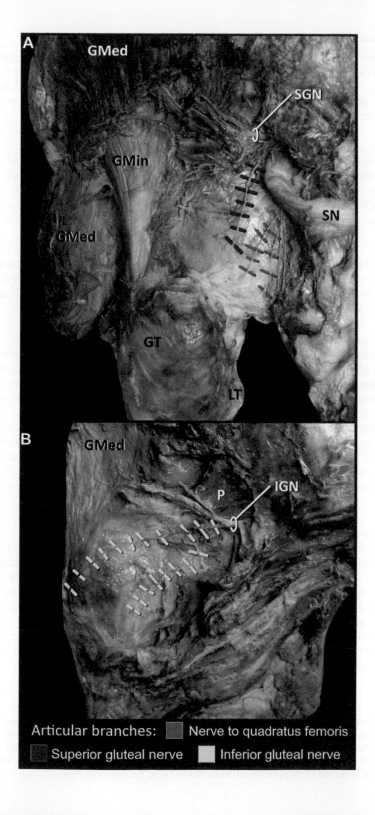

## Innervation of the Posterior Hip Joint

Seventeen cadaveric studies were found that investigated the innervation of the posterior hip joint (**Table 2**). Innervation to the posterior capsule was reported from the nerve to quadratus femoris/inferior gemellus (NQF),[1,3–5,7–11,13–15,19,23,32] superior gluteal nerve (SGN),[2,8,12–15,32] sciatic nerve (SN),[1–5,7,9,11,12,14,15,32] and/or inferior gluteal nerve (IGN).[2,15]

### Nerve to quadratus femoris

The nerve to NQF was found to innervate the posterior aspect of the capsule in 14 of 17 studies, with 4 studies reporting frequency ranging from 84.9% to 100% (see **Table 2**).

The NQF exited the pelvis via the greater sciatic notch and then coursed deep to the piriformis, gemelli, and obturator internus.[7–9,13] The NQF gave off superior and inferior articular branches, also named posterosuperior and posteroinferior articular nerves.[7,9,13] The posterosuperior articular nerve was given off the NQF at the proximal margin of the superior gemellus.[7,13] In contrast, the posteroinferior nerve arose from the NQF at the level of the inferior gemellus.[7,13–15] Both nerves further divided into smaller "twigs" to innervate the posterosuperior[7,13] and posteroinferior[13–15] aspects of the hip joint capsule (**Fig. 3**A).

### Superior gluteal nerve

The frequency of articular innervation by SGN was reported in 3 studies, varying from 4.9% to 43% (see **Table 2**). The nerve to gluteus minimus and/or tensor fascia latae, both branches of SGN, supplied the posterosuperior,[15] posterolateral,[14] and superolateral[8] regions of the hip joint capsule (see **Fig. 3**A). Branches of the superior gluteal artery and vein accompanied their corresponding articular nerves.

Articular branches from the IGN have been reported by Rüdinger[2] and Kampa and colleagues[15] (**Fig. 3**B). Capsular innervation was found by Kampa and colleagues[15] from IGN in 2 of 20 specimens that innervated the posteroinferior region of the capsule, overlapping with the area supplied by NQF. However, Poláček,[12] Dee,[13] and Sadovsky[32] commented that they were not able to isolate articular branches of IGN.

### Direct branches from sciatic nerve

Infrequently, articular branches to the posterior capsule have been found to emerge directly from the SN (see **Table 2**). Wertheimer[11] reported articular branches from SN in 3.8% of dissected specimens, and Tavernier and Pellanda[9] in 13.6%. Kampa and colleagues[15] stated that "The area of the capsule supplied by the SN overlapped with that of the SGN, with its branches traveling along the posterior margin of the capsule and entering the capsule mainly medially, but also laterally over an arc of 90° between nine and 12 o'clock." In addition, Birnbaum and colleagues[14] described articular branches from the nerve to obturator internus and Kaplan[1] from the posterior femoral cutaneous nerve.

---

**Fig. 3.** Innervation of the posterior hip joint, posterior views. (*A*) Articular branches of nerve to quadratus femoris and superior gluteal nerve. (*B*) Articular branches of inferior gluteal nerve. GMed, gluteus medius; GMin, gluteus minimus; GT, greater trochanter; IGN, inferior gluteal nerve; LT, lesser trochanter; P, piriformis; SGN, superior gluteal nerve; SN, sciatic nerve. (Reproduced with permission from Philip Peng Educational Series.)

## SUMMARY

The innervation of the hip joint is multifaceted as it receives innervation from large nerves and small muscular branches. The anterior capsule has been found to be innervated by articular branches of the FN, ON, and less frequently by AON. The posterior capsule receives innervation most frequently from the NQF, SN, and SGN.

## CLINICAL PEARLS

Thorough knowledge of hip joint innervation and the relationship between articular nerves and anatomic landmarks provides an evidence-based approach to assess nerve capture rates. Evaluation of existing radiofrequency nerve ablation procedures and development of new image-guided techniques depends on precise anatomic landmarking to improve clinical outcomes.

## CLINICS CARE POINTS

---

- The innervation of the hip joint is complex, with articular nerves originating from many sources including the femoral, obturator, accessory obturator, superior gluteal and sciatic nerves, as well as the nerve to quadratus femoris.
- The anatomical relationships between articular nerves and landmarks provides an evidence-based approach to developing novel radiofrequency ablation procedures.

---

## ACKNOWLEDGMENTS

The authors thank Dr John Tran for composing and editing the figures in this article. The authors wish to thank the individuals who donated their bodies and tissue for the advancement of education and research.

## DISCLOSURE

A.M.R. Agur is an Anatomy Faculty with Allergan Academy of Excellence.

## REFERENCES

1. Kaplan EB. Resection of the obturator nerve for relief of pain in arthritis of the hip joint. J Bone Joint Surg Am 1948;30(1):213–6.
2. Rüdinger N. Die gelenknerven des menschlichen körpers: mit sechs lithographischen tafeln. Erlangen: Verlag von Ferdinand Enke; 1857.
3. Beaunis HE, Bouchard A. Nouveaux éléments d'anatomie descriptive et d'embryologie. Première partie: ostéologie, arthrologie, myologie, angéiologie, névrologie. 3rd edirion. Paris, France: Librairie J. -B. Baillère et Fils; 1879.
4. Chandelux A. Note sur les nerfs de l'articulation coxo-femorale ches l'homme. Lyon Méd 1886;51:551–4.
5. Duzèa R. Note sur les nerfs de l'articulation coxo-fèmorale. Lyon Méd. 1886; 52:35–8.
6. Bardeen CR, Elting AW. A statistical study of the variation in the formation and positions of the lumbo-sacral plexus in man. Anat Anz 1901;19(1):209–32.
7. Billet H, Vincent G, Gaudefroy M. Les nerfs de la hanche. C. R Ass Anat 1947; 34:42–7.
8. Gardner E. The innervation of the hip joint. Anat Rec 1948;101(3):353–71.

9. Tavernier L, Pellanda C. Les nerfs articulaires de la hanche. C R Ass Anat 1949; 36:662–5.

10. Poulhés J, Planel H, Gédéon A. Recherches sur l'innervation de la hanche (Etude anatomique et histologique). C R Ass Anat 1949;590–7.

11. Wertheimer LG. The sensory nerves of the hip joint. J Bone Joint Surg Am 1952; 34(2):477–87.

12. Poláček P. The nerve supply of the hip joint and the knee joint and its features. Anat Anz 1963;112:243–56.

13. Dee R. Structure and function of the hip joint innervation. Ann R Coll Surg Engl 1969;45(6):357–74.

14. Birnbaum K, Prescher A, Hessler S, et al. The sensory innervation of the hip joint - an anatomical study. Surg Radiol Anat 1997;19(6):371–5.

15. Kampa RJ, Prasthofer A, Lawrence-Watt DJ, et al. The internervous safe zone for incision of the capsule of the hip. A cadaver study. J Bone Joint Surg Br 2007; 89(7):971–6.

16. Short AJ, Barnett JJG, Gofeld M, et al. Anatomic study of innervation of the anterior hip capsule: implication for image-guided intervention. Reg Anesth Pain Med 2018;43(2):186–92.

17. Nielsen ND, Greher M, Moriggl B, et al. Spread of injectate around hip articular sensory branches of the femoral nerve in cadavers. Acta Anaesthesiol Scand 2018;62(7):1001–6.

18. Sakamoto J, Manabe Y, Oyamada J, et al. Anatomical study of the articular branches innervated the hip and knee joint with reference to mechanism of referral pain in hip joint disease patients. Clin Anat 2018;31(5):705–9.

19. Cruveilhier J. The anatomy of the human body. New York, NY: Harper and Brothers; 1844.

20. Minne J, Depreux R. Précisions anatomiques sur l'innervation sensitive de la coxo-fémorale. C R Ass Anat 1947;357–9.

21. Kaiser RA. Obturator neurectomy for coxalgia; an anatomical study of the obturator and the accessory obturator nerves. J Bone Joint Surg Am 1949;31(4): 815–9.

22. Larochelle JL, Jobin P. Anatomical research on the innervation of the hip joint. Anat Rec 1949;103(3):480–1.

23. Locher S, Burmeister H, Böhlen T, et al. Radiological anatomy of the obturator nerve and its articular branches: basis to develop a method of radiofrequency denervation for hip joint pain. Pain Med 2008;9(3):291–8.

24. Schmidt JA. Commentarius de nervis lumbalibus eorumque plexu anatomico-pathologicus. Vindobonae 1794;82–3.

25. Eiseler P. Der Plexus lumbosacralis des Menschen. Abh Naturforsch Ges Halle 1892;17:279–364.

26. Patterson AM. The origin and distribution of the nerves to the lower limb. J Anat Physiol 1894;28:84–95.

27. Ancel P, Sencert L. Contribution à l'étude du plexus lombaire chez l'homme. Bibl Anat 1901;9:209–22.

28. Poláček P. Accessory femoral nerve, accessory obturator nerve, and their practical significance in hip joint surgery. Acta Chir Orthop Traumatol Cech 1958; 25(2):150–5.

29. Woodburne RT. The accessory obturator nerve and the innervation of the pectineus muscle. Anat Rec 1960;136(3):367–9.

30. Katritsis E, Anagnostopoulou S, Papadopoulos N. Anatomical observations on the accessory obturator nerve (based on 1000 specimens). Anat Anz 1980; 148(5):440–5.
31. Akkaya T, Comert A, Kendir S, et al. Detailed anatomy of accessory obturator nerve blockade. Minerva Anestesiol 2008;74(4):119–22.
32. Sadovsky DM. Innervation of the capsule of the hip joint. Vestn Khir 1933;31: 100–3. Cited by: Gardner E. The innervation of the hip joint. Anatomical Record. 1948;101(3), 353-371.

# Hip Ablation Techniques

Guy Feigin, MD[a,b,*], Philip W.H. Peng, MBBS, FRCPC[a]

## KEYWORDS

- Radiofrequency ablation, • Osteoarthritis, • Hip, • Articular branches of the hip

## KEY POINTS

- The innervation for the anterior capsule is from femoral, obturator, and accessory obturator nerves (FN, ON, AON).
- The 3 key landmarks for locating the articular branches for FN, AON, and ON are anterior inferior iliac spine, iliopubic eminence, and inferomedial acetabulum.
- The nociceptive fibers concentrate in the anterior capsule, and the innervation for posterior capsule is mainly mechanoreceptors.
- The targets for articular branches for FN and AON are between IPE and AIIS deep to the psoas, and for ON, the target is inferomedial acetabulum.

## BACKGROUND

Pain of the hip can be acute (eg, fracture) or chronic (eg, osteoarthritis). The prevalence of hip pain in the general population in adults over 45 years is 7% to 10%.[1] Osteoarthritis (OA) is the most common cause of chronic hip pain.[2] Rheumatoid arthritis, osteonecrosis, avascular necrosis, labral tears of the acetabulum, post-traumatic arthritis, chronic infectious coxarthrosis, and persistent postoperative pain following total hip arthroplasty (THA) are also important causes of chronic pain in the hip.[2]

Nonsurgical treatment strategies recommended for the management of hip OA include assistive devices, exercise, physical therapy, topical agents, and analgesics such as acetaminophen, nonsteroidal anti-inflammatory drugs, and opioids. Some patients with severe incapacitating disease, however, may fail to respond to these conservative measures because of either low efficacy, increased adverse effects, or severity of disease. Minimally invasive interventional techniques such as intra-articular injection with corticosteroids or hyaluronic acid often fail to provide long-term pain relief.[3] Even though surgical management is an alternative, some patients may not be candidates because of increased risk of surgery secondary to their

Conflicts of interest: None.
[a] Department of Anesthesia & Pain Management, The University of Toronto, Toronto Western Hospital, Women's College Hospital, Wasser Pain Management Clinic, Mount Sinai Hospital, McL 2-405, TWH, 399 Bathurst Street, Toronto, Ontario M5T 2S8, Canada; [b] Department of Anesthesiology, Critical Care and Pain Management the Meir Medical Center, Kfar Saba, Israel
* Corresponding author.
E-mail address: feiginguy1@gmail.com

Phys Med Rehabil Clin N Am 32 (2021) 757–766
https://doi.org/10.1016/j.pmr.2021.05.010
1047-9651/21/© 2021 Elsevier Inc. All rights reserved.

pmr.theclinics.com

comorbid diseases, or they simply may not wish to undergo surgery, which is associated with a concerning failure rate (5%–15%).[4–6]

Radiofrequency ablation (RFA) is emerging as a promising alternative treatment with few complications for patients with chronic hip OA refractory to conservative management or for patients who are not candidates for surgery.[7] Investigators examined the feasibility of ablation of the articular branch network of the hip joint by radiofrequency technique.[8] However, the clinical results were mixed, as there was no clear understanding of the anatomy, specifically the course of articular branches to the hip joint. It reflects the importance of the understanding of the anatomy of the articular branches and the pertinent landmarks.

This article summarizes the current understanding of the anatomy of the articular branches, sonoanatomy, and the suggested techniques for RFA of the hip. It also reviews the literature on the clinical studies.

## PATIENT SELECTION

The most well studied indication in the literature for RFA of hip is chronic hip pain from patients with moderate-to-severe symptomatic osteoarthritis that fails to respond to conservative measures or has limited response to therapeutic or diagnostic injections. In the past, the main option for this group of patients was total hip arthroplasty. However, there are conditions for which patients are not surgical candidates such as patients with significant comorbidities, with conditions that increase possibilities of implant failure (eg, lymphedema of lower limb), or in young patients who have symptomatic OA.[9] Young patients who have symptomatic OA are not considered good candidates for hip arthroplasty because of the limited life span of the implant.[5] Chemical ablation is described in the literature in palliative situations such as metastatic hip disease or inoperable hip fracture.

## TARGET FOR HIP DENERVATION

The anatomy of the articular branches to the hip will be detailed in another article of this issue. In brief, the innervation of the anterior capsule is supplied by 3 nerves: femoral nerve (FN), obturator nerve (ON) and accessory obturator nerve (AON) (**Fig. 1**).

Most of the femoral articular branches can be target between anterior inferior iliac spine (AIIS) and iliopubic eminence (IPE). The accessory obturator nerve courses over the pubic rami in the vicinity of the IPE. The articular branches of the obturator nerve typically pass inferior to the inferomedial acetabulum before they innervate the inferior joint capsule. Thus, the important landmarks for the articular branches for anterior hip capsule are AIIS, IPE, and inferomedial acetabulum. The distribution of these articular branches to the 4 different quadrants of the anterior hip capsule is shown in (**Fig. 2**). Although the sensory innervation for anterior capsule is mainly nociceptive, the posterior capsule is innervated mainly by proprioceptive nerve fibers.

## IMAGING TECHNIQUE

The articular branches from the AON and FN can be found in the fascia plane between the AIIS and IPE deep to the psoas tendon. Both ultrasound and fluoroscopy guidance methods have been described, and all interventions are performed with the patient in the supine position. With ultrasound, the probe is placed over the anterior superior iliac spine (ASIS). The probe is then moved in caudal direction to reveal the AIIS, which is typically deep to the sartorius. At this position, the probe is rotated to align both AIIS and IPE together (**Figs. 3A–C**). Under fluoroscopy, the target for AIIS can be easily

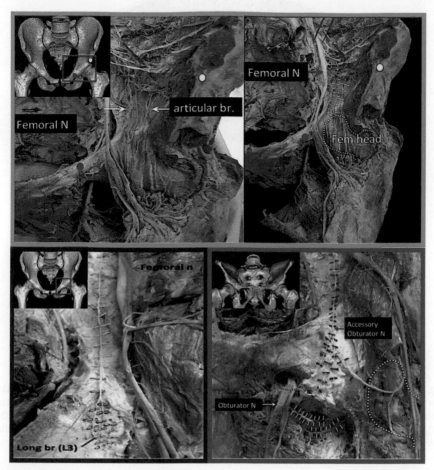

**Fig. 1.** Articular branches of the anterior hip capsule. (*Green box*) Articular branches of the femoral nerve (highlighted on the right with green sutures run between the anterior inferior iliac spine [*yellow dot*] and iliopubic eminence [*red dot*]). (*Blue box*) Accessory obturator nerve runs over the iliopubic eminence. (*Red box*) The obturator nerve comes out from the obturator foramen (circle outlined by red *dotted line*) and divides into anterior and posterior division. The obturator nerve also sends articular branches coursing deep into the inferomedial acetabulum (*) toward the hip joint. In this picture, the accessory obturator can also be seen (highlighted by black suture). The locations of the dissections are all indicated with the insert in the left upper corner. (*Courtesy of* Philip Peng Educational Series.)

discerned. However, this is where the straight head of rectus femoris originates, and the authors suggest placing the needle medial to this. The line joining the AIIS and IPE is not the same as the joint space because of the 3-dimensional shape of the acetabulum (**Fig. 4**).

The landmark for the articular branches from the ON is inferomedial acetabulum. Under fluoroscopy, it appears as a double-walled structure well known as a tear drop (**Fig. 5**). Because this landmark is deep to the femoral neurovascular bundle, the needle is inserted from the side to avoid damaging the femoral nerve and vessels. However, the needle trajectory can be difficult to be estimated, and there are also

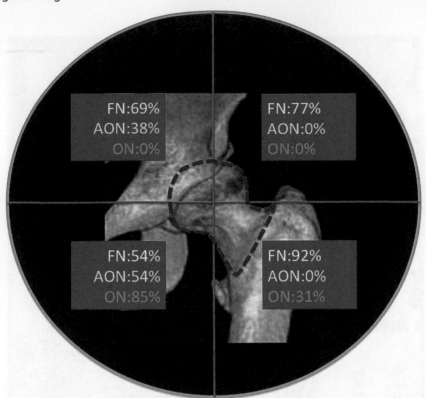

**Fig. 2.** The diagram summarized the contribution of various articular branches to the anterior hip capsule. The articular branches from FN contribute to all 4 quadrants including the weight-bearing superior (medial and lateral) quadrants. Articular branches from the ON only contribute to the lower half and that from accessory obturator nerve (AON) to medial half of the anterior capsule. (*Courtesy of* Philip Peng Educational Series.)

other different vessels in the vicinity of the trajectory such as lateral femoral circumflex artery. The placement under ultrasound has also been described. The initial probe position will be over the hip aligning the acetabulum, femoral head, and neck (**Fig. 6**). The probe is then moved in medial and inferior direction until the disappearance of the femoral head and neck. This part of the acetabulum is the inferomedial acetabulum.

### Diagnostic Block

For the articular branches of AON and FN, the ultrasound probe is placed as described previously. A 22G 3.5 inch spinal needle is inserted in-plane from lateral to medial targeting the space between AIIS and IPE deep to the psoas tendon. The authors prefer placing the needle closer to the IPE, as the AON articular branches are located in that area. After confirming the needle position using hydrolocation, 2 to 3 mL of local anesthetic (0.25% bupivacaine) is injected. An optimal injection should result in transient spread of injectate between the psoas tendon and the pubic bone (**Fig. 7**).

For the articular branches of ON, the authors prefer a combination method with both fluoroscopy and ultrasound guidance. Once the scan shows the inferomedial acetabulum under ultrasound, attention is directed to the vessel (femoral artery itself or the circumflex arteries) in the needle trajectory. An optimal path is determined by rocking the ultrasound probe. A 22G 3.5-inch needle is inserted in-plane from lateral to medial

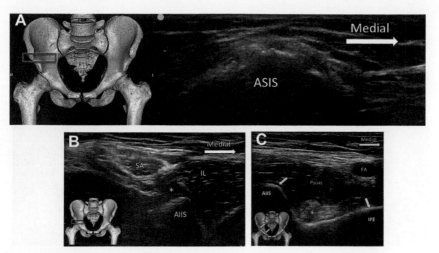

**Fig. 3.** Ultrasound imaging of the femoral and accessory obturator articular branches of hip joint. (*A*) The probe is placed initially over anterior superior iliac spine (ASIS). (*B*) By moving the probe caudally, the AIIS is revealed. The structures around it are sartorius (SA), iliacus (IL), and straight head of rectus femoris (*). (*C*) By rotating the probe to align the AIIS and iliopubic eminence (IPE), the ultrasound reveals the target which is the plane between the psoas muscle/tendon (*) and the pubic bone between AIIS and IPE (*bold arrows*). FA, femoral artery. (Courtesy of Philip Peng Educational Series.)

toward the deep part of inferomedial acetabulum. The position of the needle is assessed with fluoroscopy, and the final position is fine-tuned under fluoroscopic guidance (**Fig. 8**); 1 mL of 0.25% bupivacaine is administered upon confirmation of optimal position.

## ABLATION TECHNIQUE
### Radiofrequency Ablation

The technique is similar to that of the diagnostic block with a few differences. For the ablation of the articular branches of the FN and AON, RF needles are used, and a palisade lesion or a large lesion from cooled RF is suggested because the articular branches span between AIIS and IPE. Thus, 2 or 3 RF needles are required, and a bipolar lesion is created. For the articular branches of ON, only 1 RF needle is required. Motor testing is mandatory, especially in the location of inferomedial acetabulum to assess whether the needle is too close to the main trunk of the ON.

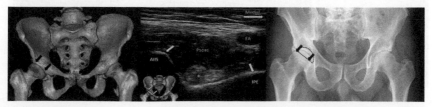

**Fig. 4.** Correlation of the AIIS and iliopubic eminence IPE in 3-dimensional computerized tomography scan reconstruction, ultrasound and radiograph. Both AIIS and IPE are indicated by *bold arrows*. (*Courtesy of* Philip Peng Educational Series.)

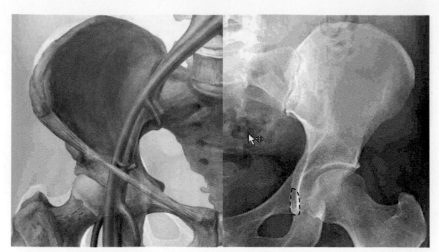

**Fig. 5.** Hybrid diagram to show the radiograph of the pelvis on the right side and pelvis bone on the left side. Note the inferomedial acetabulum (tear drop outlined by *dotted line*) is covered by femoral vessels. (*Courtesy of* Philip Peng Educational Series.)

## Chemical Ablation

Instead of creating thermal injury to the articular branches, chemical is administered instead. Currently, this technique is mainly indicated for palliative care (metastatic disease of hip or inoperable hip fracture) or for patients with significant comorbidity, as more evidence of the safety is required. Both alcohol (100%) and phenol (6%–10%) can be used. For the target between AIIS and IPE, or over the pubofemoral ligament, the authors usually put in 1.5 mL of long-acting local anesthetic first, followed by 3.5 mL of neurolytic agent. If 100% alcohol is used, the final concentration will be 75%. An additional of 1 mL of anesthetic should be injected on removal of the needle to prevent the neurolytic agent from remaining in the soft tissue track. For the target in the inferomedial acetabulum, 0.5 mL of local anesthetic is administered first, then followed by another 1 mL of neurolytic agents. The lower the volume of local anesthetics is injected, the more burning discomfort the patient will experience upon absolute alcohol injection in an exchange for a higher final alcohol concentration. A final concentration of at least 50% alcohol is commonly believed to be the minimum for a long-lasting neurolytic effect.[10–12]

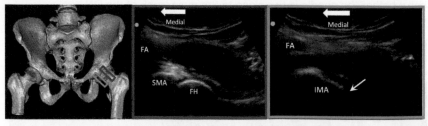

**Fig. 6.** Ultrasound scanning of the inferomedial acetabulum. The left figure shows the position of the ultrasound probes (*red* and *green boxes*). The corresponding images are shown in *red* and *green boxes*. FA, femoral artery; F, femoral head; IMA, inferomedial acetabulum; SMA, superomedial acetabulum. (*Courtesy of* Philip Peng Educational Series.)

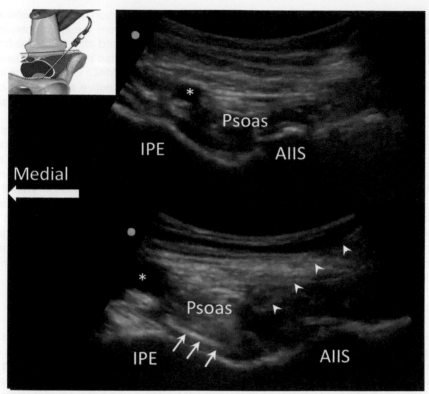

**Fig. 7.** Needle placement is performed by inserting the needle in-plane from lateral to medial toward the pubic bone between the AIIS and IPE. A successful injectate is indicated by the lifting of the psoas fascia. *-femoral artery. The needle is indicated by the *arrowheads*. (*Courtesy of* Philip Peng Educational Series.)

## EFFICACY OF HIP ABLATION

A comprehensive review of literature in RF ablation was performed by Pranab and colleagues.[13] There is no randomized controlled trial but 16 case series or reports. Of the 10-case series, 3 are prospective and 7 are retrospective. The duration of follow-up varied substantially, from 8 days to 3 years. All reported pain

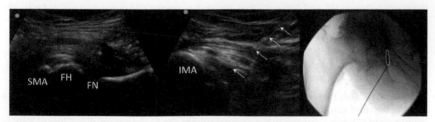

**Fig. 8.** Combined ultrasound and fluoroscopy-guided needle placement. (*Left*) The sonograph shows the superomedial acetabulum (SMA) and femoral head and neck (FH, FN). (*Middle*) Sonograph shows the needle insertion to the inferior aspect of the inferomedial acetabulum (IMA). (*Right*) Radiograph shows the corresponding needle placement. Tear drop or IMA is highlighted. (*Courtesy of* Philip Peng Educational Series.)

relief following the RFA, ranging from 30% to over 90% reduction from the baseline. Most studies did not document the opioids-sparing effect from the RF procedure. Kapural and colleagues[14] reported the use of opioids before and after the procedure but failed to find a difference. Most studies did not use validated measures for functional outcome such as Western Ontario and McMaster (WOMAC) Osteoarthritis Index, Harris Hip Score, or Oxford Hip Score, but used subjective assessment on function such as sleep or ambulation instead. For those studies including these validated scores, they usually documented meaningful improvement.

For chemical ablation, the literature is scant. The initial description of a purely ultrasound-guided pericapsular alcohol neurolysis in a patient with inoperable hip fracture was from Sasaki and colleagues in early 2018.[12] The procedure involved infiltrations of a high volume of the local anesthetic superficial to the pubofemoral and iliofemoral ligament over the hip capsule followed by the use of alcohol. With the recent understanding of the anatomy of the anterior capsule innervation, the use of chemical ablation with a much lower volume of injectate had been used in a case series of inoperable hip fractures and a patient with hip metastasis. In particular, a large case series on chemical ablation of 20 patients with inoperable hip fractures showed promising analgesic effect, with half of the cohort able to sit up within 5 days.[10]

## ADVERSE EVENTS WITH HIP ABLATION

Hip RF denervation of the articular branches of the femoral and obturator nerves is a relatively safe procedure with minimal complications; nonetheless, adverse effects of the procedure were reported in some publications. These included loss of sensation in the cutaneous distribution of the ON and FN.[15–17] Hematoma caused by blood vessel puncture and numbness in lateral thigh with RF lesioning using the anterior vertical approach for ablation of the articular branches of the ON was reported in 1 publication. However, this can be avoided with an ultrasound-guided lateral approach insertion of the needle to the inferomedial acetabulum.[18]

## CLINICS CARE POINTS

- When targeting the AON and FN, the needle entry site is close to the lateral femoral cutaneous nerve. After infiltrating the skin with a smaller needle, if the patient complains of tingling sensation down the lateral thigh, it is an indication to reposition the needle.

- Consider prognostic blocks with local anesthetics prior to RF ablation. Considering the size of the space between IPE and AIIS with that for medial branch of lumbar or cervical facet, the authors prefer a larger volume of 2 to 3 mL. This volume is not sufficient to spill to the femoral nerve, which is in the plane superficial not deep to the psoas muscle.

- With fluoroscopy, the tear drop appears to be a double-wall structure. The authors highly suggest placement of the needle on the middle or lateral aspect of the tear drop to avoid being too close to the trunk of the ON.

- Charcot joint rarely happens in RFA, as the essential elements for Charcot joint are complete denervation and vascular compromise. With the principle of partial denervation and avoidance of extensive damage to the vascular supply, the RF did not result in Charcot joint in the literature.

- A combined use of ultrasound and fluoroscopy for lateral insertion of the cannula toward the obturator articular branch to avoid damaging neurovascular structures is strongly recommended.

• Following the insertion of the needle deep to the psoas between IPE and AIIS, the authors highly suggest rotating the needle to allow piercing action on the psoas fascia. If high pressure is encountered, the needle is likely to be in the iliofemoral ligament, and the needle should be withdrawn slightly. If this maneuver does not result in lifting of the psoas fascia, the needle can be repositioned to a slightly more medial location.

## DISCLOSURES

None.

## REFERENCES

1. Bergmann G, Deuretzbacher G, Heller M, et al. Hip contact forces and gait patterns from routine activities. J Biomech 2001;34(7):859–71.
2. Battaglia PJ, D'Angelo K, Kettner NW. Posterior, lateral, and anterior hip pain due to musculoskeletal origin: a narrative literature review of history, physical examination, and diagnostic imaging. J Chiropractic Med 2016;15(4): 281–93.
3. Flanagan J, Casale FF, Thomas TL, et al. Intra-articular injection for pain relief in patients awaiting hip replacement. Ann R Coll Surg Engl 1988;70(3):156–7.
4. Hip and knee replacements: Canadian Joint Replacement Registry 2013.. Available at: https://secure.cihi.ca/estore/productFamily.htm?pf= PFC2209&lang= en&media=0. Accessed November 27, 2020.
5. Grayson CW, Decker RC. Total joint arthroplasty for persons with osteoarthritis. PM R 2012;4(Suppl 5):S97–103.
6. Belmont PJ Jr, Powers CC, Beykirch SE, et al. Results of the anatomic medullary locking total hip arthroplasty at a minimum of twenty years. A concise follow-up of previous reports. J Bone Joint Surg Am 2008;90(7):1524–30.
7. Hernández-González L, Calvo CE, Atkins-González D. Peripheral nerve radiofrequency neurotomy: hip and knee joints. Phys Med Rehabil Clin N Am 2018;29(1): 61–71.
8. Bhatia A, Hoydonckx Y, Peng P, et al. Radiofrequency procedures to relieve chronic hip pain: an evidence-based narrative review. Reg Anesth Pain Med 2018;43(1):72–83.
9. Tönnis D, Legal H, Graf R. Congenital dysplasia and dislocation of the AQ3 hip in children and adults. Berlin, Germany: Springer Verlag; 1987.
10. Kwun-Tung Ng T, Chan WS, Peng PWH, et al. Chemical hip denervation for inoperable hip fracture. Anesth Analg 2020;130(2):498–504.
11. Rocha Romero A, Carvajal Valdy G, Lemus AJ. Ultrasound-guided pericapsular nerve group (PENG) hip joint phenol neurolysis for palliative pain. Can J Anaesth 2019;66(10):1270–1.
12. Sasaki S, Chan WS, Ng TK, et al. Ultrasound-guided pericapsular hip joint alcohol neurolysis for the treatment of hip pain: a case report of a novel approach. A A Pract 2018;11(3):60–2.
13. Kumar P, Hoydonckx Y, Bhatia A. A review of current denervation techniques for chronic hip pain: anatomical and technical considerations [published correction appears in Curr Pain Headache Rep 2019 May 28;23(6):45]. Curr Pain Headache Rep 2019;23(6):38.
14. Kapural L, Jolly S, Mantoan J, et al. Cooled radiofrequency neurotomy of the articular sensory branches of the obturator and femoral nerves - combined approach using fluoroscopy and ultrasound guidance: technical report, and

observational study on safety and efficacy. Pain Physician 2018;21(3): 279–84.

15. Akatov OV, Dreval ON. Percutaneous radiofrequency destruction of the obturator nerve for treatment of pain caused by coxarthrosis. Stereotact Funct Neurosurg 1997;69(1–4 Pt 2):278–80.

16. Malik A, Simopolous T, Elkersh M, et al. Percutaneous radiofrequency lesioning of sensory branches of the obturator and femoral nerves for the treatment of non-operable hip pain. Pain Physician 2003;6(4):499–502.

17. Cortiñas-Sáenz M, Salmerón-Velez G, Holgado-Macho IA. Bloqueo intraarticular y de ramas sensoriales de los nervios obturador y femoral en cuadro de osteo-necrosis y artrosis de cabeza femoral [Joint and sensory branch block of the obturator and femoral nerves in a case of femoral head osteonecrosis and arthritis]. Rev Esp Cir Ortop Traumatol 2014;58(5):319–24.

18. Rivera F, Mariconda C, Annaratone G. Percutaneous radiofrequency denervation in patients with contraindications for total hip arthroplasty. Orthopedics 2012; 35(3):e302–5.

# Overview of Innervation of Knee Joint

John Tran, HBSc, PhD[a],*, Philip W.H. Peng, MBBS, FRCPC[b],
Vincent W.S. Chan, MD, FRCPC[b], Anne M.R. Agur, BSc(OT), MSc, PhD[a]

## KEYWORDS

• Knee joint • Innervation • Anatomy • Denervation

## KEY POINTS

• Knee joint innervation is extensive, with articular nerves originating as single or multiple branches from the femoral, obturator, and sciatic nerves.
• The innervation pattern of the anterior and posterior aspects of the knee joint capsule is relatively consistent, with some variation in supply by the saphenous, anterior division of obturator, and common fibular nerves.
• To improve nerve capture rates for diagnostic block and radiofrequency ablation, multiple target sites may be necessary.
• Further clinical research is required to assess pain relief and functional outcomes of multiple target sites.

## INTRODUCTION

More recently, image-guided diagnostic block and radiofrequency ablation (RFA) of the genicular nerves have emerged as an alternative management strategy for chronic knee joint pain. To effectively utilize image-guided diagnostic block and RFA to manage pain, a detailed understanding of the location of articular branches supplying the knee joint, in relation to soft tissue and bony landmarks, is required. This article reviews the innervation of the knee joint to describe the origin and course of articular nerves and identify bony and soft tissue landmarks, visible with image-guidance, that can be used to localize the articular nerves. Dissections documenting the innervation of the knee joint capsule in this article were carried out in the authors' laboratory.

[a] Division of Anatomy, Department of Surgery, Temerty Faculty of Medicine, University of Toronto, 1 King's College Circle, Room 1158, Toronto, Ontario M5S 1A8, Canada; [b] Department of Anesthesia and Pain Management, Toronto Western Hospital, University of Toronto, 399 Bathurst Street, McL 2-405, Toronto, Ontario M5T 2S8, Canada
* Corresponding author.
E-mail address: johnjt.tran@utoronto.ca

Phys Med Rehabil Clin N Am 32 (2021) 767–778
https://doi.org/10.1016/j.pmr.2021.05.011
1047-9651/21/© 2021 Elsevier Inc. All rights reserved.
pmr.theclinics.com

## INNERVATION OF THE KNEE JOINT CAPSULE

Previous cadaveric studies have identified numerous sources of knee joint innervation including branches originating from femoral, obturator, and sciatic nerves (**Table 1**). The innervation of the knee joint is extensive (**Figs. 1 and 2**), and the course of each nerve will be described.

### Femoral Nerve

Twelve cadaveric studies were found that reported articular branches from the femoral nerve supplying the knee joint capsule (see **Table 1**). More specifically, the articular nerves originated from muscular branches of the nerves to vastus medialis (NVM), lateralis (NVL), and intermedius (NVI), as well as from the infrapatellar branch of the saphenous nerve (IPBSN), a cutaneous branch.

#### Nerve to vastus medialis

Of the 12 studies investigating the femoral nerve, 10 studies reported innervation of the knee joint capsule from the NVM (see **Table 1**). Most studies found 2 to 3 branches of the NVM that coursed antero-inferiorly through the vastus medialis obliquus to terminate in the superomedial knee joint capsule[1–5] Horner and Dellon[6] also reported contribution of NVM to the superomedial knee joint capsule but recommended it should be termed the "medial retinacular nerve." In contrast, Gardner,[7] in one of the earliest studies, also reported that the NVM descended along the medial edge of the vastus medialis and distally gave off articular branches that coursed deep to the muscle to supply the superomedial capsule. Although the descriptions of the course of the NVM varied, the articular branches were found to supply the anteromedial/superomedial knee joint capsule in all studies (**Fig. 2C**).

The articular branches of NVM can be localized using ultrasound guidance as they course through the vastus medialis obliquus to the medial border of the patella. Thus, the identification of these branches relies on soft tissue landmarking.

#### Superior medial genicular nerve

The superior medial genicular nerve (SMGN) has been previously described as a branch of the tibial nerve[7,8]; however, in other cadaveric studies, SMGN was found to be a terminal branch of the NVM originating from the femoral nerve.[3,5] The SMGN coursed along the posteromedial surface of the vastus medialis and continued to descend along the adductor magnus tendon (see **Fig. 2C**). The SMGN gave off articular branches proximal and distal to the adductor tubercle, which supplied the superomedial knee joint capsule and medial femoral condyle.[9] These articular branches were located more posterior and inferior to the site of termination of the articular branches of NVM, which coursed intramuscularly (see **Fig. 2C**).

Along its course, the SMGN can be localized using the tendon of the adductor magnus and descending genicular artery. More specifically, the proximal branches of SMGN can be located at the junction of the femoral shaft and medial femoral condyle, whereas the distal branches can be found at or just inferior to the adductor tubercle.

#### Nerve to vastus lateralis

The NVL was reported to innervate the superolateral knee joint in 9 previous studies (see **Table 1**). In all studies, the NVL was found to course deep to the vastus lateralis and terminate in the anterolateral/superolateral capsule (see **Fig. 2B**). The frequency of innervation for the NVL was variable. Tran and colleagues[3] reported the presence of articular branches of NVL in all specimens, whereas Sakamoto and colleagues[4] reported articular branches in only 1 of 14 specimens.

**Table 1**
Previous dissection studies of the innervation of knee joint capsule

| Origin | SCN CFN | SCN SLGN | SCN LRN | SCN LAN | SCN ILGN | SCN RFN | SCN TN | SCN IMGN | FN IPBSN | FN NVM | FN/SCN SMGN | FN NVL | FN NVI | ON AON | ON PON |
|---|---|---|---|---|---|---|---|---|---|---|---|---|---|---|---|
| Gardner,[7] 1948 | Y | Y | X | X | Y | Y | Y | Y | Y | Y | Y[a] | Y | Y | Y | Y |
| Kennedy et al,[10] 1982 | X | X | X | Y | X | Y | Y | X | Y | Y | X | Y | Y | X | Y |
| Horner & Dellon,[6] 1994 | X | Y | Y | Y[c] | X | Y | Y | X | Y | Y[b] | X | Y | Y | X | Y |
| Hirasawa et al,[2] 2000 | Y | X | X | X | X | X | Y | X | Y | Y | Y | Y | X | X | X |
| Franco et al,[11] 2015 | X | X | X | X | X | Y | - | X | Y | Y | X | Y | Y | X | - |
| Kalthur et al,[13] 2015 | - | - | - | - | - | - | - | - | X | - | - | - | - | - | - |
| Yasar et al,[8] 2015 | - | - | - | - | - | - | - | Y | - | - | Y[a] | - | - | - | - |
| Burckett-St Laurant et al,[1] 2016 | - | - | - | - | - | - | - | X | Y | Y | Y | - | - | X | - |
| Sutaria et al,[16] 2017 | - | Y | Y | - | - | - | - | - | - | - | - | - | - | - | - |
| Valls et al,[12] 2017 | X | X | Y | X | X | Y | Y | X | Y | Y | X | Y | Y | X | Y |
| Tran et al,[3] 2018 | Y | Y | X | X | Y | Y | - | Y | Y | Y | Y | Y | Y | X | - |
| Sakamoto et al,[4] 2018 | X | X | X | X | X | X | X | X | X | Y | X | Y | Y | Y | X |
| Tran et al,[14] 2019 | Y | - | - | - | - | - | Y | - | - | - | - | - | - | - | Y |
| Fonkoue et al,[5] 2019 | X | Y | Y | X | X | Y | Y | Y | Y | Y | X | Y | Y | Y | X |

AON, anterior division of obturator nerve; CFN, common fibular nerve; FN, femoral nerve; ILGN, inferior lateral genicular nerve; IMGN, inferior medial genicular nerve; IPBSN, infrapatellar branch of saphenous nerve; LAN, lateral articular nerve; LRN, lateral retinacular nerve; NVI, nerve to vastus intermedius; NVL, nerve to vastus lateralis; NVM, nerve to vastus medialis; ON, obturator nerve; PON, posterior division of obturator nerve; RFN, recurrent fibular nerve; SCN, sciatic nerve; SLGN, superior lateral genicular nerve; SMGN, superior medial genicular nerve; TN, tibial nerve; X, not found; Y, found; -, not investigated.

[a] Branch of tibial nerve originating from sciatic nerve.
[b] Recommended to be named medial retinacular nerve.
[c] Recommended to be named articular branches of CFN.

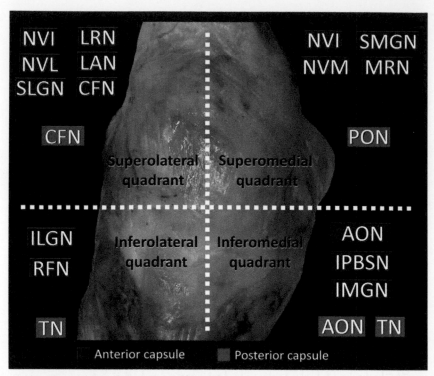

**Fig. 1.** Summary of the innervation of the anterior and posterior aspects of the knee joint capsule by quadrants. AON indicates anterior division of obturator nerve; CFN, common fibular nerve; ILGN, inferior lateral genicular nerve; IMGN, inferior medial genicular nerve; IPBSN, infrapatellar branch of saphenous nerve; LAN, lateral articular nerve; LRN, lateral retinacular nerve; MRN, medial retinacular nerve; NVI, nerve to vastus intermedius; NVL, nerve to vastus lateralis; NVM, nerve to vastus medialis; PON, posterior division of obturator nerve; RFN, recurrent fibular nerve; SLGN, superior lateral genicular nerve; SMGN, superior medial genicular nerve; TN, tibial nerve. (*Courtesy of* Philip Peng Educational Series.)

The articular branches of NVL can be localized using soft-tissue and bony landmarks. Proximal to the quadriceps tendon, the NVL can be located in a plane between the vastus lateralis and intermedius. At the level of the base of the patella, the articular branches of NVL can be localized adjacent to the lateral border of the patella (see **Fig. 2**B).

### Nerve to vastus intermedius

The articular branches of the NVI were reported by 8 cadaveric studies (see **Table 1**). Of the 8 studies found, 7 described the articular branches of NVI coursing deep to the vastus intermedius muscle along the anterior/anteromedial aspect of the femur.[3,5–7,10,11] In 1 study,[12] the nerve was described as descending along the fascia between the vastus lateralis and intermedius muscles. Tran and colleagues[3] found distinct medial and lateral articular branches of NVI. These branches coursed along the anteromedial and anterolateral aspect of the distal femur, deep to vastus intermedius, to supply the suprapatellar bursa and superomedial/superolateral knee joint capsule (see **Fig. 2**A and C). This pattern was consistent with the illustration of articular branches of NVI by Gardner.[7]

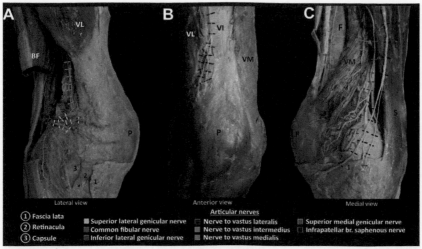

**Fig. 2.** Articular nerves supplying the anterior knee joint capsule. (*A*) Articular innervation of the anterolateral knee joint capsule. (*B*) Articular innervation from nerve to vastus lateralis. (*C*) Articular innervation of the anteromedial knee joint capsule. BF, biceps femoris (cut); F, femoral shaft; P, patella; S, sartorius; VI, vastus intermedius; VL, vastus lateralis; VM, vastus medialis. (*Courtesy of* Philip Peng Educational Series.)

Both soft tissue and bony landmarks could be used to localize the articular branches of NVI. The medial and lateral articular branches of NVI can be identified in the distal third of the thigh as they course between the deep surface of the vastus intermedius and the anterior surface of the femoral shaft (see **Fig. 2**A and C).

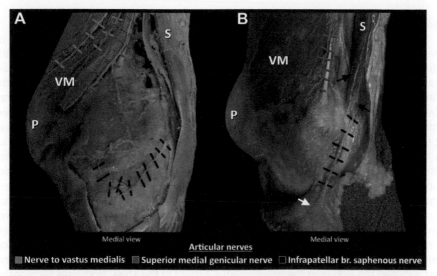

**Fig. 3.** Dissection of course and termination of infrapatellar branch of saphenous nerve (IPBSN). (*A*) Termination of the IPBSN in a knee joint capsule. (*B*) Termination of the IPBSN in subcutaneous tissue (*white arrow*). P, patella; S, sartorius; VM, vastus medialis; black arrows, IPBSN piercing the sartorius. (*Courtesy of* Philip Peng Educational Series.)

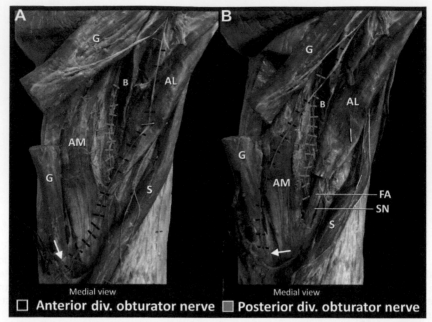

Medial view                    Medial view

☐ **Anterior div. obturator nerve** ■ **Posterior div. obturator nerve**

**Fig. 4.** Course of anterior (AON) and posterior (PON) divisions of the obturator nerve. (*A*) Course of AON showing its termination in subcutaneous tissue (*white arrow*). (*B*) Course of PON in the adductor canal. Inferiorly, note the PON coursing with the femoral artery toward the adductor hiatus. The AON has been retracted posteriorly to reveal the distal course of the PON. AL, adductor longus; AM, adductor magnus; B, adductor brevis; FA, femoral artery; G, gracilis; S, sartorius; SN, saphenous nerve. (*Courtesy of* Philip Peng Educational Series.)

*Saphenous nerve*
In 11 cadaveric studies, the infrapatellar branch of saphenous nerve (IPBSN) was investigated (see **Table 1**). The IPBSN, in 9 studies, was reported to innervate the knee joint capsule below the joint line. Hirasawa and colleagues[2] described a main branch that originated from the saphenous nerve and coursed inferiorly along the anterolateral edge of the sartorius and turned anteriorly to supply a "wide area covering the articular capsule." Horner and Dellon[6] also reported innervation of the anterior inferior knee joint capsule. Similar to these 2 studies, Tran and colleagues[3] reported the IPBSN originating from the saphenous nerve emerging anterior or posterior to the sartorius and coursed anteroinferiorly to the inferomedial aspect of the knee joint. However, Tran and colleagues[3] reported only the presence of articular branches supplying the knee joint capsule in 3 out of 15 specimens. These articular branches, when present, terminated in the inferomedial aspect of knee joint anterior to the sartorius and deep to the fascia lata/crural fascia (**Fig. 3**A). In the remaining 12 specimens, the IPBSN terminated in the subcutaneous tissue (see **Figs. 2C and 3**B). This was consistent with Kalthur and colleagues,[13] who investigated the course and branching pattern of the IPBSN in 32 specimens. The IPBSN was found to be a cutaneous nerve that supplied the skin over the anteromedial aspect of the knee; branches terminating in the knee joint capsule were not reported. Kalthur and colleagues[13] found the IPBSN can be related to the apex of the patella and tibial tuberosity. In 65.6% of specimens the division of the IPBSN was located between the apex of patella and tibial tuberosity.

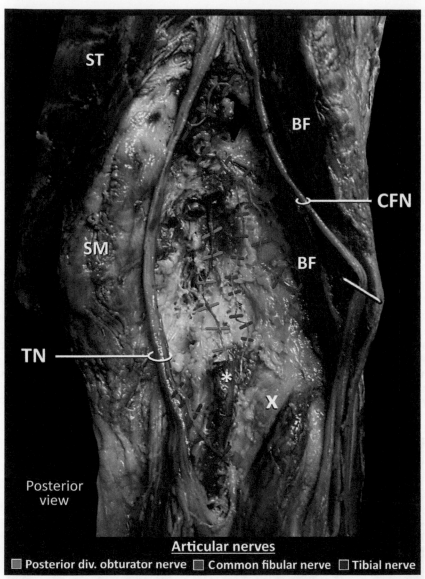

**Fig. 5.** Articular nerves supplying the posterior knee joint capsule. Asterisk, popliteal vessels; BF, biceps femoris; CFN, common fibular nerve; SM, semimembranosus; ST, semitendinosus; TN, tibial nerve; x, lateral femoral condyle. (*Courtesy of* Philip Peng Educational Series.)

## Obturator Nerve

The innervation of the knee joint capsule by the anterior and/or posterior division of obturator nerve was investigated in 10 previous cadaveric studies (see **Table 1**). Only 3 of these studies reported innervation of the knee joint capsule by anterior division of the obturator nerve (AON), whereas 5 studies found contribution from the posterior division of the obturator nerve (PON).

### Anterior division of obturator nerve

In 2 of the 3 studies reporting AON innervation, Sakamoto and colleagues[4] and Gardner[7] described innervation to the anteromedial aspect of the knee joint. Posteromedial innervation was found only by Fonkoue and colleagues.[5] The course of the articular branch of AON has been related to the adductor longus muscle.[4,5] Sakamoto and colleagues[4] described the articular branch of AON coursing "down the adductor longus after converging with the saphenous nerve" to supply the knee joint capsule. Similarly, Gardner[7] described possible innervation from an anastomosis between the AON and the articular branch of the saphenous nerve. Fonkoue and colleagues[5] described the articular branch of AON as coursing along the posterior aspect of the adductor longus, through the adductor hiatus, to enter the popliteal fossa to innervate the posteromedial capsule. Based on the descriptions by Sakamoto and colleagues[4] and Fonkoue and colleagues,[5] the posterior surface of the adductor longus, proximal to the adductor canal, may be used to localize the articular branch of AON.

### Posterior division of obturator nerve

The PON, after supplying the adductor muscles, continues distally along the anterior surface of the adductor magnus to reach the adductor hiatus (**Fig. 4**). Horner and Dellon[6] reported this distal branch coursing through the adductor hiatus, fascially bound to the popliteal artery, to enter the popliteal fossa where it "ramified about the genicular vasculature" to supply the posterior knee joint capsule. This was consistent with Tran and colleagues,[14] who reported the genicular branch of PON coursing through the adductor hiatus and descending to the level of the superior border of the medial femoral condyle, where it further divided into 2 to 3 articular branches to supply the posterior capsule.

In the 5 dissection studies that found articular branches of PON, the frequency of innervation was reported in only 2 studies.[7,14] Gardner[7] found articular branches of PON in 9 out of 11 specimens, and Tran and colleagues[14] found them in all 15

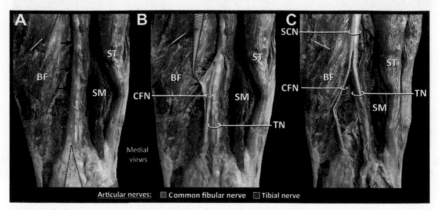

**Fig. 6.** Serial dissection to reveal origin of articular nerves from the common fibular and tibia nerves. (*A*) Exposure of fascial sheath (*black arrows*) surrounding the popliteal neurovascular structures. Fat in the popliteal fossa has been removed proximally. Note the dotted line outlines the apparent bifurcation of the sciatic nerve. (*B*) Incision and reflection of fascial sheath (*black arrow*) to reveal common fibular and tibial nerves. (*C*) The fascial sheath has been removed to expose the actual bifurcation site of the sciatic nerve into the common fibular and tibial nerves. BF, biceps femoris; CFN, common fibular nerve; SCN, sciatic nerve; SM, semimembranosus; ST, semitendinosus; TN, tibial nerve. (*Courtesy of* Philip Peng Educational Series.)

specimens. Additionally, in a dye injection study, Runge and colleagues[15] reported articular branches of PON in 10 out of 10 specimens. Articular branches of PON can be localized using their relationship to the popliteal artery at the level of the medial femoral condyle (**Fig. 5**).

## Sciatic Nerve

Previous studies have reported articular nerves originating from the sciatic nerve (SCN) and its terminal branches (ie, the common fibular [peroneal] and tibial nerves) (see **Table 1**). The course and termination of the articular nerves originating from the SCN will be described first, followed by those from the common fibular (CFN) and tibial (TN) nerves.

### Superior lateral genicular nerve

The superior lateral genicular nerve (SLGN) was found to course deep to the biceps femoris tendon and iliotibial tract and the biceps femoris toward the posterosuperior angle of the lateral femoral condyle; additionally, it shared a common trunk with articular branches of the CFN and coursed along the posterolateral aspect of the femur joining the superior lateral genicular artery (see **Fig. 2**A). Sutaria and colleagues[16] reported the SLGN gave off the lateral retinacular nerve (LRN) at the lateral aspect of the knee. Fonkoue and colleagues[5] described the SLGN divided into a transversal branch (LRN) and a longitudinal branch descending toward the femoro-tibial space. In contrast, Tran and colleagues[3] reported in 5 of 15 specimens the SLGN originating from the SCN and in the remaining 10 specimens originating from an articular nerve of the CFN (see **Fig. 2**A). In the specimens where SLGN originated from the SCN, it descended to the level of the superior border of the lateral femoral condyle to accompany the superior lateral genicular artery (SLGA). The SLGN can be localized using the SLGA at the junction of the femoral shaft and lateral femoral condyle (see **Fig. 2**A).

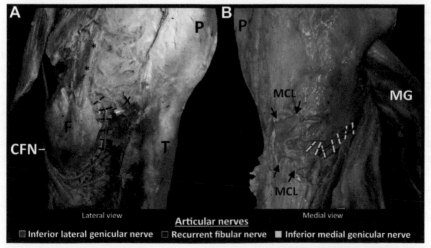

**Fig. 7.** Articular nerves supplying the anteroinferior knee joint capsule. (*A*) Branches from the inferior lateral genicular and recurrent fibular nerves. (*B*) Branches from the inferior medial genicular nerve. *Asterisk*, lateral collateral ligament of the knee; *Black arrows*, cut edge of medial collateral ligament of knee; CFN, common fibular nerve; F, head of fibula; MCL, medial collateral ligament of knee; MG, medial head of gastrocnemius; P, patella; T, tibia; X, Gerdy tubercle. (*Courtesy of* Philip Peng Educational Series.)

*Common fibular nerve*
The CFN has been found to give off articular nerves that innervated the lateral aspect of the knee joint capsule (see **Table 1**). Kennedy and colleagues[10] described a lateral articular nerve (LAN) originating from the CFN at the level of the joint line that supplied the inferior portion of the lateral capsule and lateral collateral ligament of the knee. Horner and Dellon[6] also found innervation from the LAN but recommended it should be named articular branches of the common peroneal nerve. Similarly, in 10 of 15 specimens, Tran and colleagues[3] found an articular nerve originating from the CFN just inferior to the bifurcation of SCN (**Fig. 6**). This articular nerve at the level of the superior border of the lateral femoral condyle gave off the SLGN that accompanied the SLGA (see **Fig. 2**A). The articular nerve continued to course inferiorly, where it gave off several articular branches to the lateral aspect of the knee joint and then terminated as the inferior lateral genicular nerve (ILGN) accompanying the inferior lateral genicular artery (ILGA). In this study, the SLGN and ILGN were defined based on their close relationship to the SLGA and ILGA, respectively. The articular branches of CFN can be localized at the level of the lateral femoral condyle, just posterosuperior to the lateral epicondyle (see **Fig. 2**A).

In 2 studies, articular nerves from the CFN were identified that supplied the posterior knee joint capsule.[2,14] Hirasawa and colleagues[2] described this articular nerve as descending deep to the long head of the biceps femoris to innervate the posterior and lateral joint capsule. Tran and colleagues[14] called this nerve the posterior branch of CFN, as it coursed distally, lateral to the popliteal vein, to terminate in the superolateral aspect of the posterior knee joint capsule. When present, the posterior branch of CFN innervating the posterior knee joint capsule can be localized using the popliteal vein at the level of the lateral femoral condyle (see **Fig. 5**).

The recurrent fibular nerve (RFN) originates from the CFN at the neck of the fibula and then courses superiorly to reach the anterolateral knee joint capsule.[3,6,10] Gardner,[7] Horner and Dellon,[6] and Fonkoue and colleagues[5] also reported innervation of the proximal tibiofibular joint by the RFN. The RFN can be localize anterior to the head of the fibular, posterior to Gerdy tubercle (**Fig. 7**A).

*Tibial nerve*
In the previous literature, the TN has been reported to consistently contribute articular branches to the popliteal plexus of nerves supplying the posterior knee joint capsule.[6,7,14] Gardner[7] reported these branches could emerge from the SCN before its bifurcation. Horner and Dellon[6] found the articular branches of TN to originate 10 to 25 cm above the joint line. Tran and colleagues[14] identified superior and inferior articular branches of TN emerging superior and/or inferior to the superior border of the femoral condyles. All of these studies also found contribution to the popliteal plexus from the PON. In addition, Tran and colleagues[14] reported CFN contribution in 11 out of 15 specimens (see **Fig. 5**). The articular branches of the popliteal plexus coursed medial, lateral, and/or between the popliteal vessels to innervate the posterior capsule of the knee joint. Landmarks to localize the popliteal plexus include the popliteal vessels as they coursed distally in the intercondylar region (see **Fig. 5**).

*Inferior medial genicular nerve*
Gardner,[7] Tran and colleagues,[3] and Fonkoue and colleagues[5] found innervation to the anterior knee joint from the inferior medial genicular nerve (IMGN). In 2 studies,[3,7] the IMGN was reported to originated from the TN, whereas 1 study[5] reported origin from the SCN. Regardless of its origin, the IMGN accompanied the inferior medial genicular artery to course deep to the tibial collateral ligament to supply the anterior knee

joint capsule. The IMGN can be localized deep to the tibial collateral ligament just inferior to the medial tibial condyle (see **Fig. 7**B).

## SUMMARY

The nerve supply to the knee joint capsule is extensive. The anterior capsule is innervated by articular branches originating from the femoral (NVI, NVL, NVM, SMGN, IPBSN) and sciatic (SLGN, CFN, ILGN, RFN, IMGN) nerves, whereas the posterior capsule receives innervation from the obturator (PON) and sciatic (CFN, TN) nerves.

## CLINICAL PEARLS

In the context of diagnostic block and RFA, the extensive innervation of the knee joint suggests improvements in nerve capture rates require multiple target/lesion sites. Further clinical studies are required to determine feasibility and analgesic implications.

## DISCLOSURE

Anne Agur is an anatomy faculty member with Allergan Academy of Excellence.
  Philip Peng received equipment support from Fujifilm Sonosite Canada.

## ACKNOWLEDGMENT

The authors wish to acknowledge the individuals who donated their bodies and tissue for the advancement of education and research.

## REFERENCES

1. Burckett-St Laurant D, Peng P, Girón Arango L, et al. The nerves of the adductor canal and the innervation of the knee: an anatomic study. Reg Anesth Pain Med 2016;41(3):321–7.
2. Hirasawa Y, Okajima S, Ohta M, et al. Nerve distribution to the human knee joint: Anatomical and immunohistochemical study. Int Orthop 2000;24(1):1–4.
3. Tran J, Peng P, Lam K, et al. Anatomical study of the innervation of anterior knee joint capsule: implication for image-guided intervention. Reg Anesth Pain Med 2018;43(4):407–14.
4. Sakamoto J, Manabe Y, Oyamada J, et al. Anatomical study of the articular branches innervated the hip and knee joint with reference to mechanism of referral pain in hip joint disease patients. Clin Anat 2018;31(5):705–9.
5. Fonkoué L, Behets C, Kouassi J, et al. Distribution of sensory nerves supplying the knee joint capsule and implications for genicular blockade and radiofrequency ablation: an anatomical study. Surg Radiol Anat 2019;41(12):1461–71.
6. Horner G, Dellon A. Innervation of the human knee joint and implications for surgery. Clin Orthop Relat Res 1994;6(301):221–6.
7. Gardner E. The innervation of the knee joint. Anat Rec 1948;101(1):109–30.
8. Yasar E, Kesikburun S, Kılıç C, et al. Accuracy of ultrasound-guided genicular nerve block: a cadaveric study. Pain Physician 2015;18(5):E899–904.
9. Tran J, Peng P, Agur A. Evaluation of nerve capture using classical landmarks for genicular nerve radiofrequency ablation: a 3D cadaveric study. Reg Anesth Pain Med 2020;45(11):898–906.
10. Kennedy J, Alexander I, Hayes K. Nerve supply of the human knee and its functional importance. Am J Sports Med 1982;10(6):329–35.

11. Franco C, Buvanendran A, Petersohn J, et al. Innervation of the anterior capsule of the human knee: implications for radiofrequency ablation. Reg Anesth Pain Med 2015;40(4):363–8.
12. Valls J, Vallejo R, Pais P, et al. Anatomic and ultrasonographic evaluation of the knee sensory innervation a cadaveric study to determine anatomic targets in the treatment of chronic knee pain. Reg Anesth Pain Med 2017;42(1):90–8.
13. Kalthur S, Sumalatha S, Nair N, et al. Anatomic study of infrapatellar branch of saphenous nerve in male cadavers. Ir J Med Sci 2015;184(1):201–6.
14. Tran J, Peng P, Gofeld M, et al. Anatomical study of the innervation of posterior knee joint capsule: implication for image-guided intervention. Reg Anesth Pain Med 2019;44(2):234–8.
15. Runge C, Moriggl B, Børglum J, et al. The Spread of ultrasound-guided injectate from the adductor canal to the genicular branch of the posterior obturator nerve and the popliteal plexus: a cadaveric study. Reg Anesth Pain Med 2017;42(6): 725–30.
16. Sutaria R, Lee S, Kim S, et al. Localization of the lateral retinacular nerve for diagnostic and therapeutic nerve block for lateral knee pain: a cadaveric study. PM R 2017;9(2):149–53.

# Knee Ablation Approaches

Nimish Mittal, MBBS, MD, MSc[a], Michael Catapano, BHSc, MD, FRCPC[b],
Philip W.H. Peng, MBBS, FRCPC[c],*

## KEYWORDS

- Radiofrequency ablation • Denervation • Osteoarthritis • Knee pain

## KEY POINTS

- The convention targets for knee denervation are superomedial, superolateral, and infero-medial genicular nerves.
- These landmarks have been extensively examined for the anatomic basis.
- Literature supports the improvement in pain and function after the radiofrequency ablation of those three genicular targets in patients with chronic knee pain secondary to osteoarthritis.
- Ongoing investigation is needed to explore the optimal number, types, and configuration of lesions.

## BACKGROUND

Osteoarthritis (OA) is well known to be one of the most prevalent conditions, with over 54 million people in the United States alone living with OA and an estimated productivity cost of work lost in the range of 17.5 billion dollars per year.[1,2] The knee joint continues to be the most common joint affected by OA, necessitating invasive intervention with a minimum of 60,000 total knee arthroplasties (TKAs) performed per year in Canada and an estimate of near 500,000 per year in the United States.[1] Despite its prevalence and impact, there is no cure for OA. Current conservative therapies target symptom management and pain relief and are known to have diminishing returns with repeat interventions.[3] These therapies include therapeutic exercise,[4] pharmacologic medications,[5,6] viscosupplementation,[7] corticosteroid,[8] and platelet-rich plasma (PRP).[9] Knee arthroplasty remains the treatment of choice for moderate to severe knee OA resistant to adequate nonsurgical management options; however, it carries surgical risks and adverse events that preclude or limit its availability to all

Authors' contribution: All the authors participated in the conception of the review, acquisition, analysis, interpretation of data, and drafting the article.
[a] Toronto Rehabilitation Institute, 550 University Avenue, 7-131 Toronto, Ontario M5G2A2, Canada; [b] Toronto Rehabilitation Institute, 550 University Avenue, Toronto, Ontario M5G 2A2, Canada; [c] Department of Anesthesia and Pain Medicine, Toronto Western Hospital, 399 Bathurst Street, McL2-405, Toronto, ON M5T 2S8, Canada
* Corresponding author.
E-mail address: Philip.Peng@uhn.ca

Phys Med Rehabil Clin N Am 32 (2021) 779–790
https://doi.org/10.1016/j.pmr.2021.05.012
1047-9651/21/© 2021 Elsevier Inc. All rights reserved.

patients, including those with significant comorbidities. Furthermore, a substantial proportion of patients continue to experience persistent pain, or functional restrictions after TKA, limiting its attractiveness as a definitive treatment option.[10,11]

Radiofrequency ablation (RFA) has been used by practitioners for more than half a century as a treatment for a multitude of chronic pains because of its ability to inhibit pain signals through the destruction or modulation of peripheral nerves with either high or pulsatile thermal energy, respectively.[12] In recent years, starting in 2011,[13] there has been increased interest in genicular nerve ablation to aid in pain management in either those who are not a surgical candidate for knee replacement or to prolong the function of the native knee before total joint arthroplasty. Since its initial publication describing RFA of three genicular nerves at the superomedial, inferomedial, and superolateral joints, there has been significant interest in describing and optimizing techniques to effectively denervate the sensory supply to the anterior knee joint. This review aims to summarize the available literature on the intervention of genicular nerve RFA, including different techniques and targets as well as clinical outcomes and potential complications. Clinical neuroanatomy relevant to knee RFA has been discussed in another chapter of this issue.

## INDICATIONS (PATIENT SELECTION)

Genicular nerve RFA is offered to patients with moderate to severe symptomatic knee OA with grade II to IV Kellgren-Lawrence classification refractory to conservative treatment and not the surgical candidate for joint replacement due to significant comorbidities or reluctance to pursue the surgical option.

At the time of publication of this review, there is on-going research to determine the clinical effect of genicular nerve RFA on persistent knee pain after TKA and whether genicular nerve RFA before TKA facilitates pain management and/or rehabilitation. At the current time, there is inadequate evidence to determine the effect of genicular RFA in these patient populations. Although RFA provides pain relief for patients with pain related to OA, patients with unstable knee joints will not benefit from this procedure, and a surgical option should be considered.

## TARGETS FOR DENERVATION AND TECHNIQUES

The current technique is based mostly on the original description by Choi and colleagues with slight modification.[13] The three targets that most practitioners believe are superomedial (SMGN), inferomedial (IMGN), and superolateral genicular nerves (SLGN). Since the original description of RFA in these three nerves, several anatomy studies evaluated the anatomic basis of these landmarks. These include one of the most comprehensive dissections with 3-dimensional documentation of all articular branches in the anterior knee capsule published by Tran and colleagues[14] (**Fig. 1**). So far, these publications support the anatomic landmark of these articular branches at the junction of diaphysis and epiphysis. Both Tran and colleagues[14] and Franco and colleagues[15] suggested having the needle placed slightly more posterior in the lateral plane for SMGN and SLGN. Most recently, Tran and colleagues also published an article validating the articular branches captured by the lesions in these three locations.[16] They confirmed that the superomedial and superolateral lesions capture the SLGN and SMGN, respectively. Interestingly, only the transverse deep branches of SMGN and SLGN are captured, and nerves to the posterior division of medial and lateral branches of nerve to vastus intermedius are also captured in the convention lesion (**Fig. 2**).

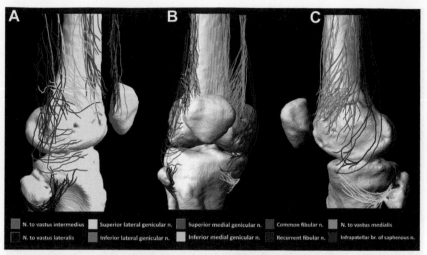

N. to vastus intermedius  Superior lateral genicular n.  Superior medial genicular n.  Common fibular n.  N. to vastus medialis
N. to vastus lateralis  Inferior lateral genicular n.  Inferior medial genicular n.  Recurrent fibular n.  Infrapatellar br. of saphenous n.

**Fig. 1.** Frequency map and distribution of the 10 articular branches of anterior knee capsule. N, n, nerve. (*Courtesy of* Philip Peng Educational Series.)

Recently, there are some additional landmarks suggested,[17,18] but the benefit of adding further site of ablation is still being investigated. Therefore, we only discuss the ablation technique for SMGN, SLGN, and IMGN, respectively.[16]

Both ultrasound (US) and fluoroscopy guidance techniques have been described for both diagnostic and ablation. Under fluoroscopy guidance, the patient is put in a supine position with a bolster or pillow to keep the knee in flexion. For the SMGN and SLGN, the target is the junction between epiphysis and diaphysis in the anteroposterior view and midpoint between anterior and posterior cortex in the lateral view. For the IMGN, the target is the junction between epiphysis and diaphysis deep to the medial collateral ligament (**Fig. 3**). Similarly, the targets for SMGN, SLGN, and IMGN are the same for the US-guided technique (**Figs. 4** and **5**). For diagnostic block, 1 mL of local anesthetic is administered to the target. For RFA, the radiofrequency (RF) needle is inserted instead. In some centers including the authors' center, a palisade lesion is preferred for the superior quadrants, especially the medial compartment given the configuration of the articular branches.

## CLINICAL EFFECTIVENESS AND SAFETY

Since the first randomized trial[13] on genicular nerve RFA, there has been outpouring interest culminating in over 35 clinical studies and 15 randomized controlled trials that are all of moderate to high methodological quality.[19–21]

The clinical efficacy of genicular RFA is best exemplified with the largest double-blind, randomized control trial of cooled RFA (CRFA) compared with intra-articular steroid (IAS) in 151 patients with symptomatic knee OA (Kellgren and Lawrence [KL] grade 2–4).[22] Despite having similar preintervention numeric pain rating scores, the mean knee pain score was less in the CRFA group than in the IAS group at every follow-up interval, including 1, 3, and 6 months after the intervention. Mean improvement in the CFRA group at 1 and 6 months was 4.2 and 4.9 points, respectively, on a 10-point numeric rating scale (NRS) compared with 3.3 and 1.3 in the IAS group. Similarly, at 6 months, 74% and 22% in the CRFA group met successful outcome criteria

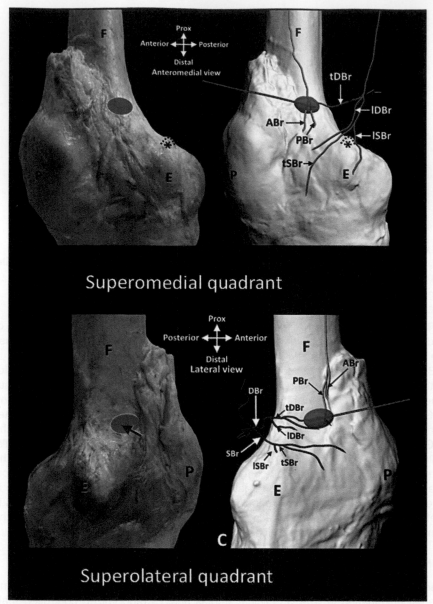

**Fig. 2.** Simulated lesion and the nerves capture. *Upper panel*, a conventional lesion in the superomedial quadrant captures the transverse deep branch (tDBr) of superomedial genicular nerve. It also captures the posterior division (PBr) of the medial branch of nerve to vastus intermedius. *Lower panel*, a conventional lesion in the superolateral quadrant captures the transverse deep branch (tDBr) of superolateral genicular nerve. It also captures the posterior division (PBr) of the lateral branch of nerve to vastus intermedius. *, adductor tubercle; ABr, anterior division of nerve to vastus intermedius medial branch; E, epicondyle; F, femur; lDBr, longitudinal deep branch; lSBr, longitudinal superficial branch; tSBr, transverse superficial branch of superomedial genicular nerve. (*Courtesy of* Philip Peng Educational Series.)

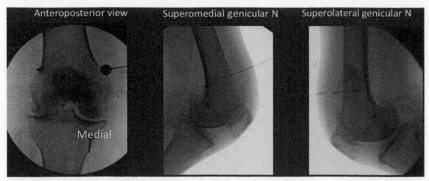

**Fig. 3.** Fluoroscopy view of the needles at the three targets of genicular nerves. (*Courtesy of* Philip Peng Educational Series.)

(>50% reduction in NRS score) and 100% pain relief, respectively, compared with only 25.9% and 4% in the IAS group. Similarly, to pain relief, where CFRA demonstrated improved and long-lasting improvement compared with IAS, functional outcomes demonstrated clinically and statistically significant improvements in the CRFA group compared with those in the IAS group.[22]

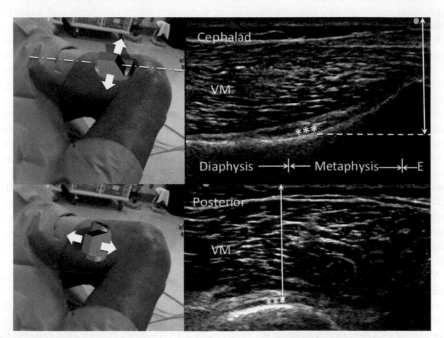

**Fig. 4.** Ultrasound image of the target for superomedial genicular nerve. The leg is put in external rotation of hip, and the orientation of the probe is in long axis of femur. The target is the fascial expansion (***) deep to the vastus medialis (VM) between diaphysis and epiphysis (*E*). The probe is then rotated 90° keeping the target at the same depth. This view allows in-plane insertion of needle from anterior to posterior orientation. (*Courtesy of* Philip Peng Educational Series.)

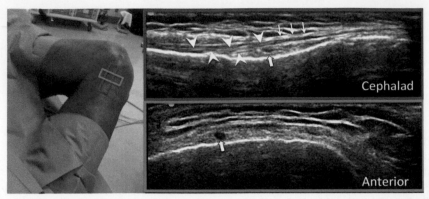

**Fig. 5.** Ultrasound image of the target for inferomedial genicular nerve. The initial position of the probe is over the medial collateral ligament (*red rectangle*). The inferior medial genicular nerve (IMGN) and vessel (*bold arrow*) is deep to the medial collateral ligament (*arrowheads*), which is deep to the crural fascia (*arrows*). The depth of the target is marked, and the probe is rotated 90° keeping the target at the same depth as the previous scan. The neurovascular bundle (*bold arrow*) was seen again. This view allows in-plane insertion of needle from anterior to posterior orientation. (*Courtesy of* Philip Peng Educational Series.)

The clinical efficacy of genicular RFA has been supported by multiple systematic reviews and meta-analyses.[19–21] Genicular RFA has demonstrated greater than 50% pain relief in 194 of 296 patients (65.5%) at 6 months when combining all available comparative studies or a pooled mean difference in the visual analog scale (VAS) of −4.196 when combining only US-guided RFA studies.[19–21] Similarly, 27 of 28 (96%) comparative studies demonstrated enhanced functionality from baseline up until 6 months[19] in those undergoing RFA or a pooled mean difference in the Western Ontario and McMaster Universities Osteoarthritis index (WOMAC) scores of 23.155 points when combining only US-guided RFA studies.[21]

The large majority of randomized controlled trials have final follow-ups at the 6-month postintervention period; however, long-term follow-up studies of these large, randomized trials have demonstrated sustained pain relief and improved function up to 24 months after the intervention.[23,24] At 18 and 24 months after the intervention, there was a demonstration of a significant decrease in NRS pain scores from 6.6 ± 1.6 at baseline to 3.1 ± 2.7(n = 25) and 3.6 ± 2.8 (n = 18) at 18 and 24 months, respectively, with 12 of 25 subjects reporting ≥50% pain relief at 18 months and 11 of 18 demonstrating ≥50% pain relief at 24 months from the baseline.[23] Similarly, there was a demonstration of prolonged functional improvement as measured by the Oxford Knee Score, with an overall mean change from baseline of 26.0 ± 9.6 points (Minimal clinically important difference = 5) at 18 months and 29.9 ± 10.4 points at 24 months.[23]

While the evidence supports the use of RFA in patients with chronic knee pain as a result of OA in the native knee, this procedure has not shown expected benefits in some scenarios: preoperative for those undergoing TKA or in those with persistent chronic TKA pain. A single-center sham-controlled prospective trial that assessed the efficacy of preoperative knee RF performed 2 to 6 weeks before TKA reported a lack of benefit in terms of postoperative pain, consumption of analgesics including opioid medications, and functional recovery.[25] The authors proposed a 26% nonresponder rate of this procedure and is probably explained by the variable course of genicular nerves and copresence of central sensitization with chronic advanced knee OA.[26] Similarly, RFA of the knee joint has not been rigorously tested in subacute and chronic persistent knee pains after arthroplasty. A retrospective comparative study of US-guided knee RFA in chronic pains secondary to TKA or advanced knee OA (KL grade III-IV) in 23 patients reported comparable benefits (67% in TKA group and 88% in knee OA group of >50% improvement in VAS pain scores) in both the groups at 3 months.[27] A few isolated case reports of knee RF in acute posttraumatic pains[28] and acute postoperative TKA pains[29] have been published, although the clinical efficacy in these conditions remains to be established.

### Comparison with Other Treatment Groups

Eight studies have compared genicular nerve RFA to common injection therapies including corticosteroid injection,[22,30,31] ozone injection,[32] hyaluronic acid (HA) injection,[33] PRP with sodium hyaluronate injection,[34] solely sodium hydrate injection,[35,36] and intra articular prolotherapy with erythropoietin and dextrose injection.[36]

All randomized control trials of RFA compared with corticosteroid injection have demonstrated significant improvements at all follow-ups for pain reduction; however, only 2 of 3 studies have demonstrated significant improvements in functional scores.[22,31,37] Similar to corticosteroid, RFA has demonstrated improvements in pain and functional scores when compared with PRP and hyaluronic acid in a randomized fashion, with the RFA group demonstrating significant improvements in VAS ($P<.05$) (RF: 4.28 ± 1.12 vs PRP + HA: 6.32 ± 1.18) and American Knee Society scores ($P<.05$) at all follow-ups.[34] Finally, compared with solely hyaluronic acid, RFA demonstrated significant improvements in VAS and function (WOMAC RF: 12.06 ± 4.03 vs HA: 59.93 ± 15.97) at all time points.[33-35]

Unfortunately, compared with nontraditional intra-articular injections, including erythropoietin plus dextrose injection and ozone injection, RFA has not demonstrated significant benefits.[32,36] The significance of these randomized control trials, despite being of moderate quality, necessitate further investigation because of the infrequent utilization of these intra-articular therapies for knee OA.[32,36]

### Comparative Efficacy of US Vs Fluoroscopy-Guided Radiofrequency Ablation Techniques

Both fluoroscopy and US have been used as imaging modalities for guiding the needle to the target position. Knee RFA was initially performed using a fluoroscopy-guided approach.[13] Later, US was suggested as an alternate radiation-free office-based technique.[38] Several studies, both cadaveric and clinical, on the US-based approach for knee RFA asserted the adjacent location of genicular arteries as a surrogate marker for localization of genicular nerves to yield better outcomes.[39,40] Yet, subsequent cadaveric studies that investigated the relationship of genicular nerves and arteries did not find this assumption to be true.[41] Clinically, a couple of RCTs have compared the efficacy of pain relief in US and RFA techniques and reported similar outcomes with both techniques.[37,42] Each technique offers a unique set of advantages. Fluoroscopy guidance can easily identify the nerve targets as they run adjacent to the periosteum and offer better needle visualization regardless of tissue depth and needle gauze. In contrast, US guidance offers the benefit of an office-based cheaper alternative with no radiation exposure and improved safety due to better visualization of adjacent soft-tissue structures. The choice of technique should be based on the availability of set up and individual experience and comfort with the imaging modalities.

### Complications/Adverse Events

Most publications regarding genicular nerve RFA have not demonstrated any significant adverse events related to the procedure. With the significant increase in the procedure rate of genicular nerve RFA, there have been reports of rare, however, significant safety concerns.[42,43] Transient hypoesthesia,[44,45] numbness,[45] and periosteal touch allodynia[13] were reported in few studies and significantly improved within a few weeks after the procedure. Rare complications including vascular injury of the knee including large subcutaneous bleeding,[44] ecchymosis,[46] hematoma formation,[47] skin burns,[48] hemarthrosis, pes anserine tendon damage,[49] septic arthritis,[50] or pseudoaneurysm as well as osteonecrosis of the patella have been described in the literature.[42] Direct comparison of fluoroscopy and US-guided knee RFA was performed in two studies and did not report any adverse effects.[37,43]

Several clinicians argue Charcot's neuropathy is a possible catastrophic side effect of knee joint nerve ablation. Nevertheless, Charcot's neuropathy has never been reported as a complication after knee RFA, even in the studies with relatively more prolonged duration of follow-up.[23,46] The reasons for the non-occurrence of Charcot's neuropathy are twofold. First, the partial nerve supply to the joint is preserved with knee RFA as the articular sensory branches to the posterior joint is spared. Second, Charcot neuropathy develops in systemic conditions with inflammatory mediators that disrupt the homeostasis of bone mineralization, causing osteolysis.[51] Owing to the rarity of these adverse events and no description in large cohort studies, it is unknown what the true prevalence of these adverse events are, nor the procedural aspects that may increase or decrease the risk of these events.

## SUMMARY

Knee RFA has quickly become one of the most promising interventions for those with knee pain secondary to OA because of its reproducible and prolonged effectiveness in reducing pain and improving function without violating the native knee joint, necessitating irreversible biomechanical changes or exposing patients to potentially serious adverse events. However, there continues to be debate regarding the true efficacy, optimal imaging technique, ideal targets, and lesion size and/or system.

Although numerous studies have been published since the original description by Choi and colleagues describing alternative descriptions of nerve supply to the anterior knee joint and potential targets for RFA, there has been no definitive evidence regarding the optimal number and location of targets.[13] Most of the published clinical studies have embraced the SMGN, IMGN, and SLGN as conventional landmarks following the first RCT[13] that adopted these landmarks. Tran and colleagues described the detailed course of articular branches in four quadrants.[14] Succeeding studies reported disparity in the sensory innervation of the knee joint,[14,52] and thereafter, a range of procedural targets to capture different nerve combinations for improvement of responder rate and magnitude of pain relief have been described.[17,18,53] The optimal location to target these nerves has also been argued based on the heterogeneity of the course of genicular nerves identified in cadaveric dissections with the suggestion of revised locations.[17,41] While there has been a suggestion to modify the conventional targets for genicular nerve ablation, clinical studies that have used conventional landmarks have reported excellent benefits.[22,48] Hence, despite the fact that recent anatomic studies may advocate a correlation of improved nerve capture with reduced arterial ablation using revised ablation points,[17,41] it remains to be determined if the correlation of these points yields either improved clinical efficacy or safety after genicular nerve RFA.

Several patient- and procedure-related factors have been debated to contribute to the success of knee RFA procedure. Clinical trials that enrolled patients with variable grades of knee OA from mild to severe (KL grade 1–4) have reported beneficial outcomes.[19,20,22] There is a lack of precise data to predict if the success of knee RFA depends on the structural severity of knee RFA. While a study reported approximately 3 times better outcomes in those with a KL grade 3 or less than KL grade 4,[54] another study in advanced knee OA (KL grade 3–4) reported at least 32% improvement in pre-treatment pain scores at 1-year follow-up.[46] The variability in success rate could likely be owing to multiple nonstructural elements such as psychological comorbidities and central sensitization that contribute to determining subjective knee pain, and these factors should be carefully assessed before making a decision to offer this treatment. Diagnostic nerve blocks have not shown any value to determine the predictive outcome of genicular nerve RFA.[48] Furthermore, authors have reported a 64% success rate of knee RFA at 6 months without a proceeding diagnostic block.[46]

In summary, knee RFA has been demonstrated to be a promising intervention resulting in prolonged improvement in pain and function. Further investigation is needed to compare and optimize technical aspects of knee RFA, including the number of neuroablative lesions, needle location, imaging technique, lesion size, and the need and effectiveness for repeat interventions.

## DISCLOSURE

P.W.H. Peng received equipment support from Sonosite Fujifilm Canada. The other authors declare nothing to disclose. The authors have not received funding for this work and have no conflicts of interest in the authorship or publication of this contribution.

## REFERENCES

1. Sloan M, Premkumar A, Sheth NP. Projected volume of primary total joint arthroplasty in the U.S., 2014 to 2030. J Bone Joint Surg Am 2018;100(17):1455–60.
2. Sharif B, Kopec J, Bansback N, et al. Projecting the direct cost burden of osteoarthritis in Canada using a microsimulation model. Osteoarthritis Cartilage 2015; 23(10):1654–63.
3. Ethgen O, Bruyère O, Richy F, et al. Health-related quality of life in total hip and total knee arthroplasty. A qualitative and systematic review of the literature. J Bone Joint Surg Am 2004;86(5):963–74.
4. Ebell MH. Osteoarthritis: rapid evidence review. Am Fam Physician 2018;97(8): 523–6.
5. Charlesworth J, Fitzpatrick J, Perera NKP, et al. Osteoarthritis- a systematic review of long-term safety implications for osteoarthritis of the knee. BMC Musculoskelet Disord 2019;20(1):151.
6. Hermann W, Lambova S, Muller-Ladner U. Current treatment options for osteoarthritis. Curr Rheumatol Rev 2018;14(2):108–16.
7. Johal H, Devji T, Schemitsch EH, et al. Viscosupplementation in knee osteoarthritis: evidence revisited. JBJS Rev 2016;4(4):e11–111.
8. da Costa BR, Hari R, Jüni P. Intra-articular corticosteroids for osteoarthritis of the knee. JAMA 2016;316(24):2671–2.
9. Meheux CJ, McCulloch PC, Lintner DM, et al. Efficacy of intra-articular platelet-rich plasma injections in knee osteoarthritis: a systematic review. Arthroscopy 2016;32(3):495–505.
10. Nashi N, Hong CC, Krishna L. Residual knee pain and functional outcome following total knee arthroplasty in osteoarthritic patients. Knee Surg Sports Traumatol Arthrosc 2015;23(6):1841–7.

11. Wylde V, Hewlett S, Learmonth ID, et al. Persistent pain after joint replacement: prevalence, sensory qualities, and postoperative determinants. Pain 2011; 152(3):566–72.

12. Shealy CN. Percutaneous radiofrequency denervation of spinal facets. Treatment for chronic back pain and sciatica. J Neurosurg 1975;43(4):448–51.

13. Choi WJ, Hwang SJ, Song JG, et al. Radiofrequency treatment relieves chronic knee osteoarthritis pain: a double-blind randomized controlled trial. Pain 2011; 152(3):481–7.

14. Tran J, Peng PWH, Lam K, et al. Anatomical study of the innervation of anterior knee joint capsule: implication for image-guided intervention. Reg Anesth Pain Med 2018;43(4):407–14.

15. Franco CD, Buvanendran A, Petersohn JD, et al. Innervation of the anterior capsule of the human knee: implications for radiofrequency ablation. Reg Anesth Pain Med 2015;40(4):363–8.

16. Tran J, Peng P, Agur A. Evaluation of nerve capture using classical landmarks for genicular nerve radiofrequency ablation: 3D cadaveric study. Reg Anesth Pain Med 2020;45(11):898–906.

17. Fonkoue L, Behets CW, Steyaert A, et al. Current versus revised anatomical targets for genicular nerve blockade and radiofrequency ablation: evidence from a cadaveric model. Reg Anesth Pain Med 2020;45(8):603–9.

18. Conger A, Cushman DM, Walker K, et al. A novel technical protocol for improved capture of the genicular nerves by radiofrequency ablation. Pain Med 2019; 20(11):2208–12.

19. Ajrawat P, Radomski L, Bhatia A, et al. Radiofrequency procedures for the treatment of symptomatic knee osteoarthritis: a systematic review. Pain Med 2020; 21(2):333–48.

20. Hong T, Wang H, Li G, et al. Systematic review and meta-analysis of 12 randomized controlled trials evaluating the efficacy of invasive radiofrequency treatment for knee pain and function. Biomed Res Int 2019;2019:9037510.

21. Huang Y, Deng Q, Yang L, et al. Efficacy and safety of ultrasound-guided radiofrequency treatment for chronic pain in patients with knee osteoarthritis: a systematic review and meta-analysis. Pain Res Manag 2020;2020:2537075.

22. Davis T, Loudermilk E, DePalma M, et al. Prospective, multicenter, randomized, crossover clinical trial comparing the safety and effectiveness of cooled radiofrequency ablation with corticosteroid injection in the management of knee pain from osteoarthritis. Reg Anesth Pain Med 2018;43(1):84–91.

23. Hunter C, Davis T, Loudermilk E, et al. Cooled radiofrequency ablation treatment of the genicular nerves in the treatment of osteoarthritic knee pain: 18- and 24-month results. Pain Pract 2020;20(3):238–46.

24. Iannaccone F, Dixon S, Kaufman A. A review of long-term pain relief after genicular nerve radiofrequency ablation in chronic knee osteoarthritis. Pain Physician 2017;20(3):E437–44.

25. Walega D, McCormick Z, Manning D, et al. Radiofrequency ablation of genicular nerves prior to total knee replacement has no effect on postoperative pain outcomes: a prospective randomized sham-controlled trial with 6-month follow-up. Reg Anesth Pain Med 2019;45:90–1.

26. Wylde V, Sayers A, Odutola A, et al. Central sensitization as a determinant of patients' benefit from total hip and knee replacement. Eur J Pain 2017;21(2):357–65.

27. Erdem Y, Sir E. The efficacy of ultrasound-guided pulsed radiofrequency of genicular nerves in the treatment of chronic knee pain due to severe degenerative disease or previous total knee arthroplasty. Med Sci Monit 2019;25:1857–63.

28. Carrier JD, Poliak-Tunis M. Genicular radiofrequency ablation for the treatment of post-traumatic knee pain: a case presentation. Pm r 2018;10(11):1279–82.

29. Sahoo RK, Krishna C, Kumar M, et al. Genicular nerve block for postoperative pain relief after total knee replacement. Saudi J Anaesth 2020;14(2):235–7.

30. Sarı S, Aydın ON, Turan Y, et al. Which one is more effective for the clinical treatment of chronic pain in knee osteoarthritis: radiofrequency neurotomy of the genicular nerves or intra-articular injection? Int J Rheum Dis 2018;21(10):1772–8.

31. Yao P, Hong T, Li G, et al. Comparing the safety and effectiveness of radiofrequency thermocoagulation on genicular nerve, intraarticular pulsed radiofrequency with steroid injection in the pain management of knee osteoarthritis. Pain Physician 2020;23(4s):S295–304.

32. Hashemi M, Nabi BN, Saberi A, et al. The comparison between two methods for the relief of knee osteoarthritis pain: radiofrequency and intra-periarticular ozone injection: a clinical trial study. Int J Med Res Health Sci 2016;5(7):539–46.

33. Ray D, Goswami S, Dasgupta S, et al. Intra-Articular hyaluronic acid injection versus RF ablation of genicular nerve for knee osteoarthritis pain: a randomized, open-label, clinical study. Indian J Pain 2018;32(1):36–9.

34. Shen WS, Xu XQ, Zhai NN, et al. Radiofrequency thermocoagulation in relieving refractory pain of knee osteoarthritis. Am J Ther 2017;24(6):e693–700.

35. Xiao L, Shu F, Xu C, et al. Highly selective peripheral nerve radio frequency ablation for the treatment of severe knee osteoarthritis. Exp Ther Med 2018;16(5):3973–7.

36. Rahimzadeh P, Imani F, Faiz SH, et al. Investigation the efficacy of intra-articular prolotherapy with erythropoietin and dextrose and intra-articular pulsed radiofrequency on pain level reduction and range of motion improvement in primary osteoarthritis of knee. J Res Med Sci 2014;19(8):696–702.

37. Sarı S, Aydın ON, Turan Y, et al. Which imaging method should be used for genicular nerve radio frequency thermocoagulation in chronic knee osteoarthritis? J Clin Monit Comput 2017;31(4):797–803.

38. Yasar E, Kesikburun S, Kılıç C, et al. Accuracy of ultrasound-guided genicular nerve block: a cadaveric study. Pain Physician 2015;18(5):E899–904.

39. Vanneste B, Tomlinson J, Desmet M, et al. Feasibility of an ultrasound-guided approach to radiofrequency ablation of the superolateral, superomedial and inferomedial genicular nerves: a cadaveric study. Reg Anesth Pain Med 2019;44:966–70.

40. Kesikburun S, Yaşar E, Uran A, et al. Ultrasound-guided genicular nerve pulsed radiofrequency treatment for painful knee osteoarthritis: a preliminary report. Pain Physician 2016;19(5):E751–9.

41. Park MR, Kim D, Rhyu IJ, et al. An anatomical neurovascular study for procedures targeting peri-articular nerves in patients with anterior knee pain. Knee 2020;27(5):1577–84.

42. Kim SY, Le PU, Kosharskyy B, et al. Is genicular nerve radiofrequency ablation safe? a literature review and anatomical study. Pain Physician 2016;19(5):E697–705.

43. Kim DH, Lee MS, Lee S, et al. A prospective randomized comparison of the efficacy of ultrasound- vs fluoroscopy-guided genicular nerve block for chronic knee osteoarthritis. Pain Physician 2019;22(2):139–46.

44. Ikeuchi M, Ushida T, Izumi M, et al. Percutaneous radiofrequency treatment for refractory anteromedial pain of osteoarthritic knees. Pain Med 2011;12(4):546–51.

45. Ahmed A, Arora D. Ultrasound-guided radiofrequency ablation of genicular nerves of knee for relief of intractable pain from knee osteoarthritis: a case series. Br J Pain 2018;12(3):145–54.

46. Santana Pineda MM, Vanlinthout LE, Moreno Martín A, et al. Analgesic effect and functional improvement caused by radiofrequency treatment of genicular nerves in patients with advanced osteoarthritis of the knee until 1 year following treatment. Reg Anesth Pain Med 2017;42(1):62–8.

47. Strand N, Jorge P, Freeman J, et al. A rare complication of knee hematoma after genicular nerve radiofrequency ablation. Pain Rep 2019;4(3):e736.

48. McCormick ZL, Korn M, Reddy R, et al. Cooled radiofrequency ablation of the genicular nerves for chronic pain due to knee osteoarthritis: six-month outcomes. Pain Med 2017;18(9):1631–41.

49. Conger A, McCormick ZL, Henrie AM. Pes anserine tendon injury resulting from cooled radiofrequency ablation of the inferior medial genicular nerve. PM R 2019; 11(11):1244–7.

50. Khanna A, Knox N, Sekhri N. Septic arthritis following radiofrequency ablation of the genicular nerves. Pain Med 2019;20(7):1454–6.

51. Papanas N, Maltezos E. Etiology, pathophysiology and classifications of the diabetic Charcot foot. Diabet Foot Ankle 2013;4.

52. Fonkoué L, Behets C, Kouassi JK, et al. Distribution of sensory nerves supplying the knee joint capsule and implications for genicular blockade and radiofrequency ablation: an anatomical study. Surg Radiol Anat 2019;41(12):1461–71.

53. Wong PK, Kokabi N, Guo Y, et al. Safety and efficacy comparison of three- vs four-needle technique in the management of moderate to severe osteoarthritis of the knee using cooled radiofrequency ablation. Skeletal Radiol 2021;50(4): 739–50.

54. House LM, Korn MA, Garg A, et al. Severity of knee osteoarthritis and pain relief after cooled radiofrequency ablation of the genicular nerves. Pain Med 2019; 20(12):2601–3.

# Overview of the Innervation of Ankle Joint

John R. Han, BPHE*, John Tran, HBSc, PhD, Anne M.R. Agur, BSc(OT), MSc, PhD

## KEYWORDS

- Ankle joint innervation • Articular nerves • Talocural joint • Nerve block
- Radiofrequency ablation • Anatomy

## KEY POINTS

- The ankle joint is innervated by articular branches from the tibial, saphenous, sural, and superficial and deep fibular nerves.
- The anterior aspect of the joint capsule receives innervation from articular branches from the saphenous, superficial, and deep fibular nerves; laterally from the sural and superficial fibular nerves; and medially and posteriorly from the saphenous and tibial nerves.
- Articular branches innervating the joint capsule have been documented from all of the nerves coursing in the ankle region, suggesting the necessity for multiple target sites to optimize image-guided nerve block and radiofrequency ablation procedures.

## INTRODUCTION

Knowledge of the sensory innervation of the ankle joint is necessary to accurately target the articular nerves for image-guided nerve block and radiofrequency ablation to treat chronic joint pain. Studies of the innervation of the ankle (talocrural) joint are scarce. Only 8 cadaveric studies documenting the innervation of the ankle joint capsule were found in the literature. Of these studies, published between 1857 to 2016, 6 investigated the innervation of the ankle joint by the tibial, sural, saphenous, and superficial/deep fibular nerves and 2 studies focused on saphenous nerve innervation (**Table 1**). The number of specimens used in studies that investigated the sensory innervation of the entire ankle joint ranged between 5 and 10 specimens. In 2 studies of saphenous nerve innervation, Clendenen and Whalen[1] and Eglitis and colleagues[2] examined 5 and 103 specimens, respectively.

In earlier studies, Rüdinger[3] and Nyakas and Kiss[4,5] reported ankle joint innervation from the tibial, sural, and deep fibular nerves (see **Table 1**). Neither study found saphenous or superficial fibular nerve innervation to the ankle joint. Studies by von Lanz and Wachsmuth,[6] Lippert,[7] and Champetier[8] reported innervation from the saphenous

Division of Anatomy, Department of Surgery, Temerty Faculty of Medicine, University of Toronto, 1 King's College Circle, Room 1158, Toronto, ON M5S 1A8, Canada
* Corresponding author.
*E-mail address:* john.han@mail.utoronto.ca

Phys Med Rehabil Clin N Am 32 (2021) 791–801
https://doi.org/10.1016/j.pmr.2021.05.013
1047-9651/21/© 2021 Elsevier Inc. All rights reserved.

pmr.theclinics.com

**Table 1**
**Summary of previous literature of ankle joint innervation**

|  | N | TN | SAN | SUN | SFN | DFN |
|---|---|---|---|---|---|---|
| Rüdinger,[3] 1857 | NS | ✓ | X | ✓ | X | ✓ |
| Nyakas et al,[4,5] 1954/1958 | NS | ✓ | X | ✓ | X | ✓ |
| von Lanz et al,[6] 1959 | NS | ✓ | ✓ | ✓ | X | ✓ |
| Lippert,[7] 1962 | 5 | ✓ | ✓ | ✓ | X | ✓ |
| Champetier,[8] 1970 | 10 | ✓ | ✓ | ✓ | ✓ | ✓ |
| Mentzel et al,[9] 1999 | 8 | ✓ | ✓ | ✓ | X | ✓ |
| Clendenen & Whalen,[1] 2013 | 5 | N/A | ✓ | N/A | N/A | N/A |
| Eglitis et al,[2] 2016 | 103 | N/A | ✓ | N/A | N/A | N/A |

*Abbreviations:* DFN, deep fibular nerve; N/A, did not study; NS, not stated; SAN, saphenous nerve; SFN, superficial fibular nerve; SUN, sural nerve; TN, tibial nerve.

nerve but did not state the number of specimens. Mentzel and colleagues[9] found saphenous innervation in 3 out of 8 specimens and Clendenen and Whalen[1] and Eglitis and colleagues[2] found articular branches from the saphenous nerve in all specimens. Ankle joint innervation by the superficial fibular nerve (n = 5/10 specimens) has been reported in one study.[8]

The number, site of origin, and course of the articular branches of the tibial, saphenous, sural, superficial, and deep fibular nerves described in the literature will be compared and contrasted first. This will be followed by photographs of dissected specimens and descriptions of the origin and course of the articular branches innervating the ankle joint. These dissections were carried out to supplement the line drawings that have most commonly been used to summarize ankle joint innervation.

### Tibial Nerve

Articular branches have been found to originate from the tibial nerve, medial and lateral plantar nerves, and medial calcaneal nerve. The number and site of origin of the articular branches varied between studies.

- Rüdinger[8]: 1–2 articular branches; originating close to the ankle joint
- Nyakas and Kiss[4,5]: (1) 2–3 articular branches; originating just superior to the medial aspect of the ankle joint. (2) Small number of articular branches; originating from the medial and lateral plantar nerves
- von Lanz and Wachsmuth[6] and Lippert[7]: 1–2 articular branches; originating proximal to the bifurcation of the tibial nerve
- Champetier[8]: (1) 3–5 articular branches; originating from the junction of the middle and distal third of the leg to the level of the ankle joint. (2) Unspecified number of articular branches; originating from the medial (n = 3/10) and lateral (n = 2/10) plantar nerves
- Mentzel and colleagues[9]: (1) 2–6 articular branches; originating in the distal one-third of the leg. (2) Unspecified number of articular branches; originating from the medial calcaneal nerve. (3) 1 to 6 articular branches; originating from the medial plantar nerve

The articular branches have been found to innervate the

- medial capsule; Rüdinger,[8] Nyakas and Kiss,[4,5] Lippert,[7] and Mentzel and colleagues[9]

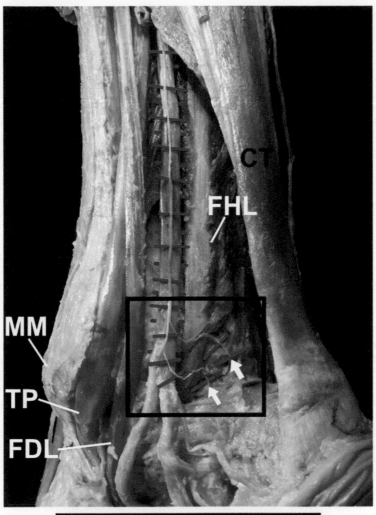

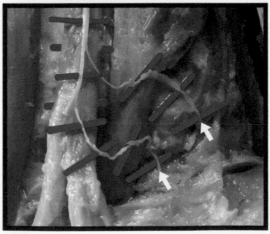

- posterior capsule; Lippert,[7] Mentzel and colleagues,[9] and von Lanz and Wachsmuth[6]

When described, the articular branches have been documented as coursing between the tendons of the tibialis posterior and flexor digitorum longus,[3–5] deep to the tendon of the flexor digitorum longus,[3,8] or superificial to tibialis posterior.[8]

In the dissection carried out in our laboratory, one articular branch was given off the tibial nerve, as it coursed inferiorly between flexor digitorum longus and flexor hallucis longus (**Fig. 1**). This articular branch coursed along the surface of the tibial nerve as far inferiorly as the medial malleolus where it gave off terminal branches that supplied the posteromedial aspect of the ankle joint. No articular branches were found originating from the medial and lateral plantar nerves. However, this could be due to the relatively inferior bifurcation of the tibial nerve in this specimen.

## Saphenous Nerve

Of the 6 studies that reported saphenous nerve innervation to the ankle joint capsule, 4 documented the number of articular branches. Three of the 4 studies found 1 to 2 articular branches from the saphenous nerve,[6–8] whereas Mentzel and colleagues[9] identified 2 to 3 articular branches. The articular branches were found to originate in the distal one-third of the leg,[9] at the level of the medial malleolus[8] or near/superior to the medial malleolus.[1] The innervation from the saphenous nerve to the medial aspect of the joint capsule was consistently found, whereas anterior capsular supply was also reported by Mentzel and colleagues.[9]

Lippert[7] and Clendenen and Whalen[1] described anterior and posterior articular branches that coursed inferiorly with the great saphenous vein. Lippert[7] reported that both anterior and posterior branches innervated the ankle joint, whereas Clendenen and Whalen[1] found innervation to the joint only from the posterior branch. In addition, Champetier[8] described the articular branches as coursing deep and posterior to the tendon of tibialis anterior.

In this dissection, the saphenous nerve as it entered the leg divided into 2 main branches, anterior and posterior, named by their location relative to the great saphenous vein. Both branches coursed in the subcutaneous tissue and approximately at the junction of the middle and distal third of the leg gave off several articular branches (**Fig. 2**A). The posterior articular branches coursed posterior to the great saphenous vein to terminate in the posterior and anteromedial aspects of the ankle joint on each side of the medial malleolus. Periosteal branches to the medial malleolus were also observed (see **Fig. 2**B). The anterior articular branches coursed distally, anterior to the great saphenous vein, to terminate in the anteromedial joint capsule (see **Fig. 2**C).

## Sural Nerve

The sural nerve, a cutaneous nerve accompanied by the short saphenous vein, is usually formed by the union of the medial and lateral sural cutaneous nerves in the

**Fig. 1.** Tibial nerve innervation of the ankle joint with enlarged inset of articular branches; posteromedial view. The tibial nerve (purple sutures) is seen coursing between flexor digitorum and flexor hallucis longus. The articular branch is highlighted with pink sutures, and its terminal branches entering the joint capsule are indicated with white arrows. CT, calcaneal tendon; FDL, flexor digitorum longus; FHL, flexor hallucis longus; MM, medial malleolus; TP, tibialis posterior.

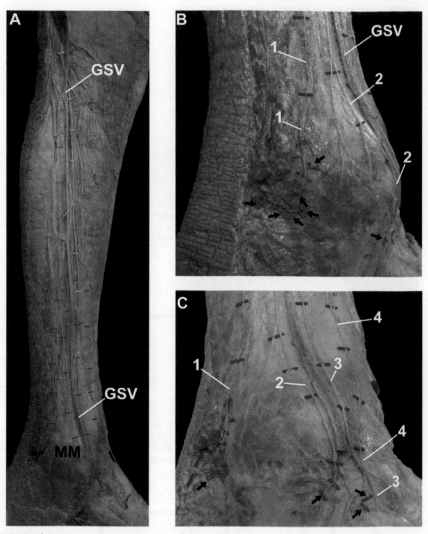

**Fig. 2.** Saphenous nerve innervation of the ankle joint; medial view. Articular branches are highlighted with pink sutures and their termination in the joint capsule is indicated with black arrows. (*A*) Overview of the course of the anterior (light green sutures) and posterior (dark green sutures) branches of the saphenous nerve. (*B*) Articular branches of the posterior branch of the saphenous nerve. Note the articular branches course posterior (1) and anterior (2) to the medial malleolus before terminating in posteromedial and anteromedial aspects of the joint capsule, respectively. (*C*) Articular branches of the anterior (3 and 4) and posterior (1 and 2) branches of the saphenous nerve. The articular branches from the anterior branch of the saphenous nerve can be seen coursing anterior to the medial malleolus to supply the anteromedial aspect of the joint capsule. GSV, great saphenous vein; MM, medial malleolus; SAN, saphenous nerve

subcutaneous tissue of the leg. Both structures pass inferior to the lateral malleolus and continue to the lateral aspect of the foot.[10]

Most of the studies found at least 1 articular branch originating both superior and inferior to the level of the ankle joint.[3,6–8] Mentzel and colleagues[9] found 2 to 5 articular

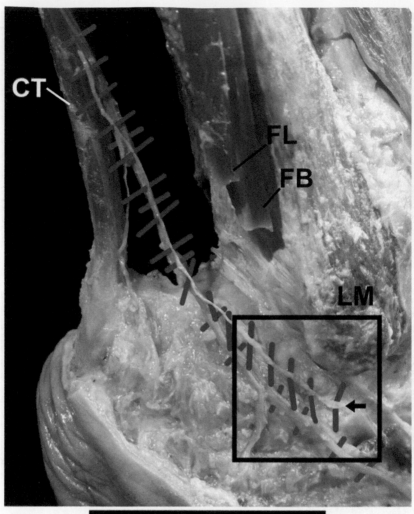

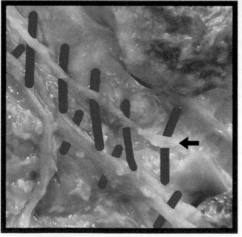

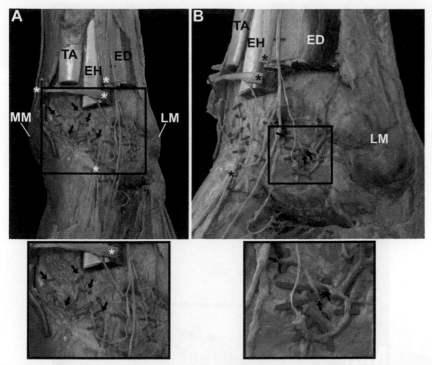

**Fig. 4.** Superficial fibular nerve innervation of the ankle joint. (*A*) Medial articular nerve with enlarged inset; anterior view. (*B*) Lateral articular nerve with enlarged inset; anterolateral view. In (*A* and *B*) the tendons of tibialis anterior (TA), extensor hallucis (EH), and digitorum (ED) longus have been transected and removed. A part of the superficial fibular nerve has been cut and reflected (*) to reveal the origin of the medial and lateral articular nerves (pink sutures) from a single branch (red sutures) originating from the superficial fibular nerve. The termination of the medial and lateral articular nerves in the anterior and anterolateral aspects of the joint capsules, respectively, are indicated with black arrows. LM, lateral malleolus; MM, medial malleolus.

branches originating from the sural nerve superior to the ankle joint, whereas Nyakas and Kiss[4,5] reported only articular innervation inferior to the level of the joint. The articular branches from the sural nerve have been reported to innervate both the posterior and anterior aspects of the capsule,[3,6,7] posterior capsule only,[9] and lateral capsule.[4,5]

When described, the articular branches originating from the sural nerve superior to the level of the ankle joint have been reported to course through the precalcaneal fat pad[6,7] and pass either deep[3] or between[8] the tendons of the fibularis (peroneus)

**Fig. 3.** Sural nerve innervation of the ankle joint with enlarged inset of the articular branch; lateral view. Note the tendons of fibularis longus and brevis have been transected and removed to expose the course of the sural nerve (blue sutures) and the articular branch (pink sutures). At the level of the ankle joint, the articular branch can be seen coursing deeply to terminate on the lateral aspect of the joint capsule, just inferior to the tip of the lateral malleolus (*black arrow*). CT, calcaneal tendon; FL, fibularis longus; FB, fibular brevis; LM, lateral malleolus.

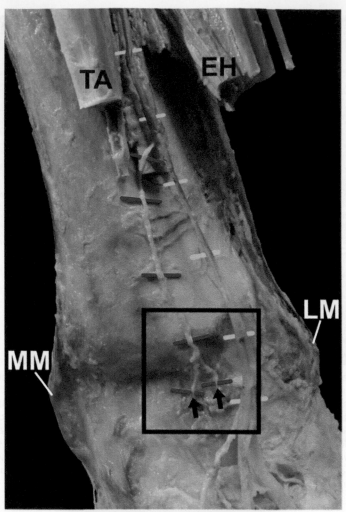

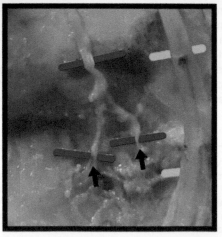

longus and brevis. The articular branches that originate inferior to the joint have been described as coursing posterior to the lateral malleolus.[3,7,8] In addition, Champetier[8] reported that these branches coursed superficial to fibularis longus and brevis tendons.

In the dissection carried out in our laboratory, the sural nerve gave rise to one articular branch in the distal third of the leg, which coursed inferiorly along the lateral surface of the sural nerve as far as the lateral malleolus (**Fig. 3**). At the lateral malleolus, the articular branch penetrated the underlying fascia and coursed deep to the tendons of fibularis longus and brevis to terminate in the lateral aspect of the ankle joint capsule.

## Superficial Fibular Nerve

The superficial fibular nerve descends in the lateral compartment of the leg, and approximately at the junction of the middle and distal third of the leg it pierces the deep fascia to enter the subcutaneous tissue where it divides into 2 terminal branches, the intermediate dorsal cutaneous nerve of the foot and the medial dorsal cutaneous nerve of the foot.

Champetier[8] was the only study found that reported ankle joint innervation from the superficial fibular nerve (n = 5/10 specimens). Both terminal branches of the superficial fibular nerve, the intermediate dorsal cutaneous nerve of the foot and the medial dorsal cutaneous nerve of the foot, were found to supply articular branches to the ankle joint. The articular branches from the medial dorsal cutaneous nerve were found to course superficial to the tendon of tibialis anterior to reach the joint capsule, whereas the articular branches from the intermediate dorsal cutaneous nerve were found to originate in the area superior to the lateral malleolus. An anomalous nerve, the deep accessory peroneal nerve, when present, was also found to innervate the ankle joint.

In our dissection, medial and lateral articular nerves were found to originate from a branch of the superficial fibular nerve. This branch of the superficial fibular nerve coursed along the medial margin of extensor digitorum longus (ED) and continued into the subcutaneous tissue of the foot, giving off medial and lateral articular nerves at the level of the ankle joint. The medial articular nerve looped and turned superiorly to ramify into fine terminal branches that supplied the anterior aspect of the joint capsule deep to the tendons of tibialis anterior and extensor hallucis longus (**Fig. 4A**). The lateral articular nerve traveled inferiorly, superficial to ED, and approximately at the musculotendinous junction of ED turned posteriorly and coursed deeply to innervate the anterolateral aspect of the ankle joint (see **Fig. 4B**).

## Deep Fibular Nerve

The deep fibular nerve has been reported to supply the ankle joint capsule in 6 of the 8 studies found in the literature (see **Table 1**). The number of articular branches originating

---

**Fig. 5.** Deep fibular nerve innervation of the ankle joint with enlarged inset of articular branches; anteromedial view. The tendons of the muscles of the anterior compartment of the leg have been transected and removed distally. Note the deep fibular nerve (teal sutures) courses between tibialis anterior and extensor hallucis longus, which has been reflected laterally. The articular branch is highlighted with pink sutures, and its terminal branches entering the anterior aspect of the joint capsule are indicated with black arrows. EH, extensor hallucis longus; LM, lateral malleolus; MM, medial malleolus; TA, tibialis anterior.

from the deep fibular nerve varied between 1 and 5.[3-9] The articular branches have been found to supply the anterior,[3-6,9] medial,[4,5] and lateral[4,5,9] ankle joint capsule.

Champetier[8] and Mentzel and colleagues[9] found articular branches that emerged from the deep fibular nerve proximally in the leg. Mentzel and colleagues[9] named one of these branches the interosseous branch, which coursed inferiorly on the anterior surface of the interosseous membrane to innervate the ankle joint capsule anteriorly. Articular branches have also been found to originate from the deep fibular nerve just proximal or at the level of the ankle joint[4-9] and from the medial and lateral terminal branches of the deep fibular nerve.[3-5,9]

In our dissection, the deep fibular nerve was traced inferiorly as it coursed between the tibialis anterior and extensor hallucis longus muscles (**Fig. 5**). In the distal third of the leg, the deep fibular nerve gave off an articular branch that coursed inferiorly on the periosteum of the tibia, posterior to the deep fibular nerve. At the inferior border of the tibia, it divided into 2 short terminal branches that innervated the anterior aspect of the joint capsule.

## SUMMARY

The ankle joint is innervated by articular branches from the tibial, saphenous, sural, and superficial and deep fibular nerves. The anterior aspect of the joint capsule receives innervation from articular branches from the saphenous, superficial, and deep fibular nerves; laterally from the sural and superficial fibular nerves; and medially and posteriorly from the saphenous and tibial nerves.

## CLINICAL PEARLS

The innervation of the ankle joint is complex. Small articular branches innervating the joint capsule have been documented from all of the nerves coursing in the ankle region, suggesting the necessity for multiple target sites to optimize image-guided nerve block and radiofrequency ablation procedures. The anatomic findings need to be corroborated with clinical studies to determine feasibility and outcomes.

## CLINICS CARE POINT

Numerous small articular branches from the tibial, saphenous, sural, and superficial and deep fibular nerves were found to innervate the ankle joint in this anatomical study. Therefore, multiple target sites would likely be needed to optimize image-guide NB/RFA procedures. Further clinical study is required.

## DISCLOSURE

Anne Agur is an Anatomy Faculty with Allergan Academy of Excellence.

## REFERENCES

1. Clendenen SR, Whalen JL. Saphenous nerve innervation of the medial ankle. Local Reg Anesth 2013;6:13–5.
2. Eglitis N, Horn JL, Benninger B, et al. The importance of the saphenous nerve in ankle surgery. Anesth Analg 2016;122:1704–6.
3. Rüdinger N. Gelenknerven Des menschlichen körpers. Erlangen: Verlag von Ferdinand Enke; 1857.
4. Nyakas A, Kiss T. Heilung Von Beschwerden Nach Calcaneusfrakturen Mittels Denervation. Zentralblatt für Chirurgie 1954;79:1273–7.

5. Nyakas A. Unsere neueren Erfahrungen mit der Denervation des Knöchel- und tarsalen Gelenks. Zentralbl Chit 1958;58:2243–9.
6. Von Lanz T, Wachsmuth W. Praktische Anatomie Bd. 1, Teil 4. Bein und Statik 2. auflage. Berlin, Göttingen, Heidelberg: Springer; 1959.
7. Lippert H. Zur Innervation der meschlichen Fußgelenke. Z Anat Entwicklungs-gesch 1962;123:295–330.
8. Champetier J. Innervation del'articulation tibio-tarsienne (Articulatio talocruraris). Acta Anat 1970;77:398–421.
9. Mentzel M, Fleischmann W, Bauer G, et al. Ankle joint denervation. Part 1: anatomy–the sensory innervation of the ankle joint. Foot Ankle Surg 1999;5: 15–20.
10. Moore KL, Dalley AF, Agur AMR. Clinically oriented anatomy. 8th edition. Philadelphia, PA: Wolters Kluwer; 2018.

# Nerve Ablation in the Foot and Ankle

Nahum M. Beard, MD, CAQSM

## KEYWORDS

- Ablation • Radiofrequency • Neuroma • Foot and ankle • Ultrasound
- Osteoarthrosis • Pain

## KEY POINTS

- The ankle and foot joint has a limited but growing body of evidence for the efficacy of nerve ablations in the foot and ankle centered on heel pain and mononeuritic states.
- The preservation of downstream proprioception and muscular innervation is compelling and unique even when compared with other body areas.
- Regional and when possible, focal approaches to pain control through denervation/ablation is the preferred approach.
- Knowledge and use of high-frequency ultrasound imaging is essential to apply technique to individual patient situations including diverse anatomic variations.

## INTRODUCTION

Denervation treatments in the region of the foot and ankle are common and have been historically in the armamentarium of the foot and ankle surgeon. Denervation of terminal nerve fibers by decompression or debridement through the sinus tarsi or through synovectomy when treating painful tendinosis and tenosynovitis are routine techniques to facilitate improvements in pain and function. They may be undertaken either as primary procedures or as part of a larger intervention. Selective neurectomy, especially of the sural in posterior lateral ankle pain or for primary sural neuritis is well established. Specific neurotomy/neurectomy of this type has been typically applied focally to a recalcitrant region or cause of lower extremity pain. However, surgical options are not indicated in all patients, even those with straightforward diagnoses. Pain from variable causes after failed surgery or even successful surgery is common, and alternate treatment options are needed. In the case of ankle joint osteoarthrosis (OA) surgical joint denervation is described as an alternative to fusion or replacement; however, even these techniques require large incisions for visualization of anatomy and to

Faculty Campbell Clinic Sports Medicine Fellowship, Department of Orthopaedic Surgery and Rehabilitation, Department of Family Medicine, University of Tennessee Health Science Center, 1400 South Germantown Road, Germantown, TN 38138, USA
E-mail address: nbeard@campbellclinic.com

Phys Med Rehabil Clin N Am 32 (2021) 803–818
https://doi.org/10.1016/j.pmr.2021.05.014
1047-9651/21/© 2021 Elsevier Inc. All rights reserved.

| Table 1 Nerve ablation by diagnosis | |
|---|---|
| **Nerve** | **Diagnosis** |
| Sural (including lateral calcaneal nerve) | Osteoarthritis (OA) ankle: lateral gutter Subfibular impingement OA lateral column foot OA subtalar joint Peroneal tendinopathy Chronic lateral heel pain Plantar fasciosis: central and lateral band Insertional Achilles tendinosis/enthesitis |
| Superficial peroneal nerve | OA ankle anterolateral and subfibular impingement OA central column Broad midfoot OA Peroneal tendinopathy Tibialis posterior tendinosis |
| Deep peroneal nerve | Sinus tarsi pain syndrome Anterolateral and subfibular impingement Painful pes planus OA lateral column foot |
| Saphenous nerve | OA ankle: med. gutter Medial impingement OA medial column foot Tarsal tunnel region incisional pain Tibialis posterior tendinosis |
| Medial calcaneal nerve | Entrapment Chronic heel pain Plantar fasciosis Subcalcaneal bursitis |
| Baxter nerve | Baxter neuritis Tarsal tunnel syndromes Chronic heel pain |
| Common digital nerve | Morton neurofibroma Stump neuroma (postsurgical) Digit arthrosis |

allow for the targeting small terminal branches while the main nerve trunks are preserved.[1-3] Complete denervation at or above the ankle joint has held historic cautionary considerations; the most notable being the potential for precipitation of Charcot changes. There is evidence that therapeutic denervation as opposed to the pathologic denervation of peripheral neuropathy or trauma does not impute the same risks.[2] Perhaps more concerning is the potential for compromise of proprioception and balance both at the ankle and downstream within the foot. Unlike the knee, where copious capsular redundancy in innervation is the rule and extracapsular innervation in the multiple periarticular myotendinous structures remains intact after ablation, the innervation of the foot and ankle is much more vulnerable. The tendons and sheaths of the foot and ankle extrinsics as well as the whole of the foot's intrinsics are intimate with the capsular branches within their region and are routinely compromised during denervation. There is concern for the potential loss of a critical amount of proprioceptive input and extrinsic/intrinsic control that may increase local limb trauma and fall risk. Balancing the need for pain control against this concern we propose a focused, selective approach to ablation techniques, based around a single nerve distribution and or region of dysfunction, emphasizing the smallest possible area of effect that improves pain and function (**Tables 1 and 2**).

The preponderance of the literature follows a similar pattern of reporting, with the emphasis on single nerve or branch treatment, and focused on a specific region and diagnosis. There is a notable lack of large trials with most evidence based in case series. Within the literature, the most commonly studied region is the heel[4–10] and Morton neurofibroma.[1,9,11–13] Specificity of application can be further refined by using targeted pathology-specific interventions as in Morton neurofibroma. Other neuritides or neuromata of traumatic or medical causes can be addressed specifically this way with good efficacy[14] (**Table 3**). This allows the sparing of a larger region of the limb despite a sometimes larger region of referred pain. Radiofrequency interventions both with needle and percutaneous surgical techniques, along with cold probe, and medical/chemical ablations can be applied with precedence but varying strength of evidence, potential complications, and skill set may affect choice of technology. Nonablative neuromodulatory interventions such as pulsed radiofrequency may have a role in many pathologies with good early evidence,[9,15] but are outside the scope of this review.

Ultrasound has become the modality of choice for real-time procedural imaging in the literature, especially in the foot and ankle.[16] Real-time high-frequency ultrasound has distinct advantages to landmark-based, nerve localization techniques by electrical stimulation, or other imaging due to its ability to quickly localize even very small nerve targets that have significant variability in both position and branch anatomy. It also assists in avoiding compromise of the often intimately accompanying vascular or tendinous structures. Direct visualization also allows accurate administration of local anesthesia, eliminating the discomfort of other techniques or the need for multiple needle repositioning.[4,7–9,11] Real-time diagnostic imaging informs and refines the diagnosis of pathology that may have not been apparent on other imaging modalities. This in turn can allow significantly more focal application of technique, especially in the case of recognized nerve injury or entrapment causing primary neurogenic pain that mimics other orthopedic causes. The techniques we review in detail are based on this imaging modality and require a basic knowledge of ultrasound-guided needle localization and diagnostic imaging of relevant structures.

## POTENTIAL COMPLICATIONS

Treatment failure and potential complications of these interventions are typical of those found in all percutaneous-based ablation techniques, as well as those inherent to treating chronic pain syndromes. The most common complications are skin related when reported.[9] Nerve regrowth with return of symptoms is a possibility and even expected in some modalities like cold probe/cryogenic techniques. Neuroma formation in the absence of Wallerian degeneration requiring a revision ablation at a further point may need to be considered. Return of symptoms over months to several years despite initial success can be attributable to worsening of the original underlying pathology, new injury, or collateralization; for example, the reinnervation of pathologic structures from adjacent or overlapping nerves that may require additional treatment. Failure of pain control even initially can be a phenomenon of anatomic variability and branching pattern in an individual nerve resulting in insufficient effective denervation. Nerve-to-nerve anastomosis or unusually extensive overlapping innervation among adjacent nerves can result in innervation patterns very different from classic distributions and present as treatment failure. When pain syndromes have a primary neuropathic/neurogenic cause, nerve overlap may present with a migrating or "distribution jump"

**Table 2**
**Nerve ablation by region of pain**

| Nerve | Medial | Lateral | Anterior/Dorsal | Posterior | Heel |
|---|---|---|---|---|---|
| Sural (including lateral calcaneal nerve) | | Lateral ankle and subfibular region | Anterolateral | Posterolateral ankle Lateral foot | Lateral heel |
| Superficial peroneal nerve | | Anterolateral ankle | Complete Anterior ankle Dorsal midfoot Dorsal hindfoot | Posterior lateral ankle (via posterior branch) | |
| Deep peroneal nerve | | Anterolateral ankle Sinus tarsi | Anterolateral ankle 1st webspace | | |
| Saphenous nerve | Medial ankle Medial midfoot Dorsal arch | | Dorsal arch | | |
| Medial calcaneal nerve | Medial heel | | | | Medial heel |
| Baxter nerve | Medial heel Proximal arch | Lateral foot (via innervation of abductor minimi digiti muscle) | | | Medial heel Plantar heel |
| Common digital nerve | | | Forefoot pain Digital pain | | |

| Table 3 Common primary nerve pathology syndromes | |
|---|---|
| Sural (including lateral calcaneal nerve) | Peroneal tendon surgery: incisional neuroma, scar entrapment<br>Post immobilization entrapment<br>Peripheral neuropathy |
| Superficial peroneal nerve | Dorsal ankle surgery: neuromata, nerve contusion/entrapment<br>Dorsal foot/ganglion incisional neuroma<br>Inversion injury causing traction injury at the fascial tunnel<br>Peripheral neuropathy |
| Deep peroneal nerve | Compression/entrapment: shoewear/repetitive motion<br>Compression/entrapment: positional<br>Peripheral neuropathy |
| Saphenous nerve | Open reduction internal fixation tibial fracture: plateau, shaft/diaphyseal, pilon, medial malleolar<br>Compression/entrapment: trauma, shoewear/repetitive motion<br>Peripheral neuropathy |
| Medial calcaneal nerve | Tarsal tunnel syndrome<br>Entrapment: post immobilization, shoewear |
| Baxter Nerve | Compression/entrapment in distal tarsal tunnel/foot intrinsics.<br>Peripheral neuropathy |
| Common digital nerve/Proper digital nerve | Morton neuroma (neurofibroma)<br>Stump neuroma<br>Compression/entrapment: shoewear/repetitive motion, forefoot deformity |

phenomenon. In these cases, adequate anesthesia in the presenting region of pain is achieved, but adjacent previous uninvolved nerves and nerve distributions become symptomatic. In this author's experience, a direct interconnection between the first (posterior) branch of the superficial peroneal and the sural when present can be particularly problematic when treating pain along the lateral ankle and foot. This kind of neural anastomosis is not well characterized in the literature nor is the exact mechanism of this phenomenon. After trauma or surgery, multiple scar neuroma can occur within an overlapping distribution with a larger or more painful lesion distracting from another. If the first is removed successfully, the second may seem to become worse and present as a migrating pain syndrome but may resolve with successful follow-up ablation (**Fig. 1**). Multiple procedures in a single or overlapping distribution with primary neurogenic pain raise concern for evolution to complex regional pain syndrome (CRPS) and must be considered carefully. There is no established causal relationship between radiofrequency ablation (RFA) and CRPS in the literature; however, the high morbidity nature of this diagnosis requires consideration.

## BASIC PRINCIPLES

Fully characterizing the pathology of treatment is essential through a thorough review of the patient history and pertinent physical findings. The mechanism and evolution of

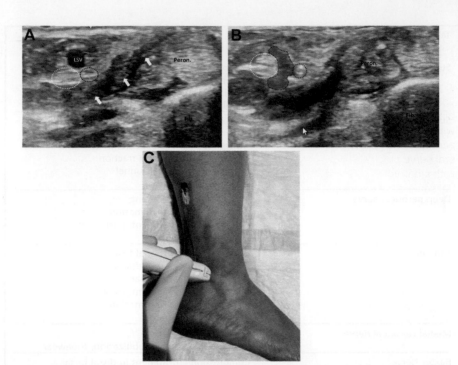

**Fig. 1.** A 33-year-old woman with persistent lancinating pain along the peroneal tendons after surgery. Previous incisional neuroma of a small branch of the superficial peroneal nerve was ablated with partial relief and change in pain syndrome. A postoperative neuroma of a branch of the sural nerve was identified on a SAX view of the posterior lateral/retromalleolar ankle region. (*A*) Sural nerve (*white hashed oval*) is identified deep to the lesser saphenous vein (LSV). A small branch (*black hashed oval*) is identified branching off and terminating into postoperatively thickened superior peroneal retinaculum; adjacent to tendinopathic peroneal tendons (Peron.). At the distal fibula/lateral malleolus (Fib.) ultrasonographic Tinel reproduced the patient's lancinating symptoms. (*B*) Local anesthetic has been injected creating space/thermal insulation between the nerve branch and the sural nerve (*shaded area*). The lesser saphenous is collapsed posterior and away from the target branch (*black hashed oval*). An out-of-plane approach for RF probe placement is used. The tip of the monopolar probe is superimposed on the target nerve branch. (*C*) Out-of-plane approach to the retromalleolar course of the sural nerve.

a pain syndrome becomes very important in the foot and ankle to direct therapy and minimize treatment failure. The combination of pathologies seen in trauma, postsurgical or long-standing disease often may include osteoarthrosis, neuralgia and nerve trauma, scarring and compression of fat pad structures, and tendinopathy. Biomechanical derangements or interventions like immobilization or late scarring that occur during a treatment course may complicate initial or referring diagnoses. Examples are entrapment of mononeuritis of superficial nerves like the medial or lateral calcaneal nerves after fracture immobilization, undiagnosed peripheral neuropathy complicating postsurgical pain, or incisional (saphenous) neuroma after tarsal tunnel release.[9,14,15,17] Full consideration may guide intervention to consider additional testing both choice of nerve, at what level or primary branch to perform ablation, and adjuvant treatments at a scar or scar neuroma.

The principle of a preprocedural nerve block or "selective block" is a key element in preparation and success of denervation therapies. However, in a recent review, only 6 of the 15 reviewed trials attempted a block before treatment.[9] In this review and in our own search of the literature, those applying this principle had an emphasis on targeting specific nerves at the medial heel and lateral ankle but did not universally report volumes used.[4,7,9,18] An additional benefit to the use of a preprocedural selective block allows for gauging of patient tolerability to an invasive procedure. Patients with elements of regional hypersensitivity or large neuromata may benefit from an alternate site "upstream" for ablation or adjuvant anesthesia with sedation or peripheral nerve blockade.[1,11] Adequate improvement in pain after a therapeutic nerve block with small volume local anesthesia is most predictive of success.[9] Pain levels on a verbal scale or visual analogue scale that are very low or have no reproducible functional element may compromise block predictive ability. In this author's experience, pain levels of a 4 of 10 or more with a reproducible functional component as in pain with ambulation or specific provocative maneuver are required to have a high confidence in an adequate block result. The volume of anesthesia should represent the approximate area of the ablation modality at the target structure or fascial plane. The compact nature of the anatomy and functional interplay of multiple potential pathologies in many patients makes a precise block with appropriate volumes essential. In needle or radiofrequency (RF) probe-based techniques, a very low volume block of 0.25 to 0.5 mL lidocaine, 0.25 to 0.5 mL bupivacaine (Marcaine) deposited with a small-bore needle directly around the target nerve or branch is most specific. A larger volume may cause diffusion of injectate across tissue planes anesthetizing overlapping nerve distributions or directly anesthetizing capsular/synovial structures, providing false reassurance of potential success.[9] Follow-up evaluation of muscular inhibition specific to the nerve or branches in the immediate region of or distal to the block may be helpful to predict the amount of potential muscular denervation. This has the potential to assist in sensory versus motor determination at the site of potential ablation.

The technology used for ablations is diverse, with continued evolution of available tools. Cryoneurolysis is described and has been used in different forms since the 1970s, with recent limited evidence of success in the foot and ankle.[18] Hwoon and colleagues[18] demonstrated relief in a small series in excess of 12 months. Monopolar needle-based RFA is the most commonly reported in the literature. Small trials, retrospective analyses, and case series focused around the medial heel region and Morton neurofibroma both with and without ultrasound guidance.[1,4,5,7–9,11,13] There is the conspicuous absence of randomized control trials at this stage for any truly ablative modality.[9] Although available as a technology, cooled RF has not been studied. A standard 22-gauge RF needle with a 10-mm active tip is commonly used. When targeting the peripheral nerves of the heel, RF parameters of 80 to 90° C for 75 to 120 seconds is described, with most using 90° C for 90 seconds with variable target impedances.[5,7–9] RFA in the case of Morton neurofibroma is much more intensive and warrants a specific description found later in this article (see section Digital Nerves). Chemical ablation treatments with phenol and ethanol have been used historically in varying concentrations. Ethanol is the most well studied in the foot, specifically in the case of Morton neurofibroma, with recent evidence supporting its use.[12] Potential limitations of injectable sclerosing or ablating agents is the diffusion along fascial lines of the agent potentially involving unintended nerves, vascular structures, or muscular tissue. Monopolar or bipolar probe use in the destruction of neuromata or peripheral nerves is rarely described and is analogous to electrocautery techniques in surgery to transect and destroy nerves.[16] These devices used focused application of intensive electrothermal or plasma discharges. Percutaneous application of these probes typically requires a small incision and advanced ultrasound technique and knowledge of anatomy. Future research is needed to establish safety and efficacy for broad use.

Local anesthesia can be applied at the time of ablation, with real-time ultrasound imaging through a small-bore needle achieving circumferential infiltration and/or fascial dilation.[11,16,18] One advantage of this approach is reduction of patient discomfort before an RF needle or probe insertion. Circumferential dissection of the anesthetic has the added benefit of a fluid buffer separating the surrounding structures from the target nerve, which is especially important when the skin, additional nerve, or vascular structures are intimate[18]; for example, the saphenous nerve and greater saphenous vein, the sural and lesser saphenous, and the dorsalis pedis artery and the deep peroneal (see **Fig. 1**). Fluid within the adjacent fascial planes can allow easier passage of the RF device from skin to target minimizing tissue trauma of introduction and thermal injury (**Fig. 2**). If additional anesthesia is added through an RF needle or probe equipped with that function, repeat visualization is best, as too large a volume can displace the target nerve sufficiently distant from the device as to cause incomplete ablation or it can compromise the technique by lowering target impedance in needle-based RFA. If the impedance falls below 100 Ω, it suggests too much fluid is present[4,5] as well, and further time for the local to disperse is required for initiation. With direct visualization with ultrasound in needle placement and a confident selective block before the procedure, traditional RFA sensory and motor stimulation is not typically required. There is some potential utility in delaying local anesthetic administration if confidence in ultrasonographic visible anatomy is low. Sensory stimulation to ensure the close proximity of a sensory nerve in the target area should be less than 1 V. Motor stimulation should ideally be less than 2.5 V[8]; however, the passage of many of the peripheral nerves sites for ablation in the foot and ankle are immediately adjacent to muscle tissue and false positive muscular stimulation is highly likely.

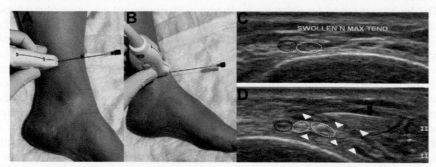

**Fig. 2.** The SN. (*A*) Common approach to the distal SN for medial ankle/foot ablation. (*B*) Approach at the diametaphysis, which is a common site of entrapment of the nerve. This site is also the preferred for medial ankle sparing dorso-medial foot ablations. (*C*) Example of entrapment of the SN at the medial diametaphysis of the left tibia 2 years after high-energy contusion with healed lacerations. Original text from clinical imaging is seen (*gray text*) noting pathology, point tenderness, and ultrasonographic Tinel. A chronically occluded greater saphenous vein (*black dashed oval*) lies adjacent to a swollen enlarged SN (*white dashed oval*) with loss of internal architecture. (*D*) Same patient during local anesthetic administration. The injectate layers between neurovascular bundle and the tibia as well as skin (*small arrowheads*) providing insulation and potential space for RF needle/probe placement. A 25-gauge needle was used (*black arrow*). Branching of the distal SN is seen on the fascial plane (*white dashed ovals*).

## THE SURAL

The sural nerve is responsible for the primary innervation of the lateral and posterior lateral ankle region and lateral foot with overlapping distribution with the superficial peroneal nerve anteriorly and dorsally.[1–3,15] Overlapping innervation with the tibial nerve (TN) occurs at the Achilles tendon.[2,3] RFA treatment of recalcitrant talo-fibular (lateral gutter crural) osteoarthrosis (OA) pain, subfibular impingement, subtalar OA pain, as well as calcaneocuboid and lateral tarsometatarsal (TMT) OA would require an ablation of the sural. The fat pad of the sinus tarsi is less likely to achieve pain relief with ablation of the sural as the bulk of its innervation is from the deep peroneal.[2,19] Chronic peroneal tendinopathy, especially in failed surgical cases can result in chronic pain, including chronic sensitization of the sural nerve.[9,15,20] The sural nerve is very superficial and vulnerable to injury, with sural neuralgia as a primary diagnosis occurring from repetitive motion trauma, external compression, internal fascial compression, surgical scar entrapment (see **Fig. 1**), systemic disease, and as a pseudo-mononeuritis presentation of peripheral neuropathy.[9,15,20,21]

The primary ablation site correlates with traditional surgical approaches, as the sural lays over the midline of the post lower leg at the gastrocnemius fascia (**Fig. 3**). As a

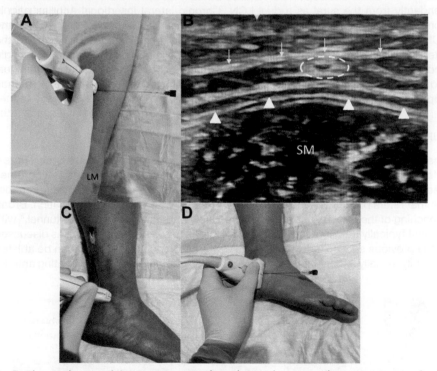

**Fig. 3.** The sural nerve. (*A*) Primary approach to the sural nerve at the gastrocnemius fascia for ablation. The sural lies midline over the broad fascia proximal to the formation of the Achilles tendon proper. The lateral malleolus (LM) is visible. (*B*) View of the sural nerve (*white dashed oval*) at this location. Superficial fascia (*white arrows*) overlies the nerve and the dense tendinous tissue of the gastrocnemius fascia (*arrowheads*) is below. The soleus muscle (SM) is seen beneath. (*C*) Approach for ablation in the retromalleolar region; the most common site of injury/entrapment. Out-of-plane approach is commonly used to avoid the peroneal and Achilles tendons (*D*) Most distal site of ablation—ankle sparing.

fairly large nerve at that level, aggressive RFA with a monopolar or bipolar probe affecting complete transection may be required to obtain complete analgesia. The lesser saphenous vein is adjacent to the nerve but can be dissected away and temporarily collapsed from local anesthetic administration easily. Failure of selective block at the gastroc fascia is suggestive of significant contributions, even plexuslike anastomoses with the initial (posterior) branch of the superficial peroneal. This may require a simultaneous additional treatment for relief. This posterior branch leaves the main trunk near the nerve exit from its fascial tunnel or even within the tunnel (**Fig. 4**). It is quite large and can be blocked/ablated independent of the main trunk in most. Ablation of the main sural nerve trunk at the tip of the lateral malleolus assuming effective selective block at that area is more ankle and heel sparing and more selective of the lateral foot (see **Fig. 3**). In specific cases, especially in peroneal tendon postsurgical situations, small segmental branch entrapment or neuromata may be identified under ultrasound visualization and ultrasonographic Tinel. If confirmed by selective block, selective site ablation can be performed (see **Fig. 1**).

The posterior-most terminal branch of the sural is the lateral calcaneal nerve (LCN), which can be easily ablated in its entirety. Shortly after leaving the sural it sends an often identifiable small branch posteriorly toward the lateral Achilles insertion, the retrocalcaneal bursa and superficial Achilles bursa (**Fig. 5**). This branch can arise independently from the sural as a dual LCN. Chronic lateral insertional Achilles pain is common even after surgery and block and ablation of the posterior branch of the LCN is possible. The LCN terminates into multiple small branches proximal to the lateral fat pad of the heel, additionally innervating the lateral band plantar fascia origin and contributes to the subcalcaneal bursa. Targeting the region of lateral (plantar) heel requires ablation of the main trunk LCN or immediately after the posterior branch departs.

## SUPERFICIAL PERONEAL NERVE

The superficial peroneal nerve (SPN) ablation has good utility for anterior and dorsal referring symptoms. Ankle OA and anterior/anterolateral impingement syndromes treated with RFA would require ablations of this nerve. Distal hindfoot and midfoot OA that refers broadly anterior can often be treated with isolated SPN ablation. Broad branching of the SPN begins almost immediately after it leaves its fascial tunnel,[2] with the first typically tracking posteriorly overlapping the sural in distribution, as discussed in the previous section (see **Fig. 4**). This posterior branch is large and can be ablated primarily, usually in conjunction with the sural. Ablation of the SPN for treating anterior

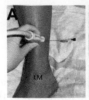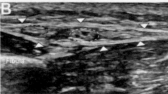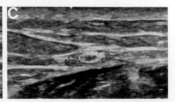

**Fig. 4.** (A) Approach to ablation of the SPN over the anterior lateral lower leg. The lateral malleolus is visible (LM). (B) The SPN (*white hashed oval*) within its fascial tunnel (*white arrowheads*) over the anterior lower leg. The posterior branch has already branched off (*black hashed oval*) in this patient. (C) Different patient: The posterior branch (*black hashed oval*) and main trunk (*white hashed oval*) branching just distal to the fibrous tunnel within the subcutaneous tissues of the lower leg.

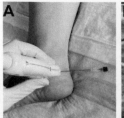
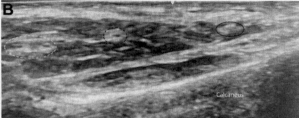

**Fig. 5.** (A) Approach to the LCN. (B) Ultrasound view of the LCN (*black dashed oval*) just below its branch point from the sural (*white dashed oval*) overlying the body of the calcaneus. The (posterior) branch to the Achilles insertion has already diverged and tracks posteriorly (*solid black oval*).

ankle or foot pain should occur immediately after the passage of this posterior branch. More distal ablations should be reserved for focal nerve lesions or neuromata clinically determined.

## DEEP PERONEAL NERVE

The deep peroneal nerve (DPN) ablation has utility in sinus tarsi syndrome or severe anterolateral impingement syndromes involving the sinus tarsi region, as is often seen in pes planus and can be adjunct to ablations of the sural for the calcaneocuboid joint or the SPN for the talonavicular.[2,19] The deep peroneal nerve branches are just proximal to the ankle joint, sending one to the extensor digitorum brevis muscle and a branch to the sinus tarsi, while the main trunk continues to the first webspace (**Fig. 6**). The dorsalis pedis artery is intimate and it is advisable to best visualize the lateral branches to their destinations under ultrasound and ablate after they have deviated from the path of the artery. Local anesthetic buffer can be injected, further lateralizing the branch to the sinus tarsi and further protecting the dorsalis pedis. Low-energy techniques using standard needle-based RFA or bipolar cautery is advisable, as any injury to the artery can be devastating in some patients.

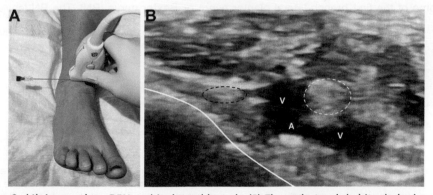

**Fig. 6.** (A) Approach to DPN and its lateral branch. (B) The main trunk (*white dashed oval*) overlying the dorsalis pedis artery (A) and veins (V) at the distal most edge of the anterior tibia (*white line*). The lateral branch (*black dashed oval*) has passed under the veins and deviates laterally.

## SAPHENOUS NERVE

Ablation of the saphenous nerve (SN) is necessary in medial ankle pain, including the medial subtalar and posterior tibialis tendon syndromes.[2,22] Primary entrapment at the ankle from trauma or shoewear (see **Fig. 2**) is common, as is neuroma formation in medial incisions. Proximal tarsal tunnel incisional pain can be a treatable neuroma of the SN.[17] Identification of the SN begins on the medial lower leg with the greater saphenous vein; variations in anatomy are common and the nerve should be tracked distal to the anterior metaphysis of the tibia to ensure the proper branch is identified. Ablation for the purposes of medial/posterior medial ankle pain should occur approximately 4 cm proximal to the medial malleolus (see **Fig. 2**). If a selective block is insufficient, a more proximal location may be needed. To more focally denervate the medial foot, ablation at the metaphysis is usually sufficient. Local anesthetic dissection of the nerve away from the vein may be helpful to prevent bruising, but temporary injury to the vessel is rarely problematic.

## TIBIAL NERVE

The TN is not primarily ablated in patients who are able to weight bear because of the loss of all plantar sensation and proprioception that would occur. Nerve destruction of the TN contributions to the posterior medial ankle need to be removed surgically,[3] as the 3 small branches involved are very short from branch point to capsule and cannot be ablated with percutaneous RF techniques without injury to the TN trunk. The primary utility of RFA within this nerve's distribution is medial and plantar heel pain.

The medial calcaneal nerve (MCN) is a viable target for RFA.[5,8] It is accessed from the middle to distal tarsal tunnel (TT) where it continues in a caudad direction as the TN often already separated into the medial and lateral plantar nerves (MPN/LPN) turn anteriorly. The MCN may branch off of the LPN/MPN or the TN before it separates. Multiple MCNs of varying origin points are described.[6] The MCN will typically puncture or pass under the inferior edge of the medial flexor retinaculum before arborization into the Achilles insertion, medial fat pad, medial band plantar fascia, and the associated bursas. It is best to perform the ablation immediately after the nerve has passed out of the TT, immediately outside or distal to the flexor retinaculum (**Fig. 7**).

Deep heel pain referring from the distal TT region without anterior referring symptoms or paraesthesias can be a sign of a common primary nerve compression syndrome of the first branch lateral plantar nerve or Baxter nerve (BN). The BN leaves

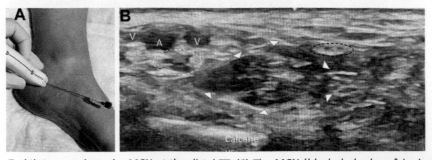

**Fig. 7.** (*A*) Approach to the MCN at the distal TT. (*B*) The MCN (*black dashed oval*) is visualized distal to the flexor retinaculum. The TN (*white dashed oval*) is below the tibial artery (A) and veins (V), with the muscle belly of the flexor hallucis longus muscle (FHL/*white arrowheads*) between the 2 nerves.

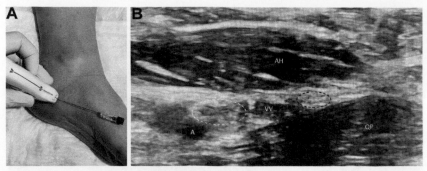

**Fig. 8.** (*A*) Approach to the Baxter/first branch LCN. (*B*) BN (*black dashed oval*) at its common entrapment/ablation site with the AH above and QP beneath. Small branching veins (VV) sit between the lateral plantar nerve (*white dashed oval*) and the tibial artery (A).

the LPN in the distal TT proximal to the arcade of the abductor hallucis muscle (AH). It is compressed either at the arcade between the AH and quadratus plantae (QP) muscles (**Fig. 8**) or between the QP and the flexor digitorum brevis cephalad of the plantar fascia. The nerve terminates into the periosteum of the calcaneus and terminally innervates the abductor digit quinti muscle (ADQ) of the lateral foot. This Baxter neuritis is often comorbid with recalcitrant plantar fasciosis and may need to be ablated with the MCN to achieve pain relief in these patients. It can be treated with ablation,[5,7] but this is usually reserved for patients who are proven recalcitrant and who have failed a surgical decompression. The ablation of BN causes loss of the ADQ, which could cause other lateral foot pain with the loss of lateral control and muscular padding. It is typically ablated after it has separated sufficiently from the main trunk of the LPN, often at its primary entrapment area of the posterior-most region of the distal arcade of the TT, that is, between the AH and QP (see **Fig. 8**).

Proximal incisional pain after plantar fascial release or TT release can derive from a posterior branch of the SN, as mentioned; however, more distal incisional sensitivity is common and can be debilitating. Small neuromata embedded within the glabrous skin scar are very difficult to see; however, standard needle-based RF treatment with the active tip within or immediately beneath the scar may be effective. Alternatively, selective block and RFA of the MCN with or without any visible posterior branches of the SN can be attempted.

## DIGITAL NERVES

The common and proper digital nerves can be ablated anywhere along their length where they can be well visualized and have an effective selective block. Low-energy techniques, like standard needle-based RF, are preferential if the ablation occurs within the digit so as to minimize trauma to the digital vessels. The most common site of ablation within the forefoot is for recalcitrant Morton neurofibroma or postsurgical stump neuroma and is typically accomplished with a long axis dorsal to volar approach (**Fig. 9**). Dehydrated alcohol is a traditional and effective treatment.[12,14] The 100% ethanol is typically diluted with local anesthetic to 4%; however, a 2012 study used a 10% concentration with a 66% success rate in resolving symptoms.[12,14] Other treatments, including nonablative (pulsed) RF and needle-based RFA may give benefit.[1,11,13] Standard RFA for Morton neurofibroma is managed very differently in the literature when compared with other peripheral nerves. In studies using

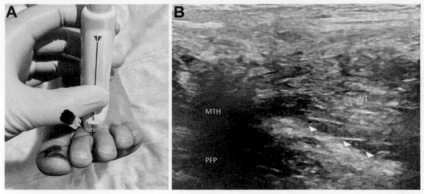

**Fig. 9.** (*A*) Common approach to the webspace for common plantar digital ablation/Morton neurofibroma. (*B*) Second webspace long axis (LAX) ultrasound view. The neurovascular bundle is seen as a bright plane (*white arrowheads*) between the interossei (INT) and plantar fat pad (PFP). It disappears into the hypoechoic tangential shadow of metatarsal heads (MTH) where the Morton neurofibroma may form. Postsurgical stump neuromas occur more proximally. RFA needle placement is typically just proximal to the shadow for Morton ablation or more proximally at site of ultrasonographic Tinel for stump neuroma with tip placement along the same plane.

ultrasound-guided needle placement, treatments were much longer using multiple cycles to reach 10 minutes at 80° C with good success.[11,13] One landmark-based trial compared 8 minutes at 90° C with 12 minutes, with 12 minutes slightly better.[1] Only 1 retrospective study suggests 90° for 120 seconds, but it had very good success as well, with near 50% of patients having acceptable relief.[14] Certainly extended times at ablation temperature seem well tolerated and may be considered. After surgical excision, symptomatic stump neuroma can be treated similarly. In some cases of stump neuroma, the pathology can be very subtle on ultrasound imaging, and block/RFA placed at the neurovascular bundle at the level of maximal symptoms/ultrasonographic Tinel is the best approach (see **Fig. 9**).

## ANKLE OSTEOARTHROSIS

Special mention of painful ankle OA is required. The complete denervation of the ankle (tibiotalar/crural) joint without unacceptable loss of distal innervation is very difficult with percutaneous means and is not well studied and should be considered only in extreme cases, including in those who cannot have a surgical denervation, which is more nerve sparing.[3] A regional approach focusing on moderating specific symptom elements in a multimodal regimen is recommended, which may require staged selective blocks. Alternatively, a theoretic maximal percutaneous denervation of the ankle joint would include ablation of the sural, SPN, DPN branch to the sinus tarsi, and SN. This preserves the plantar surface and first webspace for proprioceptive input alone. Ankle ablation with a more optimal distal functional preservation is more technically difficult and is modeled on published surgical therapies.[2,3,23] This requires the identification of the multiple variable capsular branches of the several innervations for ablation while preserving distal trunks. This technique is very time-consuming and may require multiple staged interventions. The sural main trunk is identified under ultrasound and preserved while identifying any branches between the gastrocnemius fascia and the distal tip of the lateral malleolus and for attempted ablation. This may require multiple needle entry sites. Similarly, nerve mapping under ultrasound of the SPN to establish individual patient branching patterns and ablation of any visible large branches that terminate at or proximal to the extensor retinaculum, preserving those that extend beyond this soft tissue marker. A similar technique can be applied to the SN; however, its branches tend to be very small and a complete SN RFA is usually required. The DPN branch to the sinus tarsi should be ablated, as it contributes to the anterior lateral ankle joint. The TN is preserved in entirety for the reasons we have already described. In this author's experience, partial denervations as described at the SPN, DPN, and sural are not recommended in primary nerve pain syndromes, including peripheral neuropathies, as a higher likelihood of migrating or "jump" pain syndromes and CRPS is likely. Partial denervations are best applied in OA or other true joint or tendon-based pain syndromes.

## SUMMARY

Ablation therapies in the foot and ankle are accessible adjuncts to comprehensive pain management in chronic recalcitrant pain syndromes. Techniques are best applied to individual patient anatomy with strong advantages in a working knowledge of neuromuscular real-time imaging with ultrasound. Interventionists face the unique challenge in this region of preserving balance and proprioception as well as intrinsic muscle function. A decision-making approach emphasizing selectivity by using regional and target-specific ablations is optimal. Other challenges include minimizing vascular insult and preventing progression to other chronic pain syndromes. The literature is far from comprehensive with few controlled trials; however, there is growing evidence of safety and efficacy of ablation techniques across specific regions. This field of knowledge is expected to continue to grow alongside other regional applications of peripheral joint ablation, especially as expertise in anatomic research, ultrasound medicine, and minimally invasive options grows among medical specialties. Continued collaboration between interventionists and foot and ankle surgery in order to refine and define indications, technique, and technology will open a road to better options in patient care.

## DISCLOSURE

Nahum M. Beard is clinical faculty at The Campbell Clinic and University of Tennessee Health Science Center Medical School.

## BIBLIOGRAPHY

1. Brooks D, Parr A, Bryceson W, et al. Three cycles of radiofrequency ablation are more efficacious than two in the management of Morton's neuroma foot. Ankle Spec 2018;11(2):107–11.
2. Mentzel M, Fleischmann W, Bauer G, et al. Ankle joint denervation. Part 1: anatomy - the sensory innervation of the ankle joint. Foot Ankle Surg 1999;5:15–20.
3. Mentzel M, Fleischmann W, Bauer G, et al. Ankle joint denervation. Part 2: operative technique and results. Foot Ankle Surg 1999;5:21–7.
4. Arslan A. Treatment of chronic plantar heel pain with radiofrequency neural ablation of the first branch of the lateral plantar nerve and medial calcaneal nerve branches. J Foot Ankle Surg 2016;55:767–71.
5. Cozzarelli J, Sollitto RJ, Thapar J, et al. A 12-year long-term retrospective analysis of the use of radiofrequency nerve ablation for the treatment of neurogenic heel pain. Foot Ankle Spec 2010;3(6):338–46.

6. Dellon AL, Kim J, Spaulding CM. Variations in the origin of the medial calcaneal nerve. J Am Podiatr Med Assoc 2002;92(2):97–101.

7. Yener Erken H, Ayanoglu S, Akmaz I, et al. Prospective study of percutaneous radiofrequency nerve ablation for chronic plantar fasciitis. Foot Ankle Int 2014; 35(2):95–103.

8. Liden B, Simmons M, Landsman A. Retrospective analysis of 22 patients treated with percutaneous radiofrequency nerve ablation for prolonged moderate to severe heel pain associated with plantar fasciitis. J Foot Ankle Surg 2009;48(6): 642–7.

9. Orhurhu V, Urits I, Orman S, et al. A systematic review of radiofrequency treatment of the ankle for the management of chronic foot and ankle pain. Curr Pain Headache Rep 2019;23:4.

10. Yuan Y, et al. Comparison of the therapeutic outcomes between open plantar fascia release and percutaneous radiofrequency ablation in the treatment of intractable plantar fasciitis. J Orthop Surg Res 2020;15(1):595.

11. Chuter, Graham SJ, et al. Ultrasound-guided radiofrequency ablation in the management of interdigital (Morton's) neuroma. Skeletal Radiol 2013;42:107–11.

12. Musson R. Ultrasound guided alcohol ablation of Morton's neuroma. Foot Ankle Int 2012;33(3):196–201.

13. Shah R, Ahmad M, Hanu-Cernat D, et al. Ultrasound-guided radiofrequency ablation for treatment of Morton's neuroma: initial experience. Clin Radiol 2019;74(10). 815.e9-815.e13.

14. Connors JC, Boike AM, Rao N, et al. Radiofrequency ablation for the treatment of painful neuroma. J Foot Ankle Surg 2020;59(3):457–61.

15. Abd-Elsayed A, Jackson M, et al. Pulsed radiofrequency ablation for treating sural neuralgia. Ochsner J 2018;18:88–90.

16. Beard NM, Gousse RL. Current ultrasound applications in the foot and ankle. Orthop Clin North Am 2018;49(1):109–21.

17. Kim J, Dellon AL. Pain at the site of tarsal tunnel incision due to neuroma of the posterior branch of the saphenous nerve. J Am Podiatr Med Assoc 2001;91(3): 109–13.

18. Yoon JHE, Grechushkin V, Chaudhry A, et al. Cryoneurolysis in patients with refractory chronic peripheral neuropathic. Pain J Vasc Interv Radiol 2016;27(2): 239–43.

19. Dellon AL. Denervation of the sinus tarsi for chronic post-traumatic lateral ankle pain. Orthopedics 2002;25(8):849–51.

20. Paraskevas, George K, et al. Fascial entrapment of the sural nerve and its clinical relevance. Anat Cell Biol 2014;47(2):144–7.

21. Aszmann OC, Ebmer JM, Dellon AL. Cutaneous innervation of the medial ankle: an anatomic study of the saphenous, sural, and tibial nerves and their clinical significance. Foot Ankle Int 1998;19:753–6.

22. Marsland D, et al. The saphenous nerve in foot and ankle surgery: Its variable anatomy and relevance. Foot Ankle Surg 2013;19:76–9.

23. Casagrande PA, Austin BP, Indeck W. Denervation of the ankle joint. J Bone Joint Surg Am 1951;33(3):723–30.

# UNITED STATES POSTAL SERVICE ®

## Statement of Ownership, Management, and Circulation (All Periodicals Publications Except Requester Publications)

| 1. Publication Title | 2. Publication Number | 3. Filing Date |
|---|---|---|
| PHYSICAL MEDICINE AND REHABILITATION CLINICS OF NORTH AMERICA | 009 – 243 | 9/18/2021 |

| 4. Issue Frequency | 5. Number of Issues Published Annually | 6. Annual Subscription Price |
|---|---|---|
| FEB, MAY, AUG, NOV | 4 | $322.00 |

7. Complete Mailing Address of Known Office of Publication (Not printer) (Street, city, county, state, and ZIP+4®)

ELSEVIER INC.
230 Park Avenue, Suite 800
New York, NY 10169

Contact Person
Malathi Samayan

Telephone (Include area code)
91-44-4299-4507

8. Complete Mailing Address of Headquarters or General Business Office of Publisher (Not printer)

ELSEVIER INC.
230 Park Avenue, Suite 800
New York, NY 10169

9. Full Names and Complete Mailing Addresses of Publisher, Editor, and Managing Editor (Do not leave blank)

Publisher (Name and complete mailing address)

Dolores Meloni, ELSEVIER INC.
1600 JOHN F KENNEDY BLVD. SUITE 1800
PHILADELPHIA, PA 19103-2899

Editor (Name and complete mailing address)

LAUREN BOYLE, ELSEVIER INC.
1600 JOHN F KENNEDY BLVD. SUITE 1800
PHILADELPHIA, PA 19103-2899

Managing Editor (Name and complete mailing address)

PATRICK MANLEY, ELSEVIER INC.
1600 JOHN F KENNEDY BLVD. SUITE 1800
PHILADELPHIA, PA 19103-2899

10. Owner (Do not leave blank. If the publication is owned by a corporation, give the name and address of the corporation immediately followed by the names and addresses of all stockholders owning or holding 1 percent or more of the total amount of stock. If not owned by a corporation, give the names and addresses of the individual owners. If owned by a partnership or other unincorporated firm, give its name and address as well as those of each individual owner. If the publication is published by a nonprofit organization, give its name and address.)

| Full Name | Complete Mailing Address |
|---|---|
| WHOLLY OWNED SUBSIDIARY OF REED/ELSEVIER, US HOLDINGS | 1600 JOHN F KENNEDY BLVD, SUITE 1800 PHILADELPHIA, PA 19103-2899 |

11. Known Bondholders, Mortgagees, and Other Security Holders Owning or Holding 1 Percent or More of Total Amount of Bonds, Mortgages, or Other Securities. If none, check box ► ☐ None

| Full Name | Complete Mailing Address |
|---|---|
| N/A | |

12. Tax Status (For completion by nonprofit organizations authorized to mail at nonprofit rates) (Check one)
The purpose, function, and nonprofit status of this organization and the exempt status for federal income tax purposes:
☒ Has Not Changed During Preceding 12 Months
☐ Has Changed During Preceding 12 Months (Publisher must submit explanation of change with this statement)

PS Form **3526**, July 2014 [Page 1 of 4 (see instructions page 4)]  PSN: 7530-01-000-9931   PRIVACY NOTICE: See our privacy policy on www.usps.com

---

| 13. Publication Title | 14. Issue Date for Circulation Data Below |
|---|---|
| PHYSICAL MEDICINE AND REHABILITATION CLINICS OF NORTH AMERICA | MAY 2021 |

| 15. Extent and Nature of Circulation | | Average No. Copies Each Issue During Preceding 12 Months | No. Copies of Single Issue Published Nearest to Filing Date |
|---|---|---|---|
| a. Total Number of Copies (Net press run) | | 179 | 161 |
| b. Paid Circulation (By Mail and Outside the Mail) | (1) Mailed Outside-County Paid Subscriptions Stated on PS Form 3541 (Include paid distribution above nominal rate, advertiser's proof copies, and exchange copies) | 93 | 84 |
| | (2) Mailed In-County Paid Subscriptions Stated on PS Form 3541 (Include paid distribution above nominal rate, advertiser's proof copies, and exchange copies) | 0 | 0 |
| | (3) Paid Distribution Outside the Mails Including Sales Through Dealers and Carriers, Street Vendors, Counter Sales, and Other Paid Distribution Outside USPS® | 41 | 24 |
| | (4) Paid Distribution by Other Classes of Mail Through the USPS (e.g., First-Class Mail®) | 0 | 0 |
| c. Total Paid Distribution [Sum of 15b (1), (2), (3), and (4)] | ► | 134 | 108 |
| d. Free or Nominal Rate Distribution (By Mail and Outside the Mail) | (1) Free or Nominal Rate Outside-County Copies included on PS Form 3541 | 26 | 34 |
| | (2) Free or Nominal Rate In-County Copies Included on PS Form 3541 | 0 | 0 |
| | (3) Free or Nominal Rate Copies Mailed at Other Classes Through the USPS (e.g., First-Class Mail) | 0 | 0 |
| | (4) Free or Nominal Rate Distribution Outside the Mail (Carriers or other means) | 0 | 0 |
| e. Total Free or Nominal Rate Distribution (Sum of 15d (1), (2), (3) and (4)) | ► | 26 | 34 |
| f. Total Distribution (Sum of 15c and 15e) | ► | 160 | 142 |
| g. Copies not Distributed (See Instructions to Publishers #4 (page 3)) | ► | 19 | 19 |
| h. Total (Sum of 15f and g) | ► | 179 | 161 |
| i. Percent Paid (15c divided by 15f times 100) | | 83.75% | 76.05% |

* If you are claiming electronic copies, go to line 16 on page 3. If you are not claiming electronic copies, skip to line 17 on page 3.

| 16. Electronic Copy Circulation | | Average No. Copies Each Issue During Preceding 12 Months | No. Copies of Single Issue Published Nearest to Filing Date |
|---|---|---|---|
| a. Paid Electronic Copies | ► | | |
| b. Total Paid Print Copies (Line 15c) + Paid Electronic Copies (Line 16a) | ► | | |
| c. Total Print Distribution (Line 15f) + Paid Electronic Copies (Line 16a) | ► | | |
| d. Percent Paid (Both Print & Electronic Copies) (16b divided by 16c × 100) | ► | | |

☒ I certify that 50% of all my distributed copies (electronic and print) are paid above a nominal price.

17. Publication of Statement of Ownership
☒ If the publication is a general publication, publication of this statement is required. Will be printed in the NOVEMBER 2021 issue of this publication. ☐ Publication not required.

18. Signature and Title of Editor, Publisher, Business Manager, or Owner

*Malathi Samayan*

Malathi Samayan - Distribution Controller

Date 9/18/2021

I certify that all information furnished on this form is true and complete. I understand that anyone who furnishes false or misleading information on this form or who omits material or information requested on the form may be subject to criminal sanctions (including fines and imprisonment) and/or civil sanctions (including civil penalties).

PS Form **3526**, July 2014 (Page 3 of 4)   PRIVACY NOTICE: See our privacy policy on www.usps.com

# Moving?

## Make sure your subscription moves with you!

To notify us of your new address, find your **Clinics Account Number** (located on your mailing label above your name), and contact customer service at:

**Email: journalscustomerservice-usa@elsevier.com**

**800-654-2452** (subscribers in the U.S. & Canada)
**314-447-8871** (subscribers outside of the U.S. & Canada)

**Fax number: 314-447-8029**

**Elsevier Health Sciences Division**
**Subscription Customer Service**
**3251 Riverport Lane**
**Maryland Heights, MO 63043**

*To ensure uninterrupted delivery of your subscription, please notify us at least 4 weeks in advance of move.